Cambridge History of Medicine

The science of woman

Cambridge History of Medicine

Editors

CHARLES WEBSTER, *All Souls College, Oxford*

CHARLES ROSENBERG, *Professor of History and the Sociology of Science, University of Pennsylvania*

The science
of woman

Gynaecology and gender in England, 1800–1929

ORNELLA MOSCUCCI

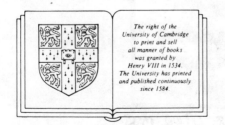

The right of the
University of Cambridge
to print and sell
all manner of books
was granted by
Henry VIII in 1534.
The University has printed
and published continuously
since 1584.

CAMBRIDGE UNIVERSITY PRESS

CAMBRIDGE
NEW YORK   PORT CHESTER
MELBOURNE   SYDNEY

Published by the Press Syndicate of the University of Cambridge
The Pitt Building, Trumpington Street, Cambridge CB2 1RP
40 West 20th Street, New York, NY 10011, USA
10 Stamford Road, Oakleigh, Melbourne 3166, Australia

First published 1990

Printed in Great Britain by Redwood Press Limited, Melksham, Wiltshire

British Library cataloguing in publication data

Moscucci, Ornella
The science of woman. – (Cambridge history
of medicine.)
1. England. Gynaecology. Obstetrics.
Gynaecology and obstetrics
I. Title
618′.0942

Library of Congress cataloguing in publication data

Moscucci, Ornella.
The science of woman: gynaecology and gender in England,
1800–1929 / Ornella Moscucci.
p.   cm. – (Cambridge history of medicine)
Originally presented as the author's thesis (doctoral – University
of Oxford, 1984)
ISBN 0–521–32741–5
1. Gynecology – England – London – History. 2. Obstetrics – England – London –
History.   I. Title.   II. Series.
RG67.G7M67 1990
618.1′00941 – dc20   89–7076 CIP

ISBN 0 521 32741 5

Contents

Plates

To my children Giacomo and Jessica

Preface

This book began as a doctoral thesis submitted to the University of Oxford in 1984. It traces the evolution of gynaecology from the elaboration of modern medical theories of femininity to the establishment of the Royal College of Obstetricians and Gynaecologists in 1929. Its geographical focus is England, and London in particular. This is not because other parts of Britain are less interesting, but because London, with its wealthy and aristocratic clientele, has led the way in gynaecological professionalism.

The history of obstetrics and gynaecology is a burgeoning field and I have learnt a great deal from the work of feminist and socialist historians. Unfortunately Frank Mort's work came to my attention after the typescript was completed. It is clearly impossible to provide a truly comprehensive account of such a vast subject. Gynaecological practice at provincial hospitals, for example, demands further research; so does the influence of gynaecological surgery on obstetrical practice. The relations between science and technological innovation in gynaecology are currently being investigated by Michael Bevan.

It would not have been possible to complete this book without the help of many people. My first debt is to Dr Ludmilla Jordanova, who supervised my doctoral thesis and read parts of the manuscript. Her continuing encouragement and unstinting help are greatly appreciated. I am grateful to the members of the Wellcome Unit for the History of Medicine, Oxford, especially to Dr Charles Webster and Dr Irvine Loudon, for their generous support and advice. My thanks also go to Dr Adrian Wilson for commenting on sections of the draft. Dr M. Jeanne Peterson and Karl Figlio contributed precious comments in the early stages of the research.

I am grateful to the Royal College of Obstetricians and Gynaecologists for granting me access to its archives and to all those people who helped with the arduous task of retrieving archival material relating to the hospital care of gynaecological patients. The Chelsea Hospital for Women and Queen Charlotte's Hospital Joint Medical Committee gave me permission to look at the case-records at the Chelsea Hospital for Women. The late Mr W. Winterton, FRCOG, allowed me to consult the records relating to the Hospital for Women in Soho Square. Miss Patricia Want, Librarian of the Royal College of Obstetricians and Gynaecologists, Mrs Claire Daunton, former Archivist of the College, and all the staff of the RCOG Library deserve a special mention for answering my queries with enormous patience and kindness. My thanks also go to the staff of the Royal Society of Medicine Library, of the Radcliffe Science Library, Oxford, and of the Wellcome Institute Library, London, for their unfailingly competent and prompt assistance.

Miss Patricia Want organised the photograph of Protheroe Smith's bust, which appears courtesy of the RCOG. All other illustrations appear by permission of the Wellcome Institute Library.

Financial support for the original research on which this book is based came from the Wellcome Trust and from a scholarship awarded by Magdalen College, Oxford. I am grateful to both these institutions for making this book possible.

My husband Christopher Bridgett helped in a multitude of ways which it would be too long to enumerate. I very much doubt that I would have completed this work without his moral and practical support. My seven-year-old son Giacomo once declared that writing a book about 'doctors and women' was 'pretty daft'. On many occasions when the strain on the whole family seemed too great, I have been close to agreeing with him. One day Giacomo and his sister Jessica will know why this book is dedicated to them.

Introduction

In 1891 the surgeon Thomas Spencer Wells launched an attack against the 'gynaecological proletarians' who, he claimed, were extirpating women's ovaries like the 'aboriginal spayers of New Zealand'. Ovaries were being removed not only for the cure of cysts, but also for the treatment of dysmenorrhoea, hysteria, insanity and epilepsy. 'The meshes of the physical, mental, and moral network of reasons why the operation should be done are so closely woven that few cases of a perplexing nature, that can anyhow be connected with the generative organs or functions, have a chance of escaping laparotomy or something more', Wells commented. 'But would anyone strip off the penis for a stricture or a gonorrhoea, or castrate a man because he has a hydrocele, or was a moral delinquent?' The answer to this rhetorical question could only be an emphatic 'no', but Wells wanted to leave no doubt in the mind of his reader as to his feelings about certain gynaecological practices. Suppose roles were reversed, and a trained corps of female specialists accorded as much attention to the male genitalia as gynaecologists did to the female's:

If we hold the mirror up to Nature, only changing the sex of the actors, the spectacle is not flattering. Fancy the reflected picture of a coterie of the Marthas of the profession in conclave, promulgating the doctrine that most of the unmanageable maladies of men were to be traced to some morbid change in their genitals, founding societies for the discussion of them and hospitals for the cure of them, one of them sitting in her consultation chair, with her little stove by her side and her irons all hot, searing every man as he passed before her; another gravely proposing to bring on the millennium by snuffing out the reproductive powers of all fools, lunatics, and criminals ... if too, we saw, in this magic mirror, ignorant boys being castrated almost impromptu, hundreds of emasculated beings moping about and bemoaning their doltish credulity ... should we not, to our shame, see ourselves as others see us? ... Should we not be bound ... to denounce such follies as a personal degradation, a crime against society, and a dishonour to the profession?[1]

Nearly one hundred years after the publication of *Epidemic of Laparotomy*, from which this passage is drawn, Wells' imaginary andrological ward has not lost its power to shock. A deeply entrenched belief in our culture holds that sex and reproduction are more fundamental to woman's than to man's nature. Puberty, childbirth, the menopause, are deemed to affect woman's mind and body in ways which have no counterpart in man. Because of her role in reproduction, woman is regarded as a special case, a deviation from the norm represented by the male. This difference is used to prescribe very different roles for men and women. The public arena of work, politics and commerce is said to be more appropriate for men, while women are held to be better suited for activities in the private sphere of the family as mothers and wives.

Since the beginning of the nineteenth century, the science of gynaecology has legitimated these views. The belief that the female body is finalised for reproduction defines the study of 'natural woman' as a separate branch of medicine; it identifies women as a special group of patients and a distinct type within the human species; it defines social roles and invites their acceptance. This book explores the social and medical context in which the idea of a 'gynaecology' has been able to take root and flourish.

Definitions of femininity and masculinity raise the question of the meaning of human nature. It is striking that gynaecology developed at the same time as the scientific study of humankind, yet the growth of gynaecology was not paralleled by the evolution of a complementary 'science of masculinity' or 'andrology'. Understanding the historical origins of this asymmetry entails questioning the autonomy of science from society. Scientific ideas of masculinity, femininity and humanity represent in a symbolic form the social relations between men and women, and between men and other men; by presenting historically specific notions about man's and woman's nature as the fruit of unbiased observation, they also conceal the social conditions in which they are produced.

The beginning of modern medical discourse on woman's nature can be traced back to the end of the eighteenth century and the development of the 'science of man'. (The use of the term 'man' to mean 'human being' has been retained in this book, as it reveals the ideological context in which both gynaecology and anthropology have grown.) The age of Enlightenment was characterised by the faith that empirically based knowledge was the key to improving human existence: by discovering the natural laws which governed human life, society could be reorganised on a just basis and human happiness secured. Enlightenment writers were interested in combating the doctrine that the original source of 'right' was from God through monarch and Church; in its place, they put forward a form of political legitimation based on the acceptance of the social contract. The appeal to the 'natural reason' of humankind served to criticise inherited property rights as the basis of political participation: reason was shared by all, thus all men had equal rights to citizenship through the franchise.[2]

Science and medicine played a crucial role in the rise of liberal political thought, because their methods seemed to be the only ones which would displace the 'artificial' notions of human nature derived from metaphysical speculation and religious orthodoxy and lead to a secular, value-free knowledge of the social and natural worlds. The study of 'natural man' took many forms, from comparisons of the physical varieties of humankind, to the analysis of mental operations and descriptive studies of behaviour, custom and law. Bio-medical writers were especially interested in the female form of man, her physiological functions, moral peculiarities and social status. Democracy had undermined the old basis for patriarchal authority, and it was consequently necessary to rethink the relationship between the sexes along new lines. Nature, not religion or metaphysics, had to define the place man and woman would occupy in the new social order.[3]

Central to the male attack on patriarchy was the separation of a private zone of familial relations from a public sphere of work and politics; this was accompanied by the elaboration of an anatomy and physiology of sexual difference. Men and women, argued Rousseau in Book V of *Emile*, were the same in everything that is not associated with sex; in everything connected with sex, they were related, but different. While the male was male 'only at certain moments', though, the female was female 'her whole life': childbearing, suckling, nurturing, constantly reminded woman of her sex.[4] All the other moral and social distinctions between men and women flowed from these basic biological differences: modesty, secretiveness, passivity and irrationality opposed woman to daring, reasoning and energetic man. Notions of biological maternity and of female physiology justified the association of women with nature in opposition to culture; they designated woman's place within the family, the most basic biological and social unit.

The family occupied a pivotal place in the science of man, for it served to explain the relationship between the individual and society in a totally naturalistic manner. The family was rooted in individual acts of sex and reproduction; it was also a microcosm of society and the foundation of the social order. This separation between private and public areas of life did not mirror the reality of women's experiences, nor did it fit across classes and cultures, but it did form the basis of a pervasive ideology which proposed a model of femininity, providing the rationale for excluding women from man's domain – politics, business, organised labour and the professions.[5]

During the course of the nineteenth century, the man/woman dichotomy developed relations with other oppositional pairs, notably the adult and the child, the normal and the pathological, civilisation and savagery. Woman was classed with the child and the primitive, and both femininity and savagery were seen to be pathological states and an arrested stage of development of the human species. Categories of sex, race and age came to define the standards of social worth.[6]

Medical writers' insistence on the difference between male and female belied the difficulty of pinning down the boundaries between the sexes. As Jordanova has observed, dichotomies operate at two levels: the use of separate terms highlights their difference, while pairing them evokes their kinship.[7] The second point is illustrated by the widespread interest in the latent hermaphroditism of the human species. Hermaphroditism was a phenomenon which spanned the terms 'male' and 'female'; it guaranteed the unity of the human species, but in so doing it threw into relief the likeness between man and woman. Similar ambiguities about the status of the 'child' as a category distinct from the 'adult' are displayed by the debates about the age at which children should be able to work or consent to sexual intercourse.

Despite the difficulty of defining gender categories in practice, the ideological opposition between male and female has played a crucial role in shaping representations of the social order. The putatively biological distinctions of sex cut across class barriers, displacing social issues onto a seemingly neutral terrain – the realm of nature. By incorporating notions of hierarchy and dependence, gender categories obscure the existence of hierarchies of class and the sources of inequality and domination in our society; they are thus crucially important to the maintenance of the established order and the integration of society as a whole. In historicising gynaecology, it is essential to turn this relationship between the 'social' and the 'natural' on its head: in our society, which is perpetuated by the simultaneous operation of class and gender relations, class must be a fundamental category for exploring the medical treatment of women.[8]

As the 'science of woman' developed within medical discourse, gynaecology must be analysed also in relation to the structure of medicine of which it was a part. Specialisation was an important feature of nineteenth-century medical practice, yet there are few general works on this phenomenon. In his pioneering study of *Specialization of Medicine*, published in 1944, Rosen argued that the emergence of specialist medicine was closely related to the elaboration of pathological anatomy by the early nineteenth-century Paris school of medicine.[9] Since then Toby Gelfand, taking issue with Rosen, has attempted a sociological analysis of medical specialisation in the light of its kindred notion, the division of labour. Noting how the notion of specialisation spanned disciplines as diverse as Adam Smith's economic theory, Darwin's biology and Durkheim's sociology, Gelfand has argued that the emergence of the concept must be explored in terms of the prevailing mode of economic organisation under industrial capitalism. In industry, the division of labour led to increased productivity; in medicine, specialisation enabled the practitioner to improve his skill.[10]

Neither Rosen's nor Gelfand's account are particularly convincing. Against Rosen, one would like to argue that not all the organs of the body have become the subject of medical specialties; some specialties, for example anaesthesia, have developed round particular techniques, while others, like paediatrics and geriatrics, cluster round the medicine of specific age groups.[11] Gelfand's notion of the division of medical labour is equally problematic: it is based on the assumption that medicine is a system with self-evident unity rather than a collection of phenomena people choose to bring together, and that there is something inevitable about the division of medical knowledge.[12] These observations are especially applicable to obstetrics and gynaecology, a specialism which is underpinned by a historically contingent notion of woman. It is conceivable that one day the rationale for differentiating gynaecology to the present degree may cease to exist, leading to the disappearance of gynaecology from medical cosmology.

A specialism is, by definition, a subdivision *of* something else. This 'something else' is medicine only in the most general and abstract sense. At different times in its history, gynaecology and its sister specialism obstetrics have been regarded as a branch of physic, a branch of surgery, a specialism of general practice and a subject in its own right on a par with medicine and surgery. Each of these definitions has been 'interested': it has depended on the power of certain groups of practitioners within the medical profession to impose their own view of the subject. The underlying motives have been invariably social and economic. For example, the struggle between obstetricians and general surgeons over abdominal surgery, which led directly to the foundation of the Royal College of Obstetricians and Gynaecologists, makes little sense unless the economic value of gynaecological operations is fully appreciated.

Originally, the early medical specialties like urology, ophthalmology and obstetrics were not a part of medicine at all: they were the province of lay people and itinerant 'quacks'. From the late eighteenth century onwards, these fields were encroached upon by upwardly mobile individuals who were in some important respects marginal to the medical establishment – for example, in London provincial origins and lack of professional connections were two of the factors which spurred certain medical practitioners onto the path of 'specialisation'. This was usually accompanied by claims to exclusive expertise and the search for professional status. Margaret Pelling and Robert Dingwall have urged historians to analyse the origins of professions as part of the history of occupations in general, and to view professionalism as a strategy for social mobility rather than as a goal. This seems a particularly useful framework for analysing the development of the obstetrical and gynaecological profession from the late eighteenth century to the present day.[13]

History can show the emergence of medical concepts and practices whose social meanings are easier to grasp from the vantage point of the present. The chief object of this study will be achieved if the reader can be persuaded to ask why, on the eve of the twenty-first century, we still need a 'science of woman'.

1

The problem of femininity

'The doctrine of the nature and diseases of women': this is how J. Craig, geologist and compiler of the *New Universal Etymological, Technological, and Pronouncing Dictionary of the English Language*, first explained the term 'gynaecology' in 1849.[1] This definition was intelligible in the light of shared assumptions about the biological foundations of femininity: as woman was dominated by her sexual functions, the physiology and pathology of her reproductive system provided the key to understanding her physical, mental and moral peculiarities.

In Craig's times, the evidence for this belief was highly controversial. With the exception of that quintessentially female attribute, the capacity to engender life, no anatomical, physiological or psychological character seemed to be the exclusive peculiarity of one sex or the other. Furthermore, social and environmental factors were thought to affect gender differences, allowing for conscious and historical change; this paved the way to the nature versus nurture controversy which has bedevilled research on sex differences ever since. Thus, if certain views about the nature of femininity were emphasised by medical writers and ultimately were crystallised by the 'science of woman', we must ask why it was so important to see women as sexual beings and why this occurred at the time it did.

Woman's sexuality and population concerns

Although the evidence about the practice of gynaecology before 1800 is not very extensive, it seems certain that the care of women's diseases was not the special concern of any one group of practitioners. Theoretically the organisation of medicine into three branches, each supervised by its own corporation – the College of Physicians, the Company of Barber-Surgeons and the Society of

Apothecaries – granted the physicians a monopoly of physic which included women's diseases; but as the advice of physicians was expensive, in practice the greater part of medical care fell to the surgeons and the apothecaries. It is thus probable that these two grades of practitioners provided gynaecological care as one of their medical tasks.

In 1664 an attempt was made by the London Surgeons to have the practice of women's diseases recognised as one of their legal prerogatives. Surgeons did all they could to strengthen their claim to prescribe, but it is not clear what made them particularly interested in the diseases of women. The physicians were quite willing to grant the request, as they hoped thereby to buy off the opposition of the Company of Barber-Surgeons to a new Charter which would have greatly extended their powers. In the event the apothecaries' vociferous objections to the Charter prevented the Physicians' Bill from going through Parliament, and nothing more was done about the diseases of women.[2]

It seems beyond doubt that gynaecology in Tudor and Stuart England was also practised by midwives. Books written for the instruction of midwives often included chapters on gynaecology. For example, in *Observations diverses sur la stérilité*, published in 1642, the French Court midwife Louyse Bourgeois (1563–1636) dealt with sterility, fecundity, the diseases of women and those of infants;[3] Mrs Jane Sharp's *The Midwives Book* (1671) contained sections on women's diseases and on the anatomy of the female reproductive organs.[4] According to the late seventeenth-century physician William Sermon, midwives took upon themselves three things: they assessed whether a woman was fertile prior to marriage; they assisted women in childbed and diagnosed pregnancy and virginity.[5] In her *Complete Practice of Midwifery*, published in 1737, the midwife Sarah Stone argued that 'all the Disorders of Teeming Women do not belong to Midwives; but they ought to commit themselves to the care of a Physician; a Midwife's business being only to be well instructed in her Profession'.[6] Arguably at least some of Stone's colleagues regarded women's diseases as a routine part of their practice.

A midwife's skill in treating women's ailments is mentioned in an episcopal licence in surgery granted to Mrs Elizabeth Frances in 1689. Women were debarred from the Universities of Oxford and Cambridge and thus were not eligible for the Licence granted by these institutions to graduates in medicine; however the episcopal licence in surgery, which had been instituted during the reign of Henry VIII, was open to both men and women. According to a testimonial signed by two surgeons, two physicians and a man-midwife, Mrs Frances was 'very well instructed and Practised in the art of Midwifery and also in the knowledge of Medicines which may be of use to women in their several Maladies'. She was granted a licence 'tam Chirurgiae quam Obstetricis'.[7] In the early nineteenth century Mme Boivin (1773–1841), one of the most famous of the Paris midwives, improved the speculum and wrote authoritatively upon a number of diseases of the uterus and ovaries.

Irregular practitioners of both sexes were extensively patronised by rich and poor women alike. Healing was part of women's domestic activities, and every housewife was expected to understand the treatment of the minor ailments of her own household, and to prepare her own drugs. Wealthy mistresses of households and wives of clergymen extended their medical services to the sick poor out of religious conviction and a sense of social responsibility. For example Prudence Potter (1612–83), wife of the Rector of Newton St Petrock in Devon, is said on her tombstone to have spent her life in the successful practice of 'physick, chirurgery and midwifery'.[8] 'Quack' doctresses did a lively trade out of women's complaints. For example, an eighteenth-century female empiric practising in London sold a powder which was a 'most certain and speedy cure for the Green-sickness, Melancholly and Spleen, and helps Stoppages and Obstructions in Women'; a 'gentlewoman' who dwelt at Blackfriars claimed she could cure greensickness and 'many other things in women not fit to mention'.

Among the male irregulars, John Wilmont (1647–80) in the seventeenth century and John Graham in the eighteenth are remembered for their involvement in the care of women's ailments. Wilmont, second Earl of Rochester and companion of Charles I, was often expelled from the Court for lampooning the King. It is said that at such times he set up a stall near the Tower of London and under the name of Alexandro Bindo he sold remedies, advice and cosmetics to a predominantly female clientele. In the late eighteenth century the London quality flocked to John Graham's Temple of Health to avail themselves of his infallible cure for sterility. This consisted of an ornate 'Magneto-Electrico' bed on which couples desirous of progeny could spend the night and, by a 'compliment of fifty pound bank note', partake of the 'heavenly joys' it afforded by causing 'immediate conception'.[9]

During the course of the eighteenth century, with the creation of dispensaries and the extension of the voluntary hospital system, medical institutions came to play an increasingly important role in the provision of gynaecological care for poor women. Out of the 843 patients treated by Sir Gilbert Blane at St Thomas's Hospital between 1783 and 1794, 256 were women suffering from gynaecological disease. Blane gave no details as to the nature of these cases, except in one instance, which was a case of vicarious menstruation from the navel. In private practice, he listed cases of *fluor albus* (white discharge), menstrual derangements, hysteria, cancer of the womb and ovarian dropsy.[10]

But by far the most important development in gynaecological care during the eighteenth century was the rise of a class of practitioners of midwifery and diseases of women and children. There were medical men practising midwifery before 1700, and occasionally these men-midwives (a term introduced in 1625) also took an interest in the diseases of women. Until the first quarter of the eighteenth century, though, the number of men-midwives was very small, since midwifery was not considered to be a medical responsibility, but a lay craft: midwives usually attended normal cases, which were the great majority of births, while medical men were generally called in an emergency, or booked in the expectation of such eventualities. The treatment of the diseases of infancy was also outside the purview of the medical man. This field was in the hands of local irregulars, especially women; as midwives looked after both mother and child during the lying-in period, they may well have played an important part in the care of sick babies.[11]

From about 1730 onwards, medical men rapidly encroached upon the territory of the midwife, extending the scope of their intervention in childbirth from the attendance of complications to the routine management of all births. The closing decades of the century saw medical men push the limits of their role even further: the biographies of men-midwives such as Michael Underwood (d. 1820) and John Clarke (1758–1815) provide evidence of an increasing tendency for medical men to become involved in the health care of women and children as an integral part of their midwifery practice. This prompts us to ask what motivated a redefinition of the medical practitioner's responsibilities to include not only the management of normal births, but also the treatment of the diseases of women and infants.

The answer to this question lies in the political and economic changes stimulated by the growth of industry in late seventeenth-century England. Beginning with William Petty (1623–87), production and labour came to the fore as essential elements in the generation of the national wealth, and attention was focussed on the 'population' as a fundamental category for economic and political analysis. Political theorists extolled the virtues of a growing population. A larger population, they argued, meant greater production and greater consumption as well as increased military strength; it was thus in the interest of the state not only to know the value and number of its people, but also to maintain and extend its human resources by encouraging fecundity and preserving life. In England, this system of thought came to be known as 'mercantilism'; similar arguments in the Germanies took the form of 'cameralism'.[12]

During the second half of the eighteenth century the focus of political arithmetic shifted, reflecting changes in the ideological and political status of vital statistics. In the statistical work of nonconformist clergymen and supporters of the French and American Revolutions, a new emphasis was placed on life-style: this was to show that where the 'natural equality' of individuals was subverted by property rights, people did not die just of old age, but from the diseases created by the vices of civil society. The population should thus be divided not into ranks and classes for statistical purposes, but according to their place of residence, and vital statistics should quantify the private behaviour of individuals as well as counting the people.[13]

By the end of the eighteenth century, the quantitative approach to the problem of population had given way to discussions about the manner in which the quality of the health of the labouring sector could lead to increased productivity. Governments were advised to give serious attention to the management of those physical and environmental conditions which were conducive to productive labour and a stable political order. With the new political and economic significance attached to issues of life, death, health and disease, the importance of medical practitioners emerged as the people who, by curing and preventing sickness, could assist in the creation and maintenance of a healthy workforce.

The natural sciences played a major role in articulating this growing interest in the population as an aggregate of individuals who live, reproduce and die. Bio-medical writers attempted to define the elusive concept of 'life'; there was a resurgence of medical interest in the processes and mechanisms by which life was generated, reproduction and sexuality gaining prominence as central objects of research for the life sciences in the eighteenth century.[14] Medical men further addressed themselves to three questions which directly impinged on the production and preservation of life: the standards of midwifery practice, the diseases of the childbearing woman and those of the infant child.

From 1739 onwards, an alleged fall in the population of England focussed attention on the high levels of infant and maternal death revealed by Parish Registers and London Bills of Mortality. It was in this context that medical men began to scrutinise the practices of midwives and the management of infancy. Doctors increasingly attributed the cause of infant and maternal death to the incompetence of midwives and criticised childrearing procedures as outmoded and injudicious. In the name of science and freedom from the fetters of tradition, they attacked the female rituals that had hitherto surrounded childbirth and the lying-in period (for example, the swaddling of infants), and recommended new 'enlightened' procedures, to be carried out by women under the watchful eye of the medical man: 'the Preservation of Children should become the Care of Men of Sense', typically argued the physician William Cadogan in his *Essay on Nursing* (1748), because 'this Business has been too long fatally left to the Management of Women'.[15]

Population concerns lay at the heart of men-midwives' growing involvement in the care of women's complaints and disorders during the second half of the eighteenth century. Men-midwives, it was argued, had special expertise to bring to the numerous aspects of women's sexual physiology and pathology that had social implications; for this reason the obstetric art was an aspect of forensic medicine, that branch of the law where putatively natural considerations were of the utmost importance in the administration of justice.[16] Because of their thorough knowledge of the anatomy and physiology of the female reproductive system, men-midwives were well qualified to assist the judiciary in matters relating to marriage and divorce, rape, abortion, illegitimacy and infanticide.

It was indeed in the title of a medico-legal treatise on sexual congress in woman that the word 'gynaecology' first appeared in its modern spelling. In the early eighteenth century Martin Schurig (d. 1733), physician of Dresden, was the first to use the term 'gynaecologia' in his analysis of various sex problems from the medical, social and medico-legal points of view. The topics discussed by Schurig in his *Gynaecologia* (1730) included nymphomania, chastity, pre-nuptial coitus, rape, vaginismus, lesbianism, buggery and bestiality. A slightly different version of the term had appeared in an earlier text by Joannes Petrus Lotichius (1598–1669), Professor of Medicine at the German University of Rinteln. Like Schurig's *Gynaecologia*, Lotichius' *Gynaicologia* (1630) was not about the diseases of women. In his dissertation, Lotichius addressed himself to the question of woman's nature and, challenging the doctrine of female inferiority propounded by the ancients, he argued that women were perfect in their physical creation.[17] These two themes – the discourse on feminine nature and the medico-legal interest in woman's sexual functions and behaviour – were to be incorporated into the scientific analysis of femininity which began to develop from the end of the eighteenth century onwards.

Woman's place in nature

The study of the nature of femininity began as a genre combining scientific findings with literary observation and philosophical aphorisms.[18] This inquiry was one aspect of research into the natural history of mankind, one of the fields which the emerging science of anthropology was beginning to define and appropriate. In the spirit of scientific enquiry fostered by the Enlightenment, biomedical writers aspired to create a new 'science of man' based on rational knowledge derived from the senses. Comparative anatomy and physiology, the methods proper to natural history, were applied to the analysis of the human species in the belief that it should be treated like any other animal species. Researchers further investigated the nature of mind and the working of the intellect and examined the influence of custom and social institutions upon human physiology, hoping that the data thus gathered might shed light on the problem of man's place in the grand scheme of the universe.[19]

The taxonomy of sexual diversity fulfilled two aims: first, it had to establish the characters of 'natural Man'; secondly, it had to determine how men and women differed in relation to each other. The science of woman, or 'gynaecology', could thus be regarded as part of a system of classification in which the study of feminine nature complemented on the one hand anthropology, the science of man, and on the other hand the study of the male peculiarities.

These themes were set out with exceptional clarity and insight by the late nineteenth-century gynaecologist, the Scottish-trained Professor of Medicine and Health Officer to the city of Melbourne, James Jamieson (1840–1916). His thoughts on the subject were contained in an article entitled 'Sex, in health and disease', published in the *Australian Medical Journal* in 1887. By that time anthropology had established its independent role as a science of race, a classification of human 'types' whose cultural differences were seen to derive from fundamental differences in physiological organisation. In 1871 anthropological research had become the business of the Anthropological Institute, which had arisen out of the amalgamation of the Ethnological and Anthropological Societies. Eschewing both the strictly somatological approach propounded by the Anthropological Society and the ethnologists' use of language as a test of race, the Anthropological Institute had set itself the task to bring together the physical and cultural analysis of mankind within an evolutionary paradigm.[20] Gynaecology for its part, already firmly entrenched in general and hospital practice, had just been given an institutional base with the foundation of the British Gynaecological Society in 1885; in due course the specialism would also find its place within the medical curriculum and on the medical governing bodies, such as the Royal Colleges of Physicians and Surgeons and the General Medical Council.

Jamieson began his article with an etymological note:

One very striking want in the English language is the absence of a word to denote the human being, irrespective of age and sex . . . We are compelled to use the word *man* with two distinct significations, both as a member of the human race, and as an adult male. When the need arose for a term to describe that branch of science which is concerned with the natural history of the human race, the word treasury of the old Greeks was drawn on, and the term *anthropology* constructed.[21]

In order to define man's place in nature, Jamieson explained, anthropologists employed various classificatory devices, depending on the special purposes of their enquiries: for example, the comparative degree of civilisation of human beings, their colour, or their speech. There was, however, he argued,

one obvious division, more fixed and definite than any of these, and that is according to sex. In addition, therefore, to general anthropology, or the study of human beings, as distinguished from animals ... we might properly enough speak of *Andrology* and *Gynaecology* as being concerned with the study of the physical and mental peculiarities of men and women respectively.[22]

This was no academic exercise. Since the end of the eighteenth century the study of sexual differences had been inextricably bound up with debates on the social function of the sexes, in the belief that science alone could provide conclusive evidence for the allocation of gender roles in society. What part men and women were to play in life would proceed from a just appreciation of their 'natural' capacities, and thus reliable criteria of differentiation were required. This concern became all the more pressing as the 'Woman Question' reached its climax in the 1860s and an increasingly vocal contingent of women challenged the bastions of patriarchal privilege and domination in the domestic and political spheres.[23] It was felt that issues such as women's entrance into the legal and medical professions, their claims to the vote and education should be submitted 'to Agassiz and Huxley, not to Kant or Calvin, church or Pope':[24] philosophical speculation and religious dogma had to give way to the seemingly unemotional and unbiased pronouncements of science. By the last quarter of the nineteenth century, other social problems were being subjected to the same treatment. From the late 1870s onwards, anthropometric and ethnographic surveys of the British population were undertaken for the purpose of identifying the social or physical attributes which could explain the origins of poverty and social inequality. Both sex and class had to be moved out of the social arena, into the realm of nature.[25]

In analysing nineteenth-century notions of masculinity and femininity, it is important to understand that for bio-medical writers sex differences were not a matter of the genitals alone, but of the total physiology and psychology of individuals. This view was summed up in 1889 by the gynaecologist James Oliver who, echoing ideas which the French physician Cabanis[26] had expressed before him at the end of the eighteenth century, wrote in these terms:

The difference between the man and the woman is not stamped on any one organ of the body, neither is it revealed in the function or group of functions manifested by the organs of generation, it is rather an association of such, and is the outcome of a peculiar molecular and molar state belonging to every organ and structure of the body. The difference is universal or constitutional; it pervades the whole mind and body of the individual.[27]

Sexuality – that is to say the *qualities* associated with masculinity and femininity – was not seen as a static essence, but as a dynamic biological process which unfolded from conception to puberty. Physicians insisted that it was often impossible to determine the sex of an individual at birth solely on the basis of its genitalia. The distinction between the male and the female of the species, they argued, could only be properly made out at the time of puberty, when the orientation of sexual desire and the secondary sexual characters (such as body hair, strength and physical conformation) became manifest; if these still left room for doubt, the habits and psychological traits of the individual should also be taken into account.[28] Both the anatomical and psychological distinctions of sex were thought to be coincidental with the period of functional activity of the ovaries and testes – a belief for which the masculine appearance of menopausal women and the effeminacy of eunuchs were alleged as evidence; there was however no consensus about the extent to which sexual characteristics were determined by gonadal activity as opposed to environmental and social factors.

Granted that sex differences were not limited to the reproductive organs, it remained for the physiologist to establish which characters were sex-specific and which were common to both sexes and thus standard of the species. Secondly, it had to be demonstrated whether the man or the woman should be regarded as the more typical representative of humankind. On both scores bio-medical writers displayed a degree of ambiguity which the lay reader may well find astonishing. The difficulties which beset research into sex differences stemmed in part from the comparative approach itself, with its subtle interplay between difference and similarity: laying too much emphasis on the difference between man and woman might obscure racial categories and undermine the unity of the human species in relation to the lower animals. The mid-Victorian scientist George John Romanes (1848–94) narrowly avoided this pitfall when discussing the mental differences between men and women: 'While within the limits of each species the male differs psychologically from the female', he wrote in an article first published in *Nineteenth Century* for May 1887, 'in the animal kingdom as a whole the males admit of being classified, as it were, in one psychological species, and the females in another'. By this it was not meant 'that there is usually greater psychological difference between the two sexes of the same species than there is between the same sexes of different species', he wrote. 'I mean only that the points wherein the two sexes differ psychologically are more or less similar wherever these differences occur.'[29]

During the Victorian period, attempts to reconcile the concept of sexual difference with the idea of a human nature common to both sexes typically took the form of a widespread fascination with the latent hermaphroditism or bisexuality of humankind. While the notion of difference emphasised the incommensurability of male and female, hermaphroditism brought into relief their similarity and continuity. Within the deepest recesses of their bodies, men and women were neuter persons, undifferentiated parts of a society which in theory recognised the equality of all its members: the genderless substratum of humanity became the last refuge of the ideals of the French Revolution. A useful parallel may be drawn here between the notion of hermaphroditism in anatomy and physiology and the concept of 'degeneration' in nineteenth-century anthropology. Negative though it was, the belief that savage man was a pathological deviation from the standard represented by the civilised European contained within it the possibility that the process might be reversed, either by interbreeding with a 'superior' race, or by migration to the temperate zones inhabited by the white race; it thus served to underline the fundamental kinship between civilised white and savage black man. For the monogenist school in anthropology, this was proof of the common origins of humankind and the basis on which programmes for social amelioration could be legitimated. In contrast, those anthropologists who believed in the plurality of human species, for example Paul Broca, denied that physically dissimilar races were interfertile (or 'eugenesic'), while others disputed that miscegenation led to an improvement in the quality of hybrid offspring. The association of polygenism with conservative and racist politics has been noted by a number of historians of anthropology.[30]

The science of embryology exemplifies one of the many ways in which ideas about the essential bisexuality of humankind were articulated. For nineteenth-century physiologists, the identity of male and female was recognisable at the embryological level: the penis and the clitoris, the scrotum and the labia, the testes and the ovaries, and so on, shared common origins in foetal life. During the course of the development of an individual from conception to adulthood, sex organs became differentiated in structure and function, but to each organ in the male, there corresponded a homologous structure in the female. The belief that the male and the female reproductive organs were comparable in their form, number and function had its roots in ancient medicine; by the middle of the nineteenth century, the homologies between male and female had been recast in the language of history.[31] Some organs became fully developed in the adults of one sex only, but could also be discerned in the other sex in the embryonic state: the Wolffian ducts in the female and the cornua of the male utriculus were examples of embryonic structures which became fully evolved in the adults of one sex only, the one developing into Fallopian tubes, the other into *vasa deferentia*. Other organs were functionally specific to the adult of one sex only, but were also present in the other in a rudimentary type of structure: such, for instance, was the case of the breasts[32] and indeed of the uterus. According to the obstetrician Arthur Farre, this organ was not 'altogether peculiar to the female'; it had 'its representative in the male, though only in a rudimental state'.[33]

Belief in the kinship of male and female can be fruitfully explored by looking at nineteenth-century theories of menstruation. The Victorian period saw a revival of the Greek conception of menstruation as a form of elimination or cleansing. It was widely thought that menstruation was a sort of physiological blood-letting by which women rid themselves of a superfluous quantity of blood. In cases of amenorrhoea, other organs would take over the work of the uterus and periodic haemorrhages 'vicarious' of the menstrual flux would ensue from other parts of the body – for example, the nose, the anus, the gums, the kidneys or the nipples.[34]

Given that any form of bleeding could be seen as a case of vicarious menstruation; given also that this phenomenon was allegedly observed in women whose uterus was congenitally absent,[35] it is not surprising to find that bloody discharges from the penis were also regarded as instances of vicarious menstruation. This was an idea of great antiquity which mid-nineteenth-century physicians re-interpreted in the light of new 'scientific' theories – notably the 'law of periodicity', discussed below. The well-known obstetrician

Alfred Wiltshire discussed male menstruation in an article published in the *Lancet* for 1885. Wiltshire cited a number of English
and foreign cases. The French physician Chopart, for example,
mentioned a young soldier who had a monthly discharge of bloody
urine, accompanied by all the symptoms characteristic of the menstrual flux; his fellow countryman Rayer cited two similar cases,
one of which was that of a butcher of Sedan, 'whose infirmity,
becoming known, inspired so great disgust that no one would
purchase meat from him'. Wiltshire himself knew of a surgeon who
had bleeding from his penis every three weeks.[36]

A first-hand account of a 'case of menstruation in the male' was
provided in 1867 by the American physician V. O. King. The
subject was a twenty-two-year-old youth of a lymphatic temperament who 'periodically performed the simulated functions of menstruation', though 'not possessed of the usual organs'. King had
personally witnessed this phenomenon on many occasions and
described it with abundance of anatomical detail. The menstruating
male, a fellow student at the University of Louisiana medical
school,

had been the victim of this vicarious function for a period of three years,
eliminating an apparent catamenial secretion, with the same regularity,
and attended by the same indications by which it is characterised in the
human female. The fluid exuded, flowed from the sebaceous glands of the
deep fossa behind the corona glandis, and was of a sanguineous appearance, homogeneous and thick. The quantity of this exudation varied from
one to two ounces during each haemorrhagic period, and the duration of
the periods from three to six days.[37]

King had considered the possibility that the discharge might be
caused by venereal disease, but he was emphatic that his friend had
never suffered from such afflictions.

In order to explain the occurrence of vicarious haemorrhages in
the male, mid-Victorian physicians drew on the immensely popular theory of 'vital periodicity'. First proposed by the renowned
English neurophysiologist Thomas Laycock (1812–76) in the early
1840s, this doctrine was subsequently elaborated by a number of
eminent scientists, from Charles Darwin to Sigmund Freud and
Havelock Ellis, the late-nineteenth-century pioneer in the study of
sexology.[38] Laycock's view was that all physiological phenomena
were governed by regular temporal cycles, which he ascribed to the
influence of the sun, the moon and the seasons. Vicarious haemor-

rhages and menstruation itself, he maintained, were nothing more than manifestations of this fundamental law of periodicity.[39] As the law affected all living beings, regardless of their sex, men, too, were liable to suffer from haemorrhages analogous to the menstrual flux in woman. 'All periodical haemorrhages in the human species', wrote Alfred Wiltshire,

are under the dominion of the primal law of periodicity, which it inherits in common with all animals; only in the female we see, as a matter of observation, that the influence of periodicity is most markedly displayed.[40]

The difference between male and female was thus merely one of degree. In illustration, Wiltshire mentioned the case of a distinguished London surgeon, who from the time of puberty had invariably had a crop of herpes on the left side of his penis every three weeks.

It was on the basis of such evidence that in 1897 the Viennese laryngologist Wilhelm Fliess (1858–1928), one of Freud's closest collaborators, posited the existence of two biological cycles, lasting twenty-eight and twenty-three days each. Both periods were present in both sexes, he argued; but while the first was dominant in woman, the second was more marked in man. On the basis of this 'discovery', Fliess formulated his theory of the essential bisexuality of human beings:

These two groups of periodic processes . . . have a solid inner relation with male and female sexual characteristics. And it is only in accordance with our actual bisexual constitution if both – only with different stress – are present in every man and woman.[41]

His friend Sigmund Freud was very much struck with this idea. Freud described it as 'the most significant for my subject since that of defence';[42] and the notion of bisexuality was indeed to play a very important role in his theory of the aetiology of psychoneuroses.

The well-known Edinburgh obstetrician Sir James Young Simpson (1811–70) addressed himself to the question of hermaphroditism in an influential treatise published in the late 1830s. Simpson focussed on the development of the breasts, arguing that it could not be regarded as unique to the female. He pointed out that this character had been noted in hermaphrodites in whom the *male* type predominated; sometimes it had been observed even in those males whose reproductive organs and functions were perfect. This led the eminent obstetrician to conclude that the development of the breasts was not confined to the female, but was common to both sexes and thus proper to the species in general.[43]

Instances such as this strengthened Simpson's conviction that the only true representative of a species was the hermaphrodite: 'the natural characters of any species of animal', he wrote,

are certainly not to be sought for solely either in the system of the male or in that of the female; but . . . they are both to be found in those properties which are common to both sexes, and which we have seen combined together by nature upon the bodies of an unnatural hermaphrodite, or evolved from the interference of art upon the castrated male or spayed female.[44]

Simpson believed that the secondary sexual differences depended on the ovaries in the female and the testes in the male. People in whom the activity of these organs was in abeyance closely approximated the type of the species: the individual in the pre-pubertal state and the menopausal woman provided examples of natural hermaphroditism, while castration produced hermaphrodites artificially.[45] For Simpson it was the male who at puberty departed from the androgynous state common to the young of both sexes and became more highly developed as an individual. However, he claimed that the adult female was more perfect in relation to the species, precisely because she was closer to the hermaphroditic type.[46]

By 1871 Charles Darwin had joined the debate with his *Descent of Man and Selection in Relation to Sex*, where he argued that sexual divergence was an integral part of the evolutionary process.[47] Darwin's main point was that the survival of the fittest could be of no lasting value to the evolution of the species if the fittest did not reproduce. He thus posited a mechanism independent of natural selection, whereby the fittest males had succeeded in conquering the females. Following the German comparative anatomist Carl Gegenbaur (1826–1903),[48] Darwin claimed that the progenitor of the vertebrate kingdom was androgynous. By division of labour and specialisation of function, organisms had developed a variety of bodily structures and mental qualities which gave them a reproductive advantage over other individuals of the same sex. This was the meaning Darwin attached to the term 'sex characters'.[49] Thus the males had acquired, for example, plumage, musical organs, strength and pugnacity – attributes which subserved either courtship or the struggle among the males for the possession of the females. The success of the better-endowed males in the contest for wives had gradually caused the male to vary and diverge from the female; in this way, Darwin argued, he had become her superior in terms of strength, pugnacity and mental powers.[50]

The medical profession was very slow to notice Darwin's controversial theories, but Robert Lawson Tait (1845–99), the famous Birmingham gynaecological surgeon, stood out amongst the rest in having professed himself a 'disciple of Darwin' soon after the publication of the *Origin of Species* in 1859.[51] This was congruent with his anti-establishment tendencies, which made him many enemies both within and outside the medical profession: a Gladstonian in politics, he was a committed anti-vivisectionist as well as being a fanatical Darwinist. Tait had read the *Origin of Species* while still a student in the early 1860s.[52] In 1869, he published a controversial paper on natural selection in the *Dublin Quarterly Journal of Medicine*; he was chuffed when Darwin cited it in the first edition of the *Descent of Man*.[53] By the mid-1870s, Tait was preaching Darwin's doctrines in Birmingham to the ladies who attended his biology classes. About the same time he began a correspondence with Darwin, whom he was to supply with information which he thought Darwin might find interesting. Keen to grab any opportunity to apply the theory of the survival of the fittest, Tait speculated amongst other things on the origin of tails: he was rumoured to have examined many patients at the Birmingham Hospital for Women in search of a dimple on the coccyx, which he believed to be the vestige of a lost tail.[54]

Not all late-Victorian gynaecologists were as enthusiastic about Darwinism, but it was clear that they had read the *Descent of Man* and considered its implications, especially where the theory of sexual selection led to discussions about the relative superiority of the sexes. James Jamieson for example accepted its premises, but firmly rejected its evaluative conclusions. Thus he argued that, of the two sexes, the one which showed least tendency to vary either for better or for worse was the more stable and hence the more developed. As far as it was the female who varied least, then the female body was 'more perfect, as well as more completely developed than that of the male.'[55]

Sexuality and the environment

In the *Descent of Man*, Darwin focussed on the way in which instincts were modified by new habits in order to show that the inheritance of acquired characters could help account for evolutionary change. Organisms continually interacted with their environment; in the course of time, their responses to external stimuli were incorporated into their biological make-up. Through the notion of habit, Darwin implicitly acknowledged that the distinctions between men and women were bound up with the history of the human species; as such they were not 'given in nature', but subject to the modifying influence of social and political change.

The idea that health and disease were affected by a wide range of physical and social factors had its roots in the traditions of ancient medicine, particularly the works of Hippocrates and Galen. Some of these factors were comparatively unchangeable, others were amenable to human intervention. At one end of the spectrum, one found the natural *milieu* of the organism, its geographical and climactic conditions, with which the organism was constantly interacting. At the other end there were those surroundings which human beings had purposefully created through the domination of nature, that is to say civilisation.[56] Climate, temperature, latitude and longitude formed a distinctive habitat which influenced each individual's temperament, thus shaping his or her physiology in a unique way, as an integrated totality. A similar effect was attributed to life-style, a notion which fused physical, moral and psychological considerations while also containing the idea of social change. In gynaecology, close attention was paid to climate, diet, occupation and education as factors influencing, for example, the age of menarche and the onset of the menopause.[57]

Environmentalism had an anthropological dimension which was well exemplified by the interests of the physician John Roberton (1797–1876). His enquiry on the period of puberty in Eskimo women, published in 1845, started off with an account of the geography of Labrador and of the physical and moral nature of its inhabitants, whom he described as thievish, blood-thirsty and deeply degraded. Roberton then went on to discuss how the moral changes induced by religious teaching had altered the physiological processes of puberty and the menopause.[58] These descriptions of exotic people struck a note which was much closer to home: in the second half of the nineteenth century, the equation of the criminal, pauper and work-shy at home with the savage abroad formed a theme common both to anthropological speculation and to social investigations of life in the urban slum.[59] Roberton's Eskimo female strongly evoked the degenerate inhabitants of the metropolitan bantustans described by Henry Mayhew in his study of *London Labour and the London Poor* (1861).[60]

The anthropological approach to gynaecology culminated in 1885 with Hermann H. Ploss's *Das Weib*, a book which was for many years the standard reference work on woman. Ploss, a practising gynaecologist who established the first midwifery clinic in Leipzig, envisaged his study as a 'natural history of woman' from puberty to childbirth. After his death in 1885, the book was partly rewritten by a number of editors, who were quick to perceive both its erotic potential and its originality as the beginning of a new branch of science called 'anthropological and ethnographical gynaecology'. By the time the first English edition of *Das Weib* appeared in 1935, the book had been expanded to include the history, anthropology and gynaecology of woman from birth to death, and several pictures of naked women had been added.[61] Ploss's intention in writing *Das Weib* was to illustrate 'the characteristic life and personality of woman' by means of 'facts' taken from natural and cultural history. After analysing the anatomical and psychological attributes which allegedly typified the female sex, Ploss went on to review all the legends, myths and rituals which affected women's lives. What gave such an enterprise its meaning was the underlying assumption that certain biological characters defined 'woman' as a category for anthropological inquiry. A vast array of different races could be lumped together on the basis of sex, in the belief that every aspect of woman's physiology and social life displayed her specialisation for the sexual functions.

The researches on menstruation carried out by the English physician John Power (active 1820s) in the early part of the century evinced a different aspect of the notion of environment – the idea of civilisation. John Power described the 'extraordinary periodical phenomena' which characterised the female in a collection of *Essays on the Female Economy* (1821). The title indicates his emphasis on the body as a purposeful whole, in which functions were so co-ordinated as to promote the healthy working of the organism. It was in fact to the question of the use and purpose of menstruation in the female organism that Power addressed his attention. Power had little doubt that childbearing was the only natural and hence also morally proper end for which woman had been destined: in the state of nature, such as obtained in uncivilised societies, he argued, menstruation was wholly unknown because women cyclically conceived, bore forth children and lactated without interruption. By contrast in civilised societies, where 'habit, education, moral restraint, and the customs of society' interfered with nature, pregnancy had become the exception rather than the rule. The ovum, which Power believed was spontaneously released by the ovary, was not fecundated by the male as frequently as it was in primitive cultures; it was instead expelled every month, together with the blood produced by the uterus for the nourishment of the embryo. By such a process, the unimpregnated state had become a 'second nature' produced by habit and education; subsequently the menstrual function had set in to relieve the female of the excess blood produced by the uterus.[62]

Later in the century the French zoologist Félix-Archimède Pouchet (1800–72), one of the chief proponents of the 'ovular theory' of menstruation, would invoke the action of civilisation in order to explain the development of the menstrual function in the human species. Starting from a supposed analogy between menstruation in woman and the 'heat' or 'oestrus' in the lower animals, Pouchet argued that menstruation signalled the bursting of the ovarian follicle. What difference existed between menstruation in woman and the oestrus in the female animal was quantitative rather than qualitative. In woman the frequency of the oestrus and consequently her chances of being fecundated had *increased* thanks to the influence of civilisation: living conditions in civilised societies were more favourable to the maintenance of offspring, Pouchet argued, hence civilisation must have improved women's biological capacity to bear children.[63]

This teleological argument was echoed by Alfred Wiltshire in his 'Lectures on the comparative physiology of menstruation', published in 1883. Writing in the light of Darwin's *Descent of Man* and *Variation of Plants under Domestication* (1868),[64] in which Darwin examined the variations induced in animals and plants under changed environmental conditions, Wiltshire maintained that menstruation indicated the higher evolutionary stage of the reproductive function in the human female as compared with the other mammals: he argued that the menstrual function was due to an increase in the frequency of the oestrus and attributed this change to the action of civilisation.[65]

A sexual character such as menstruation was thus conceived of as the product of an interaction between historical and environmental change and a relatively stable biological background. Other sexual differences were similarly conceptualised, although opinion differed as to the relative weight that should be assigned to biological and to social factors. The lectures on sexual differences delivered by the obstetrician John Braxton Hicks (1823–97) in 1877, running as they did the whole gamut of explanations from biological determinism to environmental relativism, are especially interesting in this respect.[66] In his first lecture Hicks wondered whether sex differences were caused by changes in the primary sex organs at puberty, or whether both primary and secondary characters were 'the common result of a primary force extending to the whole body' during the embryonic phase. In the second lecture, however, the balance shifted from nature to nurture. He observed that in terms of 'mental sensitiveness' men varied much amongst themselves, 'nearly, if not quite, as much as men differ from women', and attributed men's greater control over their nervous system to 'their mode of bringing up, their more invigorating pursuits, their rougher contact with the world ... besides the differences of a similar kind derived by descent'.[67] Exposure to the same social conditions eroded the differences between the sexes: 'Sooner or later', Hicks argued,

ill health, overwork, watching, anxieties, long-continued pain, failure in his pursuits, and many other things, singly or in combination, will bring man into a state so similar to that of woman under the same circumstances, that it must be acknowledged that it is only in degree that the sexes differ.[68]

Other late-Victorian writers struggled with the dilemmas posed by the dialectic between nature and culture. The surgeon William R. Williams, for example, considered whether the greater longevity and lower mortality rates of women were qualities inherent in the female or historical artefacts. In his opinion the higher death-rates of males during infancy, 'when the dress, food, and general treatment of both sexes are alike', showed that 'some constitutional condition inherent to sex' was probably at work. But some of the evidence pointed in other directions, for instance to the influence of occupation. Noting that there had been a comparative increase in the value of female life over a period of years, Williams commented that this was 'apparently owing to the conditions of female life being easier', for where women engaged in hard labour the mean duration of their lives was considerably shorter.[69]

Similar views were expressed by the gynaecologist James Jamieson. Women's lower mortality rates during childhood proved that this 'higher vitality' was a natural female quality, he contended, yet in the same breath he argued: 'There is good reason for believing that it is only in civilised communities that the average duration of life is greater in women than in men'.[70] For his part the gynaecologist James Oliver, commenting on the 'delicate frame' typical of the female, maintained that this was largely due to civilisation, which had 'done much to modify the physical and mental state of woman – habit in time works wondrous results'. However, it also seemed to him that there existed in woman 'a something which determines a greater structural and functional delicacy'.[71]

If nature and culture were so inextricably bound up together, how could one distinguish gender characters that were 'in nature' from those which were acquired? What hope was there of finding entirely natural justifications for the sexual division of labour? In his exhaustive study of *Man and Woman*, published in 1894, Havelock Ellis took a pessimistic view of this matter. After reviewing all the existing literature on sex differences in more than 400 densely written pages, Ellis summed up the state of the art with these discouraging remarks:

We have examined Man and Woman, as precisely as may be, from various points of view ... It is abundantly evident that we have not reached the end proposed at the outset. We have not succeeded in determining the radical and essential characters of men and women uninfluenced by external modifying conditions ... We have to recognise that our present knowledge of men and women cannot tell us what they might be or what they ought to be, but what they actually are, under the conditions of civilisation. By showing us that under varying conditions men and women are, within certain limits, indefinitely modifiable, a precise knowledge of the actual facts of the life of men and women forbids us to dogmatise rigidly concerning the respective spheres of men and women.[72]

A theory of femininity

Despite these ambiguities, there were certain ideas to which medical writers returned again and again. Physicians tended to emphasise that sex differences were not qualitative, but quantitative: they derived from the relative proportion of mutually opposed attributes in the individual. The higher intellectual faculties played the dominant role in man: this was signified by the allegedly greater cranial capacity and larger brain of the male, which nineteenth-century craniological research assessed on the basis of complex and controversial indices.[73] Woman, on the other hand, was more physical, instinctual and emotional because more powerfully dominated by the sexual functions: as the late nineteenth-century gynaecologist W. Balls-Headley enthused, the sexual instinct was the

essence and the *raison d'être* of woman's form, the expression of the cause of her existence as a woman; it is the evidence of her ancestral debt; of the instinctive necessity that the female reproductive cell must meet the male fecundating cell; the object is the propagation of the race, the production of the ensuing generation.[74]

Indeed for the Victorians 'sex' and 'woman' were interchangeable terms: the use of the phrase the 'Sex Question' to mean the 'Woman Question' is illuminating in this respect.

By contrast, man's emotions and instinctual functions, including the sexual ones, were more firmly controlled by the brain: thus head injuries were liable to cause impotence and 'wasting of the testicles', cretinism and lunacy arrested the development of the testes and suppressed the 'venereal appetite'.[75] According to the surgeon T. B. Curling (1811–88), author of the standard Victorian work on the pathology of the testicles, two officers in Vienna had become impotent in consequence of blows from fire-arms which had grazed the nape of their necks. In another case, a man 'of strong constitution and vigorous passions' had received a sabre wound which had cut off the convex part of the occipital bone and exposed the *dura mater*; within a few days of the injury he had lost the senses of sight and hearing and his testicles had become reduced to the size of beans.[76]

It is crucial to understand that the medical construction of male and female as dichotomous terms had no foundation in 'nature': it was based on ideological oppositions which are deeply entrenched in western thought. Physical and mental, feeling and thinking, tradition and science, country and city, nature and culture, all contain allusions to gender differences. Despite their deceptive clarity and the ease with which they can be used to make sense of our world, they are no more than stereotypes which do not mirror the complex reality of people's lives. In practice many intermediate stages lie between opposites, just as a variety of hamlets and villages stands between the city and the country. Gender differences were a problem for medical science precisely because of the way in which they could become blurred.[77]

During the twentieth century, theories of hormonal functioning have come to govern our understanding of sexual differentiation, but the central issues remain unresolved: as Victor Medvei writes in his history of endocrinology, the seeming 'ambivalence of sexuality' continues to puzzle contemporary endocrinologists. Medvei lists several examples. In 1935 it was found that the testicles of stallions are the richest source of oestrone, one of the female hormones. Oestrone is present in men's urine; conversely, the amount of androgenic substances found in women's urine is similar to that found in men's. Quoting the eminent endocrinologist Sir Alan S. Parkes, Medvei thus comments:

The present wonder, therefore, is not that intersexual conditions occur, but that the balance of endocrine factors usually comes down on one side or the other to produce a recognisable male or female.[78]

But what makes a human being a 'recognisable' male or female? Perceptions of masculinity and femininity in our culture are deeply informed by the ideas of 'nature' and 'culture'. It is important to understand that these are not universally valid concepts: their meanings have shifted over time, signalling changes in the way human beings have conceptualised their relationship to the natural world. To appreciate this complexity is to recognise the cultural specificity of our notions of sexual differences.

Modern ideas of nature and culture are rooted in the debate initiated by the writers of the Enlightenment, for whom an opposition between nature and society was a means of understanding and criticising the political order.[79] 'Nature' was an ambiguous term of challenge which the *philosophes* opposed to a variety of other ideas – to reason and the sciences, to law, society in general, the corrupt manners of the upper classes and civilisation. It evoked the healthy life of simple country folk, yet it could also symbolise people's unenlightened allegiance to religion and tradition. Of particular relevance to our discussion is the use of the term to signify the internal processes of the body, especially the instincts and the emotions, but also the reproductive function. Because of their biological properties as reproducers of the species, women could be readily seen as closer to nature; but by a process of metaphorical association, the concept of femininity developed relationships with the many other ideas 'nature' signified. Female vulnerability and male strength, for instance, went together with distinctions between women's activities in the private domestic sphere and man's work in the competitive sphere of waged employment; the opposition between woman's wayward brain and man's capacity for abstract thought was suggested in the struggle between tradition and science.

The message conveyed by medical science was that woman's physiological peculiarities affected her capacities more markedly than was the case in men, restricting the sphere of activity for which she was fitted. A typical example of this belief was provided by James Jamieson:

The average male and female member of the human race resemble each other more closely at the extremes of life than in the middle period. Mere differences of habit and mode of life, which are most distinct during the adolescent and early adult periods, may go some way to account for the greater diversity then; but probably, it is chiefly due to the influence of motherhood, actual or potential, on the physical and mental economy of women. The reproductive function undoubtedly has a larger place, for good or evil, in the life of woman than in that of man.[80]

Now, this was precisely the view expressed by Lawson Tait when he set out to account for the rise of the gynaecologist:

The great function of a woman's life has for years made her the subject of specialists, male and female, the obstetricians. The subsidiary relations of her special organs and the special acquirements of her physique, based upon these, have necessitated the establishment of another class of specialist, the gynaecologist.[81]

Tait's words found resonance in the views of Robert Barnes (1817–1907), a key figure in the history of obstetrics and gynaecology, to whom we owe perhaps the most lucid statement of the meaning and scope of gynaecology. Writing in the 1882 edition of Quain's *Dictionary of Medicine*, Barnes explained that

the word 'Gynaecology' ... embraces far more than is expressed in the term 'diseases of women'. In its full etymological meaning it is comprehensive beyond the strict domain of medicine . . . Without accepting the doctrine of Michelet, that the life of woman is a history of disease, it is undeniable that to appreciate justly the pathology of women we must observe her in all her social relations, study minutely her moral and intellectual characteristics – that we must, in short, never for a moment lose sight of those physical attributes which indelibly stamp her as a woman, which direct, control, and limit the exercise of her faculties. This collateral study is of infinitely more importance in the pathological history of woman than it is in that of man.[82]

Barnes was not prepared to endorse Michelet's view that woman was a pathological specimen of the human race because menstruation itself, as the French historian maintained, was an illness;[83] but he argued that knowledge of 'natural woman' was the necessary foundation of gynaecological pathology and therapy. It was not simply a question of learning what diseases peculiarly affected women: it was a matter of realising that, because women were entirely finalised for the sexual functions, mind and body, their sexual physiology and pathology affected their behaviour, and thus had social and moral consequences which had no parallel in the pathology of the male. The leniency with which women were treated in infanticide cases is one example of how this principle was applied in practice: at times of heightened sexual activity such as childbirth and the puerperium, women became physically and psychologically vulnerable and could not be regarded as criminally responsible for their actions.[84]

Thus, starting from ideological assumptions about the dominance of the sexual functions in women, nineteenth-century gynaecology went on to analyse the whole of the female organisation by focussing on the mediating links between women's reproductive organs and their minds, be it the blood – a vestige of ancient humoral theories of disease – or the complex notion of reflex action, which significantly emphasised the lack of control exercised by the higher regions of the brain on the psycho-physiology of the female. This task involved an evaluation of the balance between instinct and reason, of the senses and the moral faculties, of the relationship between organisation and environment – the very themes round which the natural history of man, one of the chief components of the science of anthropology, was organised.

There was however a crucial asymmetry between gynaecology and anthropology. Through images of physical delicacy and psychological instability, gynaecologists equated woman to the

child and made her social dependence explicit. Women were irre-
sponsible creatures in need of protection and guardianship; like
children, they were incomplete adults. By contrast the word 'man'
carried two meanings, signifying both the adult member of the
human species regardless of sex and the human male. This ambiguity was reflected by the use of reason as a criterion of sexual as
well as anthropological classification.

The degree of complexity of the intellectual faculties, as signified
in particular by brain size and cranial capacity, had played an
important role as a taxonomic device since the end of the eighteenth
century, when comparative anatomists had developed the idea of a
graded scale of intrinsic animality and intelligence. After falling
into disfavour in the early part of the nineteenth century, this notion
was revived in the mid-Victorian years within an evolutionist
framework. Races were seen to form a hierarchical chain of being,
starting from the type of nervous organisation exemplified by the
small brain and incoherent mind of the savage and culminating with
the white European male: because of his greater ability to co-
ordinate sense-impressions and his capacity for abstract thought,
white man was the pinnacle of creation and the universal standard
of social worth.[85]

Thus from the classificatory point of view, anthropology and the
science of andrology envisaged by the gynaecologist James Jamieson overlapped: as the male was the standard of the species, he could
not be set apart on the basis of his sex. This does not mean to say
that there were no diseases which were peculiar to the male. Men,
too, were liable to suffer from disorders of their sexual apparatus,
such as an inflamed or enlarged prostate, erectile impotence and
hydrocele of the testes, to name but a few. But the physiology and
pathology of the male sexual system simply *were not seen* to define
men's nature. Although gynaecology does have a male counterpart
in genito-urinary medicine, it is perhaps no coincidence that attempts to redefine urology as the 'science of masculinity' have been
unsuccessful in the past.

Both in Britain and in America, the redefinition of urology as
'andrology' was partly inspired by a desire to raise the status of a
specialty which had long been closely associated with quackery.
The first attempt was made at the 1891 Congress of American
Physicians by a committee of urologists, who formed themselves
into the Section of Andrology. The results were disappointing:

Congress participants greeted the neologism with scorn and ridicule, and the term subsequently fell into disuse.[86] Three decades later, the English urologist Kenneth Walker proposed to separate the study of the diseases of the male organs of generation from those of the urinary tract; the new specialism, which was to be a definite branch of medical science comparable to gynaecology, was to be named 'andrology'. 'Andrology clinics' were also created in the 1920s and 1930s to investigate the causes of infertility in men, a problem which had emerged in the wake of anxiety about the decline in the birth rate. As had been the case in the United States, though, the term andrology did not catch on.[87] It was not until the 1970s that this word was revived to designate a specialised area of endocrinology – significantly, the study of those hormones which are thought to determine the masculine sexual characters.

As well as drawing on prevailing ideologies of femininity, the medical construction of womanhood was also indebted to the rich literary and mythological legacy of western civilisation. Woman's seemingly mysterious capacity to bring forth and nurture life evoked ancient beliefs about the moon and the sea, which biomedical writers translated into the language of science. In the mythology of a number of cultures the lunar deity was represented as female and was related to the fertilisation of the earth, the harvesting and planting of crops and the cycle of seasons. The moon also moved the tides to its ebb and flow, and was thus linked with water and the sea. Sometimes the sea itself was perceived as female, conveying two images of the feminine principle, one positive and beneficent, the other negative and destructive: the sea could produce its own life within its depths without being planted, but it could also become a threat and swallow up lives.[88] These beliefs were suggested in the second half of the nineteenth century by the theory that the periodicity of menstruation and ovulation followed lunar periods like the tides. The intimation was that science, as the undertaking of the reasoning male, would penetrate the dark interiority where woman's sexual organs were lodged and pry open their secrets: physiologists hoped, wrote Alfred Wiltshire in 1883, that one day the physiology of reproduction 'may be brought within the domain of science, and cease to be a wonderment and a mystery'.[89]

As the search was on for the ultimate cause of woman's otherness, from the 1840s onwards increasing attention was focussed on the function of the ovaries. By the 1850s, the 'ovular theory' of menstruation provided the chief scientific explanation of the biological basis of femininity. According to the theory, it was the spontaneous release of the egg which caused menstruation, and the onset of menses coincided not only with the fertile period, but also with the peak of sexual desire in woman.[90] With the redefinition of the ovaries as autonomous control centres of sex and reproduction in the female, it rapidly became a virtually undisputed tenet of gynaecological theory that the ovaries, the 'grand organs of sexual activity'[91] in woman, were the essential difference from which all others flowed. In 1844 the French physician Achille Chéreau (1817–85) proposed to change Van Helmont's (1577–1644) dictum 'Propter solum uterum mulier est id quod est' into 'Propter solum ovarium mulier est id quod est'.[92] The same idea was vividly conveyed by Robert Barnes and his son Fancourt (1849–1908) through a political metaphor, in which the ovary was depicted as a tyrant relentlessly trying to submit the female body to its imperious laws: 'In the ordinary state', the Barneses wrote in 1884,

the active or dominant organ of the sexual system is the ovary. The reign of this organ is expressed by menstruation, the part taken by the uterus being secondary, or in obedience to the impulse of the ovary. The ovary reigns supreme until conception takes place; then the uterus succeeds, and rules until the child leaves it. Then it is deposed, and yields its place to the breast. The breast rules until it is more or less supplanted by the ovary, which is ever struggling for supremacy, and cannot long be kept in subjection.[93]

While the uterus and breast symbolised woman's maternal role, the ovaries were woman's tie with nature: they were the seat of the sexual instinct, 'the drive that most firmly binds man to the animal level'.[94] Negatively, the ovaries linked woman to a world of instincts and automatic behavioural responses that belonged to a more primitive phase of human development – a stage of consciousness which had been left behind by the progress of Reason and the advance of civilisation. Positively, the ovary made woman eager to procreate and desire the male; it thus guaranteed the continuation of the species and the cohesion of the marital relationship, for it was mutual sexual attraction which bound man and wife into an exclusive society of interests and affections.[95]

The conflation of the biological, social and moral aspects of women's sexual nature found its expression in the aesthetic appreciation of the female body:[96] 'The relations of woman', claimed an anonymous writer on 'Woman in Her Psychological Relations' in 1851, 'are twofold; material and spiritual – corporeal and moral. By her corporeal nature she is the type and model of BEAUTY; by her spiritual, of GRACE; by her moral, of LOVE.' In this article the female form was exalted as the 'model of the good and the beautiful'; it was 'during the period of activity of the reproductive organs, peculiar to her physical construction', argued the author, 'that the frame of woman is most pleasing and most beautiful'.[97] Of all the female characteristics, the beauty of the pelvis was underlined:

It is in that portion of the body in immediate connexion with those parts peculiar to her organization, that the greatest beauty of form is found in woman, as though they were the *fons et origo* of corporeal as well as mental loveliness . . . The contours of the back are of the most admirable purity; the region of the kidneys is elongated, the scapulae scarcely visible; the loins grandly curved forwards, the haunches prominent and rounded; in short, the posterior surface of the torso in woman is unquestionably the *chef d'oeuvre* of nature.[98]

No less than a 'Divine Idea' of beauty and perfection was developed 'in the encasing of the procreative organs and centre of procreative activity'. The beauty of the pelvis was equalled by that of the bust, with its 'voluptuous contours and graceful inflexions': while the one was 'the manifestation of the instinct', the other expressed the sentiment of love which bound the mother to her offspring.[99] Softness and roundness, two of the defining qualities of living things, were emphasised as the features which endowed woman with her charms, for they signified her life-giving capacities. By contrast sharpness and angularity, proper to inanimate objects, were antithetical to the idea of beauty.[100] Thus menopausal and ovariotomised women, whose sexual functions were in abeyance, lost the softness and roundness of the female form, becoming the least beautiful and also the least moral women of all:

With the shrinking of the ovaria . . . there is a corresponding change in the outer form . . . The form becomes angular, the body lean, the skin wrinkled. The hair changes in colour and loses its luxuriancy; the skin is less transparent and soft, and the chin and upper lip become downy . . . With this change in the person there is an analogous change in the mind, temper and feelings. The woman approximates in fact to a man, or in one word, she is a *virago* . . . This unwomanly condition undoubtedly renders her repulsive to man, while her envious, overbearing temper, renders her offensive to her own sex.[101]

Such was the fate of the typical 'Old Maid'.

Physiology and social roles

One theme which has emerged so far from our discussion concerns the way in which sexual differences designated social roles and created hierarchical relations between men and women. Historians have taken Victorian gynaecologists to task for typifying women as frail and dependent creatures, whose biological peculiarities debarred them from education, politics and waged work.[102] Medical ideas about woman's social destiny, however, were far more complex than has generally been assumed. They evince a degree of uncertainty about women's functions in society and indicate that the nature of the relationships of power and authority between men and women were perceived to be problematic.

Belief that the social subordination of women proceeded from their physiology was neatly expressed in an editorial published in the *Obstetrical Journal of Great Britain and Ireland* in 1874. By virtue of their intellectual abilities, it was maintained, men had gained eminence over women; as for women, their allotted task in life was to be the 'reproductive servants of the race'.[103] But other writers disagreed: they argued that there were alternatives to childrearing, although these were still conceived of as an extension of woman's functions within the family. The physician John Roberton, for instance, observed that motherhood was circumscribed to a relatively short period of a woman's life, hence nature itself indicated that her social role was not limited to reproducing and nurturing the species. The continuation of life after the menopause was proof that

> woman is destined to other duties than belong to the mere animal; that her day is not to close when the offices of mother and nurse have been fulfilled, but rather than now, when ripe in knowledge and experience, it remains for her to *train* those to whom she has given birth . . . herself, meanwhile, continuing to shed on domestic society that benign, humanising influence, which her moral constitution, when purified and elevated by Christian religion, is so eminently fitted to exercise.[104]

These sentiments were echoed by other contemporary writers. Women were portrayed as the repository of traditional wisdom and knowledge: this made them fit for employment as *sage-femmes*, and

[margin note: socially not only capable of bearing children]

particularly suited to those occupations which required dedication and a sense of altruism, such as the care of the sick.[105] The love which woman expressed as mother and wife was said to be the type 'of that higher and more fervent emotion, which fills the whole soul of woman when devoted to religion'; maternal love was commingled 'although imperfectly, with the fundamental doctrine of Christianity, the love of God to man'.[106] This elevation of womankind was part and parcel of the nineteenth-century revival of chivalry, which had brought the queenly woman back into fashion. The rhetoric of the noble woman at whose feet men knelt in adoration, rapturously expressed by Ruskin's *Sesame and Lilies* (1865), was an important facet of the Victorian iconography of femininity: here the dangerousness of women's sexuality became defused and refined by the alchemy of love and marriage, commanding men's tenderness and devotion.[107]

If man was intellectually superior, woman was so from the moral point of view; yet both hierarchies could be turned on their heads. While for some writers women's intuitive powers were evidence of intellectual inferiority, for others they were a higher instinct based on the perfection of reasoning. For Darwin, for instance, woman's intuitiveness was also typical of the child and of the lower races.[108] James Jamieson on the contrary believed that it was akin to the diagnostic genius shown by some physicians: it was a rare talent which went to make up men of the stature of a Sydenham or of a Boerhaave. Indeed in Jamieson's view woman's specialisation for the sexual functions, although associated with defects and dangers, like all specialisation was 'both a cause of complexity and a mark of perfection'.[109]

Woman's morality had positive connotations when identified with maternal love; at other times, however, it was seen negatively as an allegiance to backward modes of thought that were antagonistic to male science and the values of a secular society. The gynaecologist Robert Barnes, for instance, thus commented when women were campaigning for entrance into the medical profession in the 1870s:

Why is it that women have selected medicine as the special point of attack, is not quite clear. They are better fitted, by natural aptitude, to shine in the pulpit and at the bar . . . But medicine, whilst demanding physical power no less than other professions, is essentially based upon science. Now . . . there seems to be a natural incompatibility between science and the female brain.[110]

The opposition between science and the female brain, men's ration-
ality and women's religiosity, had wider echoes in a social struggle
for dominance between scientific medicine on the one hand, and the
Church and the law on the other: 'The clergy of all denominations,
and lawyers, as a rule, assume a direct antagonism to science',
Barnes continued:

They set themselves above it; they trample it down as something in
chronic rebellion against their authority. In this antagonism they resemble
the women; in this they find their most useful allies. The Church and the
law, then, are the professions most congenial to the somewhat arbitrary
character of the female intellect.[111]

These words portrayed the relationship between man and
woman as a battle, but at other times their opposition took on a
positive meaning: it could become a productive difference between
equivalent terms, which harmoniously complemented each other.
This is indeed what Robert Barnes himself, with his son Fancourt,
suggested elsewhere, in their discussion of pelvimetry and of the
pelvic index.

While craniometry has long attracted the interest of historians,
the study of pelvimetry remains to date totally unexplored. Anthropologists had elaborated it in the first half of the nineteenth
century to complement craniometry, as a means of classifying races
on the basis of pelvic and cranial capacity respectively. The size of
the pelvis was relevant to the question of skull measurements. It
correlated with the size of the foetal head, and this in turn was
thought to indicate the size of the brain and the development of the
intellectual faculties by which races could be ordered. But while
craniometry was believed to be applicable to the classification of
men, in the female the dimensions of the pelvis were deemed to be
more appropriate. Thus the cranial index was paralleled by the
pelvic index, a parameter devised by combining together the different diameters of the pelvis. According to the cranial index, the
white European male was invariably found to occupy the highest
place in the order of races. The European woman for her part was
also thought to be more highly developed than her 'primitive'
sister, but her superiority was indicated by the greater capacity of
her pelvis.[112]

Pelvimetry interested Robert and Fancourt Barnes mainly from
an obstetric point of view: they hoped that the study of pelvic
conformation might enable obstetricians to determine the relation

ship between pelvis and foetal skull, and thus to predict the likelihood of a difficult delivery. With this end in view, they considered the more general, anthropological aspects of pelvimetry. Drawing on the researches of comparative anatomists such as Gerardus Vrolik (1775–1859) and J. G. Garson, the Barneses commented that pelvic differences between men and women were caused by the functions the pelvis had to perform in each sex. Both sexes shared certain features which were due to the erect posture, and which differentiated the human pelvis from that of the lower animals. But while the male pelvis was built for strength and 'powerful exertion', in the female it was modified for the sexual functions: it was therefore more capacious and its bones were lighter.[113] Taking the pelvic index as a gauge of the progressive rise in the scale of mammalia, 'man, the noblest ape', showed 'an advance upon the gorilla', but this progress was not as marked as that of the female: the 'highest pelvic type' was found in the European woman. 'Does this prove that man is the inferior animal?' the two gynaecologists wondered. 'Man, perhaps, would appeal to another index – the cranium. If woman excels by the pelvis, man excels by the head.'[114]

Men and women were thus specialised for different functions, but this did not indicate the superiority of one sex or the other: each sex was perfect in its own way. It was characterised by attributes which, although opposed, were equivalent and harmoniously complemented each other. A strikingly similar view was expressed by the American physician Edward Clarke (1820–77), Professor of Materia Medica at Harvard College and author of the misleadingly titled essay *Sex in Education: or, a Fair Chance for the Girls*, in which he argued *against* widening women's educational sphere. The book was denounced by American feminists; it was widely debated in Britain as well, where it sparked off a famous controversy between the physician Henry Maudsley and Elizabeth Garrett Anderson, the first English woman doctor.[115]

Clarke contended that the struggle for the improvement of women's educational opportunities implicitly conceded that woman was inferior to man, and that her condition could only be bettered by making her a man. Although Clarke did emphasise that the sexes were widely different, he stressed that their relationship was one between equivalent terms:

Man is not inferior to woman, nor woman to man. The relation of the sexes is one of equality, not of better and worse, or of higher and lower.

By this it is not intended that the sexes are the same. They are different, widely different from each other, and so different that each can do, in certain directions, what the other cannot.[116]

It was a misconception to equate difference of organisation and function with difference of position in the scale of beings, as this was

equivalent to saying that man is rated higher in the divine order because he has more muscle, and woman lower because she has more fat. The loftiest ideal of humanity, rejecting all comparison of inferiority and superiority between the sexes, demands that each shall be perfect in its own kind.[117]

This for Clarke meant keeping gender roles distinct: the education of women was desirable as long as it remained a preparation for womanhood, that is to say marriage and the family. Any other form of education would have masculinised female students, undermining the separation of men and women and threatening social stability. The champions of women's education, Clarke argued, had 'missed the symmetry and organic balance that harmonious development yields' and 'drifted into a hermaphroditic condition'. This was also the fate that would befall the educated woman. Quoting the English physician Henry Maudsley, Clarke wrote:

While woman preserves her sex, she will necessarily be feebler than man, and, having her special bodily and mental characters, will have, to a certain extent, her own sphere of activity; where she has become thoroughly masculine in nature, or hermaphrodite in mind, – when, in fact, she has pretty well divested herself of her sex, – then she may take his ground, and do his work, but she will have lost her feminine attractions, and probably also her chief feminine functions.[118]

By holding up to woman an aesthetic ideal of femininity, Clarke conjured up a set of assumptions about the moral goodness of her biological functions. There was a necessary relationship between women's biology and their social activities: the penance for contravening the 'natural' order of society was ugliness in mind and body.

A well-developed gynaecological science supported Clarke's views. Physicians had constructed a theory of femininity which could prescribe social roles without raising opposition, because it had the validation of science: it could appear as the objective appreciation of 'natural facts' – an activity unmediated by the observer's political interests and value judgments. Thus ideologically charged beliefs about the biological foundations of femininity ensured that medical men became chief protagonists in debates over women's social duties and responsibilities. These ideas defined gynaecology as a medical specialism, providing the organising concept round which the 'science of woman' grew as a theory of femininity and a therapeutic art.

2

Men-midwives and medicine: the origins of a profession

We have histories of gynaecological techniques and analyses of gender ideology in gynaecology, but no comprehensive account of the development of the gynaecological profession. Yet nineteenth-century gynaecologists were not merely technicians or males bringing cultural constructs of femininity into the gynaecological encounter; they were also individuals pursuing an occupation for financial gain, and as such they should be studied as part of a network of social and economic relations.

Practitioners of gynaecology were held in low regard by the medical élite, partly because of the taboo nature of the subject, partly because gynaecology was bound up with midwifery, a traditionally female occupation. These difficulties were compounded by a third critically important factor – the centrality of obstetrics and gynaecology to general practice. As an integral part of general practice, obstetrics and gynaecology became caught up in the thorny question of medical reform. The rejection of obstetrics by the medical corporations in the last century stemmed in large measure from the struggle between general practitioners and the Royal Colleges over the regulation of the profession. Historians of gynaecology have generally underestimated the extent to which issues such as social background and aspirations, training, career patterns, intra- and inter-professional alliances shaped the activities of gynaecologists, influencing the clinical and institutional development of the specialism. Many aspects of gynaecology – from the foundation of special hospitals for women to debates over the propriety of gynaecological techniques – cannot be fully understood unless the historical setting of gynaecologists as individuals and as a collectivity is examined.

Midwives and accoucheurs

Until the early eighteenth century childbirth and the lying-in period were a kind of ritual collectively staged and controlled by women, from which men were usually excluded. Expectant mothers turned to a few trusted friends and relatives for aid and support during one of the most critical moments of their lives. The term 'gossip', which referred to the women attending the birth, is quite revealing of the context in which childbirth took place: originally it meant a formal witness to the birth, but by the seventeenth century it was used to describe 'a woman's circle of close female friends'. After the birth, the gossips took over the household chores for a few weeks, thus providing the mother with an opportunity to 'lie in', to recuperate her strength in bed while she devoted herself to the care of the new child.[1]

One woman stood out amongst the rest and held a position of authority: the midwife, although the extent to which she dominated the proceedings depended on her reputation and character. Midwives generally received no formal training, but learnt about the processes of childbirth through having themselves borne children and witnessed friends and neighbours give birth; indeed, right to the end of the seventeenth century personal experience of childbirth was considered an essential requirement for midwifery practice. The better class of midwife would work as 'deputy' to an experienced woman for a period of time before setting up practice on her own account. This form of training was more common in towns than in rural areas, since it was an expensive route to midwifery practice and was worthwhile as an investment only where midwifery cases commanded high fees.[2]

In England there was no formal system for the control of midwives until 1512, when a group of university men close to the Court managed to have a bill introduced which put the licensing of medical practitioners throughout England in the hands of the Bishops. Although midwives were not mentioned in the 1512 Act, a midwifery licence was established soon afterwards under its terms.[3] The ecclesiastical authorities were empowered to implement the Act because they possessed the necessary administrative machinery, but in practice the episcopal licensing of midwives was not intensively enforced. The Church already had a direct interest in midwives because of their social and religious functions. The midwife had to report cases of infanticide, to baptise the baby in an emergency and to certify its paternity. If the mother was unmarried and was keeping the father's name a secret, the midwife had to prise it from her, so that the father might not evade his duty to maintain his child; she was thus a key witness in bastardy cases when they came up for judgment before the Church's law courts (popularly known as the 'bawdy courts'), where sexual offences were punished.[4] At a time of great anxiety about sorcery and witchcraft, the midwife also had to swear to the religious authorities that she would not practise witchcraft. The caul, after-birth and still-born foetus were important elements in magical rites, so midwifery was an obvious target for the Church's attempts to stamp out the practice. As the witch-craze gathered momentum during the course of the fifteenth century, midwives were occasionally accused of witchcraft and put to death, but this was very rare in England.

Midwives seeking a licence were required to apply to the Bishop's Court with supporting testimonials as to their moral rectitude and professional competence. Candidates had to bring to the hearing six 'honest matrons' whom they had delivered and who were willing to guarantee their skill; occasionally, senior midwives would testify to a colleague's ability.[5] If the licence was granted, the midwife had to take an oath which bound her to the exercise of her profession 'faithfully and diligently'. The oath prohibited her from giving abortifacients, concealing information about birth events or parentages and practising magic rites. The midwife also had to promise that she would baptise infants in emergencies, according to the rites prescribed by the Church of England.[6]

Assessing what skill midwives actually possessed raises enormous problems, first of all because the evidence is unreliable. The 'matrons' who testified to a midwife's skill for the licence were likely to be selected cases or fellow midwives, thus hardly objective witnesses. Seventeenth- and eighteenth-century surgeons for their part often complained about the inability of midwives to cope with difficult births, but as they were usually called in an emergency, they were inevitably biased towards asking what the midwife had *not* done rather than what she could do; besides, it was in their interest to present midwives as incompetent. The other, and more fundamental, question is that judging the competence of midwives presupposes definitions of 'skill' in which a particular point of view is necessarily endorsed. Modern accounts of the history of obstetrics have tended uncritically to accept accoucheurs' own ideological views about what constituted 'good' midwifery practice. The medical practitioners who colonised childbirth in the eighteenth century characterised themselves as bringing rational knowledge to an area dominated by ignorance and tradition; beginning with James Hobson Aveling's *English Midwives* (1872), the history of obstetrics has been seen mostly through their eyes.[7]

One example drawn from early twentieth-century Britain will suffice to demonstrate how 'skill' could mean different things to different people. In his autobiography, the gynaecologist Aleck Bourne recollects how as a young medical student at St Mary's Hospital, London, in the early 1900s he was sent out on his own to attend his first delivery in the Paddington district. He found his way to a room of indescribable squalor where a 'typical fat old gamp' was in attendance, with no training in cleanliness and no knowledge of antisepsis. Bourne confesses that he had no idea what to do, and that he watched in amazement nature's remarkable process of birth. When the baby appeared he got up to leave, but the midwife called out ''Ere, doctor, what abhat the after-birth?' The student Bourne had completely forgotten about the most dangerous part of childbirth, when fatal haemorrhages may occur.[8] Bourne however recalled the episode without realising that it could have been taken to reflect badly on his skill at the time, because 'competence' to him meant attention to cleanliness and antisepsis; by contrast, for the midwife it was a question of accumulated experience and observation.

Our knowledge of the practice of midwives in the sixteenth and seventeenth centuries is culled from the obstetrical case-histories written by medical practitioners of midwifery; it is therefore patchy and of indirect derivation, two reasons why historians must be open-minded about the activities of midwives. We know that some midwives saw their role as merely that of bystanders, while others employed some form of manual intervention – for example, they might seek to 'help' the birth by stretching the cervix in the first stage and pushing on the mother's belly in the second stage; sometimes magic charms and herbal remedies were used.[9] It seems certain that midwives had techniques of their own for reviving a faint newborn baby or the mother after delivery;[10] they also managed mothers through the lying-in period, gave gynaecological advice and possibly also dealt with the diseases of the newborn.[11]

They were probably on the whole unable to deliver obstructed births – cases in which pelvic abnormalities prevented the passage of the baby past the brim of the pelvis – although some could deliver the dead foetus by craniotomy, and others seem to have specialised in difficult births.[12] Given the unregulated state of midwifery, standards varied widely: many midwives distinguished themselves locally for their knowledge and care,[13] some women were probably more notable for their incompetence and rudeness.

Male midwifery practice before 1730 was most commonly associated with the attendance of emergencies. In practice, as Wilson has shown, there were at least eight different routes by which the surgeon could get into the lying-in chamber, all of them connected with the presence or expectation of abnormality. There were advance calls, in which a pregnant woman booked the practitioner to reside with her, to advise her during the pregnancy and take charge of the delivery and the post-partum period. There were also onset calls, which summoned the practitioner as soon as labour started, and emergency calls, which were made when a difficulty arose. Both onset and emergency calls could be booked or unbooked, and with or without the midwife. The responsibility of deciding whether and when to summon a medical man was shared by the participants in the birth, but agreement was by no means automatic. An emergency had to be defined, and this depended on the judgment of a number of people in distinctive social roles. The definition of an emergency was thus not a biological 'given', but a highly complex and problematic social act; there was often argument between mother and midwife as to whether the surgeon was required.[14]

The most frequent causes of difficulty in childbirth were malpresentations, placenta praevia and contracted pelvis. In the first two cases, the surgeon would usually attempt to turn the baby and extract it by pulling down a leg (podalic version), plunging his hand through the placenta if it obstructed the mouth of the womb. Whenever birth *per vias naturales* was impossible because of abnormalities in the mother's pelvis, the surgeon was forced to perform the operation of craniotomy, or embriotomy, in order to save the mother: this procedure consisted in fixing a crotchet in the head of the foetus and removing it piece by piece. Usually the foetus was dead, but sometimes the crotchet was used to extract a living child in an attempt at saving the mother's life.[15] The practice was vehemently condemned on religious and moral grounds by contemporary French obstetricians who, as we shall see in chapter 5, preferred to carry out a caesarean section instead. The first documented caesarean section in Britain was performed about 1738 by Mary Donnally, an Irish midwife, who was 'eminent among the common People for extracting dead Births'. Donnally cut the mother's belly with a razor and held the parts together until silk and needles were found; the baby died, but the mother amazingly survived and was able to walk a mile within four weeks.[16]

After 1730 the forceps came to be employed in cases of obstruction. The story of this instrument has been told many times, but it is relevant to recapitulate its chief episodes here, since the ascendancy of the man-midwife has often been attributed to its introduction into midwifery practice. Invented by the Chamberlen family in the early seventeenth century, the forceps was kept a family secret until about 1700, when it became known to various medical practitioners; they immediately set about improving it, and a staggering number of variations on the original design were produced from about 1735 onwards. After knowledge about Dusée's short forceps with articulated branches was made public in 1733, this instrument began to be used in normal and lingering labours when the head was lying low in the pelvis.[17]

As a method of delivery, the forceps was much more humane than craniotomy, because it increased the chances of delivering the baby alive. This may initially have improved the public image of the surgeon-accoucheur: his arrival was dreaded and held off as long as possible, since it normally signified the loss of the baby and the prospect of a painful and dangerous operation for the mother. But much stronger claims have been made about the role of the forceps in the development of obstetrics. It has been maintained that the forceps was 'the key to the lying-in room'[18] for the medical practitioner, polarising the practice of midwives and that of accoucheurs – the one committed to respecting the laws of nature, the other irretrievably set on the path of surgical intervention.

There are two problems with this view. First, there was no legal prohibition against the use of instruments by midwives. In *Observations in Midwifery*, the seventeenth-century accoucheur Percivall Willughby (1596–1685) advised midwives not to employ makeshift implements to extract the foetus and gave them instructions about the use of the crotchet.[19] In the early eighteenth century, the well-known midwife Sarah Stone reported using instruments (probably the crotchet) in four out of three hundred cases.[20] Margaret Stephen, a midwife who delivered Queen Charlotte, ran a school of midwifery in London in the 1790s where she demonstrated the forceps on a wooden manikin, and it is possible that she may have employed the forceps herself.[21] Indeed, the practice of surgery in general was not restricted to men. Before 1800, a number of women worked as 'surgeonesses', and a few of them were formally accredited practitioners. Until 1745, when the Company of Surgeons broke away from the Barber-Surgeons' Company, women could be admitted to the freedom of the Surgeons either by apprenticeship or by patrimony; other 'surgeonesses' were licensed by the Bishops, a practice which continued until the end of the eighteenth century.[22] It is a puzzle why the majority of midwives, as far as we know, did not use the forceps. Perhaps the high cost of the instrument restricted its use to the tiny élite of fashionable and affluent urban midwives who could afford it. Secondly, a conscious and massive swing away from instrumental intervention occurred about 1770, just at the time when men-midwives were on the ascendancy. One might have expected male accoucheurs in this period at least to maintain their tendency to use instruments; what one finds instead is a widespread *rejection* of the forceps, made famous through the remarks of William Hunter, one of the leading men-midwives in mid eighteenth-century London: 'A thousand pities they were ever invented', he said; 'Where they save one, they murder twenty.'[23]

New evidence is beginning to challenge current ideas about the history of the forceps. According to Wilson, between 1730 and 1750 the development of this instrument, and indeed of midwifery itself, was entirely caught up in professional and political battles *between* men-midwives[24]. These were mainly centred in London, but they also spawned treatises published in provincial towns. Forceps practitioners, like the Chamberlens themselves, were surgeons and high Tories. Their rivals were the Whig men-midwives and followers of Hendrik van Deventer, the Dutch man-midwife, who claimed he could deliver obstructed births by the head without using any instruments, by exerting pressure on the sacrum with the back of the hand in order to enlarge the pelvic outlet.[25] The Deventerians, however, reserved the right to perform craniotomy – cases such as hydrocephalus would have required this – although they might have referred this kind of work to another practitioner. This was probably the practice of the surgeon John Douglas, brother to the well-known man-midwife James Douglas, and author of *Short Account of the State of Midwifery in London, Westminster, &c.* (1736).[26]

The Deventerians were physicians and opposed to the forceps. This attitude was shaped by their experience of childbirth. As the Deventerians' practice was mainly onset calls among wealthy mothers rather than emergencies, most of the births they witnessed were normal and did not call for instrumental interference. It is also probable that earlier access to cases of obstruction may have increased their chances of success with Deventer's manoeuvre, thus strengthening their belief that the forceps was unnecessary. John Maubray, who is remembered by Donnison for his denunciation of the surgeons' rashness in using instruments (i.e. the crotchet), was also the author of a book on midwifery published in 1725 which plagiarised Hendrik van Deventer.[27] The argument obstetric technology versus non-intervention in childbirth was already an ideological weapon in the battle for professional and political hegemony.

After 1742 the great Smellie (1697–1763), a second-generation forceps practitioner, was to teach the judicious use of the forceps. His views were, so to speak, a synthesis of Whig and Tory positions. Smellie had experimented with non-instrumental methods of delivery as a substitute for the forceps and concluded that the instrument was essential; at the same time, though, he believed that it had been over-used by the first generation of forceps practitioners and argued that only ten out of one thousand cases required instrumental delivery.[28]

Later men-midwives – most notably William Hunter – would take issue with Smellie's recommendations and strenuously oppose the midwifery forceps. Hunter's stance was a further shift in the direction that separated Smellie from forceps practitioners. As man-midwifery moved away from emergency to onset-call practice, the surgeon-accoucheur had an opportunity to attend an increasing number of normal births: this influenced the way he saw both the processes of birth and his role at the delivery. Hunter's aristocratic practice was made up predominantly of onset calls and, as Wilson has argued, it is in the light of his 'profile of practice' that his opposition to the forceps must be seen. William Hunter's adamant non-interventionism was also dictated by the social class of his clientele: touching a lady, he argued, was indelicate, thus any

man-midwife worth his salt should refrain from carrying out certain operations (such as examinations *per rectum*) if he wanted to stay
in business. Gaining the confidence of the upper-classes was a
question of knowing the correct form of 'dress and address' as
much as of having a good obstetrical track-record.[29] Thus the
surgeon-accoucheur gradually shed his uncouth image and, model-
ling himself on the gentlemanly Physician, he turned into the
well-mannered professional who could socialise with the aristoc-
racy as a peer.

The 'obstetric revolution' and eighteenth-century medical politics

Accoucheurs characterised themselves as the carriers of rational,
scientific expertise to an area hitherto dominated by allegedly backward and dangerous practices. They contrasted the 'incompetent'
midwife with the enlightened medical practitioner of midwifery,
claiming that accoucheurs were the only people who could conduct
mother and baby through to a safe delivery. Between about 1730
and 1770, men-midwives managed to undermine public confidence
in the midwife's capacities. The upper-classes were the first to seek
his services; by 1800, rank-and-file surgeon-apothecaries were delivering babies as a routine part of their practice, a sign that the
midwives' monopoly of childbirth was being broken lower down
the social scale. Men-midwives had also extended their sphere of
intervention beyond the delivery alone: they were now managing
pregnancy and the post-partum period and treating the diseases
incidental to women and children as well.[30]

The reasons why men-midwives succeeded in persuading the
public of the value of their skill are still the subject of keen historical
debate. The term 'medicalisation' has been used to denote the
process by which childbirth was made subject to the power and
authority of doctors, but this idea provides an unsatisfactory ex-
planatory framework for the rise of the accoucheur. Its underlying
assumption is that the dichotomy between the 'traditional', super-
stitious practices of midwives, incapable of learning from observation and experience, and the 'modern' scientific era of the male
accoucheur was a historical reality rather than an ideology constructed by men-midwives in their interest.[31] As one commentator
on childbirth in contemporary Britain has observed, ritual is all but
dead in the delivery suites produced by modern obstetric tech-

nology: for example, the emphasis placed on order and cleanliness during birth is commonly explained in terms of the need to reduce the risk of infection, yet it can also be seen as relevant to the notions of purity and pollution that surround childbirth in many societies, including our own.[32] The eighteenth-century men-midwives' onslaught on the female ceremony of childbirth must be read as an attempt to substitute women's customs for new medical rites masquerading as scientific practices founded on 'objective' knowledge.

Many of the top men-midwives employed in fashionable society became actively engaged in teaching and research in an effort to propound their own approach to childbirth. It was Scotland which inaugurated the teaching of midwifery at university level: in 1726, the first professorship of midwifery in the United Kingdom was established at Edinburgh University, but the first two professors never gave any lectures. The man who introduced a proper course in midwifery was Thomas Young, professor between 1756 and 1783. His lectures were supplemented by illustrations from printed books, demonstrations with human bones, wet anatomical preparations and wax models. Students also had the option of attending the lying-in ward, which had been established at the Edinburgh Royal Infirmary in 1755 at Young's instigation.[33]

In London instruction in midwifery flourished in the second half of the eighteenth century with the proliferation of private schools run by the most famous practitioners of midwifery, both male and female. By the 1760s London had replaced Paris as a centre of obstetrical teaching. Smellie's work was continued in Wardour Street by John Harvie in the 1760s; in the 1770s the celebrated obstetrician William Hunter gave lectures at his house in Covent Garden. The private school of midwifery set up by William Osborne (1736–1808) and Thomas Denman (1733–1815) dominated the teaching of obstetrics in the 1770s and 1780s. Lying-in hospitals and wards were founded from the mid-1700s, and these also began to provide instruction in midwifery.[34] In London, the lying-in hospitals and wards were probably an attack against Smellie and his followers, second-generation forceps practitioners who were beginning to criticise, but had not quite yet abandoned, the use of the forceps in obstetric practice. The maternity hospitals were Whig, anti-forceps and often Deventerian initiatives: the very existence of such institutions was an argument against the forceps, as a vast array of normal births was displayed within a lying-in hospital. The foundation of the London Lying-in (later Royal Maternity) Charity was an antagonistic development: it seems to have been a Tory counter-attack on behalf of midwives, which was designed to produce, and did indeed produce, highly trained midwives.[35]

How then was this new phenomenon, the man-midwife, seen by his medical and surgical colleagues, and what was his position in the eighteenth-century medical world? From the very beginning man-midwifery was caught up in the social and political relationships between practitioners. Their structure provided strategies of upward social mobility for the aspiring man-midwife as well as placing obstacles on his way to social and economic success. For the medical corporations, midwifery practice proved both an embarrassment and an asset in the professional stakes. The eighteenth century initiated what was to become a tradition in which competing groups *within* the medical profession either used obstetrics as a means to achieve further ends or shirked it as a threat to their power and privileges.

The structure of medical practice in eighteenth-century London was very different from the one we know, in which entry to the profession is regulated by the universities through the granting of one single qualification common to all practitioners. At the formal level medicine was split into three hierarchically ordained branches, similar to 'estates'. Physicians, who saw themselves as the élite of the profession, were regulated by the College of Physicians. They were university educated and drew their clientele from the higher echelons of society. Their tasks centred on the cognitive appraisal of disease and on the prescription of internal medicines.[36] Surgeons belonged to the Corporation of Barber-Surgeons until 1745, when the link with barbers was severed and the corporation renamed the Company of Surgeons. They differed from the physicians in that they were apprenticed rather than trained at universities, and practised the manual part of medicine: it was their job to carry out surgical operations, dress wounds and use any other mechanical means of treatment.[37] Apothecaries, the third branch of the profession, were apprenticed like the surgeons. They were responsible for supplying, compounding and dispensing drugs and ranked with tradesmen. The onus of controlling their activities rested with the Society of Apothecaries.[38]

The three corporations – the College of Physicians, the Company of Surgeons and the Society of Apothecaries – had the legal task of policing their membership, suppressing unlicensed practice and making sure that the division of labour between practitioners be duly observed. Members of the College of Physicians were not allowed to practise surgery or dispense drugs, and mixed practice was prohibited to the élite of the Company (later College) of Surgeons, the Council, and to the select group of Freemen who governed the Society of Apothecaries. In the provinces, physicians could take out the extra-licentiate of the College of Physicians, but the College did not have enough muscle to police medical practice and it was the Church which exercised this function under the terms of the 1512 Act. In Scotland the structure of the medical corporations differed: Glasgow had a Faculty of Physicians and Surgeons; in Edinburgh medicine was regulated by the Royal College of Physicians of Edinburgh, while the functions of surgeon and apothecary were fused and placed under the control of the Incorporation of Surgeons (renamed Royal College of Surgeons in 1778).[39]

The tripartite organisation of medicine in England had arisen at the beginning of the sixteenth century as a result of attempts by a group of London physicians to entrench a monopoly of physic in the hands of the few medical graduates who lived in the capital. It was to this end that medicine and surgery had been separated and the Barber-Surgeons' Company created in 1540 with exclusive powers to control surgical practice within one mile of the City of London. The ambitions of the monopolistic physicians, however, had never been fully realised, for the vast majority of the population could not afford to pay for the services of a physician and were forced to look elsewhere for medical attention. Furthermore, when legal actions were brought for unlicensed practice of medicine, the Courts often proved very sensitive to the arguments in favour of medical freedom put forward by the defence.[40]

The reality of medical practice, therefore, had never conformed to the tripartite model. Surgeons were notorious for diversifying in the direction of physic;[41] there was a large majority of apothecaries, who attended the poor and middle classes, and they combined the practice of physic with surgery and the dispensing of drugs. After the Rose case went against the Physicians in 1703–4, the apothecaries were legally empowered to prescribe drugs, although they were not permitted to charge for them.[42] Physicians for their part were not unknown to practise surgery and some made up their own medicines. The ease with which William Hunter in 1756 was disenfranchised from the Corporation of Surgeons and became a licentiate of the Physicians is a corrective to the view that practitioners were separated by impermeable divides.[43]

The wider context of eighteenth-century man-midwifery was thus extremely complex; in England, and in London especially, other factors exacerbated an already intricate situation. There were political tensions between men-midwives – the rivalry between forceps practitioners and the followers of van Deventer has already been mentioned. There was the problem of the influx of Scottish medical graduates, many of whom were successful men-midwives, which the College of Physicians strove to contain. Licensing initiatives and the corporations' response to man-midwifery should not be seen in isolation from the wider arena of contemporary medical politics. For example, after the dissolution of the Barber-Surgeons' Company in 1745, the new Company of Surgeons approved a by-law excluding all those who were engaged in the apothecary's trade or practised midwifery from election to the Court of Examiners. This rule had been designed to place the control of the Company in the hands of the hospital surgeons, who could afford to practise pure surgery; most of the other members of the corporation, as was noted earlier, were not in that enviable position, and were forced to eke out a living by dispensing drugs and working as accoucheurs.[44]

The question of Scottish medical degrees complicates the picture of eighteenth-century obstetrical practice. Scottish-trained practitioners had flooded London after the Union, and several of them practised successfully as men-midwives. The Fellows of the London Colleges resented their ambition, particularly at a time of Jacobite agitation, and mistrusted their qualifications: St Andrews and Aberdeen granted postal MD degrees on the recommendation of a medical practitioner, and the system was open to abuse. Scottish graduates could not be admitted to the Fellowship of the College, which was restricted to holders of the Oxford or Cambridge MD. As licentiates they enjoyed limited rights within the College – a particular complaint was that they were not allowed access to the College buildings.[45]

By the 1760s the numerical and political strength of the licentiates had increased. After unsuccessful attempts at having their status amended legally, the licentiates resolved to take action and in 1768, with William Hunter in their number, they stormed the College headquarters in Warwick Lane.[46] The episode heaped ridicule on the heads of the rebels, who by their action had proved their inferior status; however, after three of the licentiates had brought up the question of their rights in court, the College was advised to revise the statutes. This it did in 1771, when new rules for the admission of members were approved. Although more liberal in one respect (licentiates of seven years' standing could be proposed as candidates by any Fellow), the entrance requirements were made more stringent in other ways. Candidates were to have studied for two years at a university and Greek was to be one of the subjects for examination; nobody practising midwifery or the apothecary's trade was eligible for admission. These provisions were aimed not at midwifery *per se*, but at those Scottish graduates who had obtained degrees without residence: they were known to be shaky in Latin and Greek, and it so happened that many of them were also men-midwives.[47]

Until the early 1780s the College of Physicians took no interest in those practitioners who limited themselves to man-midwifery. Occasionally a man-midwife would be summoned by the censors of the College, but the purpose was to establish that he was not engaged in the practice of physic; the men-midwives who were brought before the censors were usually excused from taking examinations and licences, unless of course they were of the wrong political persuasion. In 1727 for example Middleton Walker, who was related to the Chamberlens and possessed the forceps, was summoned by the censors on suspicion of practising medicine illegally. The President of the College at the time was the Whig Sloane who, as a rival of the Tory forceps practitioners, had a vested interest in hindering Walker's activities. In his defence Walker argued that 'as man midwifery was his profession, he thought himself exempted from being incorporated into the body of physicians', but the censors refused to accept his apology. Walker was summoned again and told that if he disobeyed he would be forbidden to practise medicine and, after that, no member of the College would be allowed to consult with him. He then wrote to ask for a year's grace before being examined; nothing more was heard of him and it is thus unclear whether he continued in practice.[48] By contrast

John Birch, who seems to have been a successful Whig man-midwife, was put forward in the same year by Sloane for an Honorary Fellowship.[49]

Historians have blamed the College's lack of concern on the 'low status' of midwifery and the 'marginality' of its practitioners. It is an explanation which begs one fundamental question: lowliness and marginality are relative concepts and their terms of reference must be made explicit.[50] Man-midwifery may have not been very attractive to the eighteenth-century Oxford or Cambridge medical graduate, who had other ways and means of making his money – the perceived messiness and immodesty of childbirth rendered man-midwifery unpalatable, and besides, anyone wishing to engage in this traditionally female occupation was regarded as unmanly.[51] But in prosperous London man-midwifery was a quick way to professional success for those who started in practice with, for example, a Scottish degree and few social connections. The individual biographies of men-midwives, such as William Hunter, Sir Richard Manningham and Thomas Denman, disprove the notion of the obstetrical cowboy and clearly indicate that the corporations were largely irrelevant to their careers. Despite this, membership of the College of Physicians had cachet and was sought after by the socially ambitious man-midwife. Being a physician carried gentlemanly status and set the standards by which the upwardly mobile practitioner would be judged; for this reason the exclusion of many licentiates from the Fellowship of the College was bound to provoke resentment.

Professional marginality, in other words, could be relative to the practitioner's career cycle: what we need to bear in mind is the possibility of an evolution within the practice of an individual. Midwifery was often used as a route from surgery to physic. The ambitious man-midwife started with emergency cases and progressed to onset-call practice. This had two important consequences: his experience of labour shifted in the direction of normal births, and thus his intervention in childbirth became less surgical and more medical. At the same time the man-midwife climbed the social ladder. He acquired a wealthier clientele, was able to charge higher fees and attained the status of a physician: he learnt a social role and turned into a gentleman. William Hunter's meteoric career conforms to this pattern. Hunter himself consciously helped the process by his well-known cultivation of bedside manners and non-Scots accent.[52]

Thus there was a discrepancy between the social and the legal status of men-midwives: they might hold court positions and hospital appointments, write influential books and amass fortunes by their practice, and yet have little contact with the corporations. In 1783, however, the College of Physicians finally resolved to grant a licence in the *ars obstetrica* only. The new statute was not intended to make unlicensed practice illegal, but to offer a distinction to those practitioners who could satisfy the examiners as to their knowledge and character.[53] It may well have been a clever strategy aimed at limiting men-midwives to obstetric practice, while bringing prestigious accoucheurs within the fold of the College.

Three men immediately applied for the licence: two were the proprietors of a famous school of midwifery, Thomas Denman – a graduate of Aberdeen University and a successful accoucheur to the Middlesex Hospital – and Dr William Osborne – another Scottish graduate, physician to the General Lying-in Hospital in Store Street. The third was Michael Underwood, physician to the British Lying-in Hospital and a member of the Corporation of Surgeons (he later took his doctor's degree). Apothecaries were discouraged from applying – the 1789 resolution that applicants should be examined in Latin took care of this – and there were only ten admissions between 1783 and 1800.[54] All of these men-midwives held Scottish or foreign degrees; they had typically started off in practice under difficult circumstances but, astutely taking up midwifery, they had made a reputation for themselves, gaining the patronage of the wealthy and the esteem of the medical profession.

The nineteenth century: obstetrics, gynaecology and general practice

The distinguished holders of the Physicians' licence in midwifery honoured their leaders by the high standards of their practice and the excellence of their reputation, but in 1804 the College began to repeal the regulations that had created their status. Although no reasons were stated, other sources documenting the preoccupations of the College in those years can shed some light on this obscure point. By 1800, midwifery had become established as an entrée into general practice: the young man-midwife would start by delivering a baby and attendance on the whole family would ensue. The Physicians looked upon the trend with alarm. They were well aware of the fact that the College's own licentiates in midwifery, blatantly transgressing the regulations, were engaging in mixed practice: as the report of the outgoing censors revealed in 1805, all the midwifery licentiates had had to be summoned because they carried on the 'general practice' of physic.[55] From the Physicians' point of view, the midwifery licence gave its holders an unfair advantage over the Fellows of the College; the august body could hardly have tolerated a state of affairs which seriously undermined its once-undisputed monopoly of the best-paid medical practice.

The Company of Surgeons proved just as unsympathetic. In 1797, while the Company was busy negotiating for a new charter, a group of its members requested the Court of Assistants to institute a qualification in midwifery; at the same time, they applied for the abolition of the by-law which excluded practitioners of midwifery from the prestigious Court of Assistants, the governing body of the Company. The Surgeons argued that if the Company had granted these requests, nothing could have stopped midwives from becoming eligible for election to the Court of Assistants, and the scheme was turned down.[56]

Men-midwives were thus left with no corporate affiliation. In an attempt at altering the Colleges' policy, in 1808 a deputation of accoucheurs headed by Dr Denman approached the College of Surgeons and the College of Physicians to see if either body would set up a qualification in midwifery for both men and women. But the corporations courteously declined to consider the problem. The Surgeons declared to be concerned about Denman's request, but contended that they had 'no Authority to interfere'. The Physicians argued that man-midwifery combined a manual part – the delivery – with a medical part – the management of the pregnant woman and the post-partum care. While they had jurisdiction over persons prescribing medicine, they had none over those practising the 'Manual Part of the Profession'.[57] Thus by pedantic adherence to the legal distinction of roles within medicine – one which, as was pointed out earlier, in practice carried little force – the Physicians managed to evade the issue in a further attempt at corporate self-preservation.

Rejected by the Colleges, midwifery had found its place in general practice. By the beginning of the nineteenth century, it was widely accepted that keeping up a practice without any midwifery was impossible. General practice was centred round the delivery of the baby, and the subsequent attendance on mother and baby hinged upon the success of the first client contact.[58] I should like to argue that this is how the concept of the general practitioner as the 'family doctor' originated. Medical men generally used the term 'family' to indicate the mother-child dyad, a social and biological unit to which fathers were peripheral;[59] it is also worth noting here that popular medical advice books addressed to the family often were mostly about women and children.

The centrality of midwifery and gynaecology to nineteenth-century general practice holds the key to understanding the development of the obstetrical and gynaecological profession in the 1800s. Although hospital practice was beginning to demarcate a class of specialist (this was true of London especially) there was no sharp distinction between the general practitioner and the obstetrician and gynaecologist – indeed, obstetrics was regarded by some as a specialism of general practice. It was for this reason that the regulation of midwifery was believed to be an integral part of the organisation of medical practice as a whole.

At the beginning of the nineteenth century medical practice in the United Kingdom was regulated by twenty-one licensing bodies. These included the medical colleges and corporations of London, Edinburgh, Glasgow and Dublin, together with the universities of England, Scotland and Ireland, and the archbishop of Canterbury. The organisation of the profession throughout the country was governed by confusing and obsolete rules: for example, a licence granted in Edinburgh was of no value in Glasgow and the East of Scotland; a Glasgow licence was not recognised in the east. With the exception of the few physicians and surgeons who could live solely by the practice of physic or surgery, the vast majority of medical men practised 'generally', and many of them entered the profession without having any formal training – let alone qualifications. This kind of practice was almost the rule in the provinces, yet none of the corporations was either willing or able to act against it.

Although in 1800 the surgeons had been reorganised into a new body with the status of a royal college, they still lacked monopoly of title and coercive powers comparable to those enjoyed by the College of Physicians. The Society of Apothecaries was in a similar position, in that it too had no legal right to prosecute unlicensed practitioners. The College of Physicians alone had that power under a statute dating back to the reign of Henry VIII, but its authority had always been weak outside London and by the beginning of the nineteenth century it was waning in the capital. Support for the principle of free trade had been growing since the middle of the eighteenth century and the law had progressively whittled down the monopolistic powers of the physicians. The process of bringing an action for unlicensed practice had become lengthy, costly and uncertain in its outcome – which goes a long way to explain why there were only two prosecutions between 1735 and 1858, the year in which Parliament stripped the College of its disciplinary powers.[60]

The agitation to reform the regulatory system of the profession was begun by the apothecaries, the largest order of medical practitioners. They wanted protection from the competition of unqualified rivals, notably the chemists and druggists, who were fast encroaching upon their practice. Most medical men favoured legislation that would restrict the practice of medicine to qualified practitioners, but were divided over the precise nature of reform. Legislative action was hindered by the conflict between two major interest groups: general practitioners and provincial physicians on the one hand, and the Royal Colleges and the graduates of Oxford and Cambridge on the other. The former urged the creation of a national register that would abolish the old distinctions of rank within the profession; the latter were unwilling to give up their privileges and they opposed the idea of a single national certification enforced by the state.[61] As Cowen has shown, the wider context of this struggle was a debate over liberty and laissez-faire. Even the harshest critics of unqualified practice were reluctant to call for repressive legislation, since this would have interfered with one of the most basic liberties of the subject – the right of anyone to practise whatever trade he chose.[62] This principle was adopted by the Bill for the regulation of the medical profession that was finally passed in 1858, the seventeenth introduced in Parliament since 1840 under Whig and Conservative governments. The Medical Reform Act did not make provisions for the suppression of unqualified practice; it merely defined a 'qualified medical practitioner', leaving the public to choose between the qualified practitioner and the unqualified.[63]

Proposals for the licensing of male and female midwives were contained in one of the first schemes for the reform of medical practice. In 1804 the Lincolnshire Benevolent Medical Society commissioned one of its members, the practitioner Edward Harrison (1766–1838), to undertake an inquiry into the state of medical practice in the county. Harrison found that the empirics outnumbered the regular profession by nine to one. Much alarmed by these figures, the Society sought the help of its patron, Sir Joseph Banks, who as president of the Royal Society wielded considerable power in London medical and political circles. At the same time, Dr Harrison enlisted the sympathy of a number of eminent London surgeons and physicians. They all met at Sir Joseph Banks's house under the title of the 'Associated Faculty', and in 1806 they put forward their proposals 'for better regulating the Practice of Physic'. The Faculty envisaged a national register to which all those who had complied with certain requirements would be admitted without further examinations. The regulations laid down for men-midwives stipulated one year of lectures and one year of practical instruction; for female midwives, a certificate from one or more practitioners would suffice. In the event, the plan proved too radical for the College of Physicians, and in 1811 Harrison and his confederates had to resign themselves to failure.[64]

The following year the matter of reform was taken up again by a group of London apothecaries. The immediate cause of their discontent was the increased tax on glass bottles, a burden on dispensers of bottled medicines, but it wasn't long before they widened the scope of their agitation and began to campaign for the suppression of unqualified medical practice and the regulation of midwifery. With George Man Burrows (1771–1846) at their head, the London apothecaries formed themselves into the Association of Apothecaries and Surgeon-Apothecaries, and in 1813 they introduced a Bill which provided for a committee to control the practice of apothecaries, surgeon-apothecaries, midwives and druggists. After much opposition from the physicians and the surgeons, who saw the plan as an infringement of their prerogatives, a modified version of the Bill was finally approved by Parliament in 1815. The Apothecaries' Act extended the authority of the Society of Apothecaries to the whole of England and Wales and made it a punishable offence to practise the profession without a licence; however, it made no provisions for the regulation of midwifery. The Associated Apothecaries had proposed an enactment to control the practice of female midwives, but the Committee of the House of Commons that considered the matter 'would not allow any mention' of them.[65]

While Parliament debated the Apothecaries' Bill, the Surgeons attempted to push through legislation by which they hoped to secure control of surgical practice in England and Wales. The Bill was read in the Commons for the second time on 19 June 1815, but then came an unexpected difficulty. The Associated Apothecaries objected that the proposed law failed to deal with the regulation of midwifery, and asked that this should be included in the Surgeons' Bill; a further request concerned the fees that would be charged for the surgical diploma. Fearing that the Associated Apothecaries might block the scheme if their demands were not met, the Surgeons agreed to include a clause in their Bill limiting the practice of midwifery to those who had obtained a diploma in that subject; the diploma was to be instituted by the College of Surgeons. The Surgeons' Bill passed the Commons and was given a second reading in the Lords, but it ran aground at the committee stage and was withdrawn. A new and more ambitious Bill was drafted shortly afterwards; it too had to be dropped in the face of widespread opposition from the Irish and Scottish licensing bodies.[66] Voicing the principles of free trade, the Commons criticised the Surgeons' Bill as an attempt to establish a monopoly and refused to give it a second reading.[67]

Another licensing initiative was spearheaded in 1826 by a group of London midwifery lecturers led by Dr Augustus Bozzi Granville (1783–1872), a graduate of Pavia University who had gained his obstetrical experience in Paris. The lecturers formed themselves into an Obstetrical Society and once again they appealed to the Colleges of Physicians and Surgeons to give their branch a regular constitution. In a petition signed by Charles Clarke, brother to the well-known man-midwife John and himself an obstetrician of repute, the Society argued for the establishment of midwifery qualifications in order to distinguish the medical man who had gained special knowledge of the obstetrical art; it went so far as threatening to refer the matter to the Home Secretary in case of a negative issue.[68]

In response to the Obstetrical Society's pressures, in 1827 the Society of Apothecaries began to demand evidence that candidates for its diploma had received some training in midwifery.[69] The other corporations proved more obdurate. The Physicians resurrected their old argument about the dual nature of man-midwifery. When the Obstetrical Society appealed to the Home Secretary, Sir Robert Peel, the Physicians produced a plethora of historical evidence to prove that the object of their College was to restrict Fellows to the pure practice of physic. This was reminiscent of the phrase 'pure surgery' which marked off the governing body of the College of Surgeons, but it did not correspond to any distinction between two classes of physicians.[70] It was a preposterous argument, particularly in view of the fact that in the eighteenth century some of its Fellows (for example, Nesbit and Morley) had practised obstetrics. Defending the ban on accoucheurs from the Fellowship of the College, its President Sir Henry Halford commented that midwifery, being a manual operation, was 'foreign to the habits of Gentlemen of enlarged academical education'.[71] He was to reiterate this opinion in 1834 when he was called to explain the College policy on obstetrics before the Committee on Medical Education: 'We should be very sorry', he said,

to throw any thing like a discredit upon the men who had been educated at the Universities, who had taken time to acquire their improvement of their minds in literary and scientific acquirements, by mixing it up with manual labour. I think it would rather disparage the highest grade of the profession, to let them engage in that particular branch, which is a manual operation very much.[72]

The fatuity of this argument was exposed by Charles Clarke, who thus retorted: 'Midwifery is a branch of physic, a branch of surgery . . . [it] is the superintendence of a function of the human body: it is either medicine, or it is surgery, or it is both: it cannot be nothing.'[73]

The Council of the College of Surgeons for its part told the Obstetrical Society that 'however much disposed' it was, it did not have sufficient powers to intervene in the matter.[74] This was an excuse by which the College, already troubled by internal problems, hoped to avert the danger of another crisis. In 1826 a controversy had broken out over the surgeons' decision to recognise only certain surgical schools – in London, Dublin, Edinburgh, Glasgow and Aberdeen – for the purpose of training. The leaders of the profession were being sternly criticised by the teachers of surgery at the excluded provincial schools: they simply had enough trouble as it was without adding the question of obstetrical licensing, which may well have turned out to be a can of worms.[75] When the Obstetrical Society returned to the attack, the Surgeons argued that as the Surgeons' Court of Examiners excluded men-midwives, it could not conduct any examination in midwifery. However, as a concession the College agreed that as from 1 January 1828, every candidate for the membership of the College should attend two courses of lectures on the obstetric art and science. At the same time the Surgeons resolved to set up a Board of Examiners in Midwifery, but nothing happened until 1829 when, after a letter of inquiry from Robert Peel, the Court of Examiners was finally empowered to consult with the obstetricians.[76]

In 1833 the regulations for the new diploma were approved, but the College to its surprise discovered that it did not have the legal powers to institute the exam. It did not occur to anyone to seek them by applying to the Government until 1838, but again the Council took no action, this time it seems out of apathy rather than antipathy.[77] Developments within the College of Surgeons indirectly turned the scales in favour of obstetrics. In 1851 the College was negotiating for a new charter with the Home Secretary Sir George Grey: there was great discontent about the criteria of election to the Fellowship and the Council was under pressure to change them. Grey, however, was reluctant to grant the new charter, as he did not approve of the restrictions which prevented Council members from practising midwifery and pharmacy. James Moncrieff Arnott (1794–1885), President of the College of Surgeons, cunningly saw an opportunity for compromise: he promised Grey that the Council would abolish the restrictions if the Home Secretary would approve the charter. Six days after the meeting the restrictions were lifted. In 1852 the charter was approved and immediately afterwards the Board of Examiners in Midwifery was formed. The new Midwifery Licence qualified examinees for medical practice and was open to anyone, male or female, although in practice all the candidates were already members of the College of Surgeons. The first exam was held in December 1852. During the first year ninety-five candidates were tested, and only three were rejected.[78]

No sooner had the Surgeons instituted the Midwifery Licence than the Physicians proposed to introduce their own examination in obstetrics. But it was moved that a medical degree should be required as a condition for the licence and the scheme was defeated on the grounds that the moment was inopportune.[79] The proposals for the diploma, of course, made the Physicians vulnerable to attack from the radical wing of medical reform, for they were bound to be read as an attempt to restrict obstetrical practice to a higher grade of medical practitioner, under the aegis of the College. This was fundamentally at variance with the aspirations of people like Thomas Wakley (1795–1862), who wanted to abolish all distinctions of rank within the profession and pressed for the establishment of a common medical register, where all qualified practitioners would be listed regardless of their former legal status.[80]

In the meantime the College of Physicians had taken the decision to open its Fellowship to men-midwives, while the Surgeons had elevated some distinguished obstetricians to the Council of the College.[81] Lectureships in midwifery had also been established at all the London and provincial medical schools, and in 1860 midwifery was introduced in the syllabus for the medical degree at Oxford University.[82] Other midwifery practitioners who were devoted to general practice from 1861 onwards began to hold the new Licentiateship of the Royal College of Physicians, a diploma which implied far more than the title might suggest, as it included examinations in surgery and midwifery as well as physic.[83]

Educated accoucheurs

Despite the claims made by medical men about the superiority of their knowledge, the mere existence of courses and licences was no guarantee of the quality of the obstetric teaching that was provided. Even by mid-nineteenth-century standards the quality of obstetric education was regarded as poor. In 1842, for instance, a disgruntled student from Manchester who signed himself 'One of the Class' reported to the *Lancet* the erratic arrangements for the teaching of obstetrics and gynaecology at the medical school: it was mid-January and the lecturer in midwifery had not yet resumed teaching after Christmas; he had delivered not more than twelve lectures since the beginning of the winter session, and none on the diseases of women and children in the summer session.[84] At the St Marylebone Infirmary in London the midwifery department was not open to the physician's students unless they paid him a separate fee – hardly an incentive to further knowledge.[85]

While the medical journals continued to carry articles exposing the incompetence of midwives, manslaughter cases brought against practitioners for failing to exercise due care and skill in childbirth showed that parturient women were no safer in the hands of a medical man than they were in the midwife's. Medical commentators were always ready to excuse bungling colleagues, but they took a different line when the 'disembowelling accoucheurs' were unqualified.[86] As the debate on the reorganisation of the profession entered its most virulent phase in the late 1840s, horror stories about such practitioners were given great prominence in the medical journals in order to justify the need to restrict midwifery practice to qualified men and women.[87] The *London Medical Gazette* for August 1845 criticised the government's laissez-faire policy in this matter and the exaggerated notions of individual liberty which underlay it.[88] But the Act which finally regulated the medical profession in 1858 remained true to the principles of liberty and laissez-faire. The Act was a complete disappointment for Wakley and his supporters: it did not eliminate the Royal Colleges, it did not penalise quacks and it did not require registered practitioners to hold a licence in midwifery. Further, it gave no political representation to general practitioners on the General Medical Council (commonly known as GMC), the new body that was set up under the Act to oversee licensing arrangements.

In 1859, shortly after the passage of the Medical Act, a group of radical obstetricians and general practitioners took up the cause of obstetrics and gynaecology by founding the Obstetrical Society of London. Some of these men were already involved in medical politics: the obstetrician William Tyler Smith (1815–73), who had recently joined the staff of the newly established St Mary's Hospital and Medical School, and Robert Barnes, then a general practitioner in Notting Hill, London, were engaged in editorial work for Wakley's *Lancet*, a journal that was notorious for its attacks on the power of the corporations and its calls for greater political participation for the rank-and-file of the profession. Another sympathiser, the Sheffield practitioner James Hobson Aveling, would shortly play a prominent role in the controversy over midwife regulation and in 1884, with Robert Barnes, he would found the British Gynaecological Society to assert the obstetricians' right to operate in gynaecological cases.[89]

The Obstetrical Society of London had two aims: first, that of strengthening the position of obstetricians and secondly, that of diminishing the post-natal and maternal mortality. The two questions were seen to be directly related: they were deemed to be crucial to the advancement of obstetricians in relation to the midwife. The founders of the Society claimed that the untrained and unsupervised midwife was responsible for much of the maternal mortality, and argued that the solution to the problem of unsafe childbirth was to employ 'educated accoucheurs'.[90] For William Tyler Smith, the first President of the Obstetrical Society, the improvement of the obstetricians' social and professional standing depended on the recognition that obstetrics was an integral part of medicine. This was important in order to avert the danger of competition from partly qualified practitioners as well as from midwives. Throughout the nineteenth century, general practitioners were obsessed with the fear that an inferior grade of medical practitioner, similar to the French *officier de santé*, might arise to undermine them from below; the Midwifery Licence of the Royal College of Surgeons, which entitled anyone holding it to enter their name into the medical register, might have led to the emergence of such a cadre of partly qualified practitioners. Smith was indignant at the way in which obstetrics was under-represented in the governing bodies of the Colleges, but saw little hope from the 'pure' surgeons and physicians for an improvement in the position of midwifery: his wish was to establish a College of Obstetrics, but the political wind was not yet blowing in favour of such a plan.[91]

In the years that followed the Society worked for an extension of midwifery instruction in the medical schools and for the integration of obstetrics into the syllabus required for the licences in medicine and surgery. The rivalries between different interest groups within the medical profession, however, prevented the Obstetrical Society from achieving all of its aims, the teaching provisions for obstetrics and gynaecology being its most notable failure. This issue, as we have seen, was of the greatest importance because it was bound up with the regulation of general practice.

The 1858 Medical Reform Act allowed practitioners to register after passing a variety of qualifying examinations, yet none of these was a complete test for general practice. Medical practitioners could enter the profession after taking partial examinations such as that for the Midwifery Licence; the LRCP was no test of surgical knowledge, although the Physicians claimed that they could examine in

surgery if they wished; the MRCS made no provision for an examination in either medicine or midwifery. The GMC expected these
deficiencies to be corrected by a combination of examinations
through a conjoint board, but because of the competing interests
that were involved it took the conjoint examination twenty-five
years to evolve. Negotiations for such an examination were started
by the two Colleges in 1859; when they broke down, the College of
Surgeons attempted to make their own exam a complete qualifying
examination. In 1866 the Council agreed that every candidate for
the MRCS must pass an examination in medicine; three years later,
regulations were drawn for the midwifery part of the MRCS examination. No sooner had the College succeeded in countering the
criticism that the MRCS was an incomplete qualification for general practice than the GMC began to discuss plans for the formation
of conjoint boards. Thus in 1868 the GMC requested all the lecturers in obstetrics, medicine and surgery to investigate how the
teaching of their subject might be improved with a view to restruc-
turing medical training.[92]

At the suggestion of Robert Barnes, the teachers of obstetrics at
the London hospitals gathered together to discuss the matter. Their
recommendations were published in the *Lancet* for November
1868: they stated that the time allotted to obstetrics and gynaecology in the regulations of the licensing bodies should be extended
from three to six months, and that students should attend at least
twenty clinical lectures on the diseases of women and children. The
course had to cover all that related to pregnancy, parturition and
lactation, the functions and diseases of the female sexual system and
the diseases of childhood.[93] Practical training got a brief mention,
but it was not a priority at this stage. Obstetricians believed that
attendance at a systematic course of lectures was by far the most
important part of midwifery training and argued that the place for
gaining obstetrical knowledge was in the classroom, by means of
preparations, fresh specimens and drawings. This emphasis drew
its significance from the professional rivalry between obstetricians
and midwives. Practical experience was the area in which midwives
justly claimed superiority, thus one way of challenging the midwife's dominance of obstetrics was to stress the importance of
formal instruction, moving the debate on obstetrical practice into a
scientific terrain which midwives could not enter.[94]

Nothing, however, had come of the midwifery lecturers'

'decided opinion', Robert Barnes scornfully commented in 1875. The indefatigable campaigner for the improvement of obstetrics and gynaecology took a dim view of the situation. He regarded the scanty teaching provisions in these specialties as the measure of the estimation in which they were held 'by those who govern our hospitals, who frame our educational curricula and examinations for diplomas, and who generally legislate for the profession'. Students, he claimed, utterly neglected the subject, as it did not 'pay' at examinations: obstetrics and gynaecology were of no use, except for the licence of the Royal College of Physicians and the degree of London University. Furthermore, obstetrics was under-represented in the General Medical Council, in the Senate of the University of London and in the College of Surgeons; there were eleven teaching hospitals to which an obstetric physician was attached, and with one exception none appointed an assistant obstetrician. To sum it up, the position of gynaecology and obstetrics could only be defined as 'a scandal to the profession, and a grievous injury to the public'.[95]

One of the problems that had to be tackled was the huge disparity in the requirements laid down by the licensing bodies for their midwifery examinations. For example, in the Scottish universities medical students studied midwifery for six months, during which they had one hundred lectures on obstetrics and gynaecology; in London the course lasted three months and comprised only twenty-five lectures.[96] In 1879, while plans for the establishment of the conjoint board examinations were again being considered, the Obstetrical Society sent a memorial to all the medical licensing bodies in which it was proposed to standardise the teaching of obstetrics and gynaecology throughout the country. The Scottish universities were to provide the model, but there was great resistance to the plan from the GMC. The university teachers and clinicians who made up the GMC were anxious to encourage the study of the natural sciences and the acquisition of laboratory skills in an attempt at fostering the scientific image of the profession; they were thus unwilling to extend the length of midwifery courses at the expense of other subjects.[97]

During the inquiry carried out by the Select Committee on the Medical Act (1858) Amendment Act in 1879, it was suggested that the lot of midwifery would have been rather different if general practitioners had been better represented on the GMC, the *sancta sanctorum* of the profession. As obstetrics and gynaecology were predominantly the province of general practitioners, it would have been in their interest to raise the standards of obstetrical training. The reply from the president of the Council, Dr Acland, was uncompromising: the GMC was unwilling to have specialties represented.[98] The background to this statement was a long-standing war of attrition between the general physicians and surgeons who dominated the GMC and the profession, and the young specialties which had been developing since the beginning of the century – for example ophthalmology, dermatology and laryngology.[99] But midwifery was not a specialty for general practitioners, retorted Mr Waters. He was the representative of the British Medical Association, which had grown up in order to assert the independence of provincial medical practitioners from the capital and the Colleges. Speaking on behalf of this large body of medical men, Waters stated:

A general medical practitioner is the midwife of the district; it is the most important part of his practice; he attends the wife and the children, and therefore attends the family, and so it is that men even of position in the country are obliged to attend midwifery when they would rather not.[100]

Thus, claimed the Professor of Midwifery at King's College Hospital, London, if the young doctor was sent out in the world ill-equipped to carry out his work, the responsibility for his ignorance had to be laid squarely on the GMC.[101]

In the mid-1870s the plight of obstetrics and gynaecology was complicated by the growing enmity between midwives and accoucheurs and the accessory question of midwife regulation, which was then reaching a crescendo. Despite their best efforts, medical men had not succeeded in gaining a monopoly of childbirth. There are no precise data about the proportion of cases that were attended by midwives in this period, but it is safe to say that in many areas of the country medical men had managed to extend their practice among the wealthier classes. A report published by the Obstetrical Society of London in 1870 and in 1871 stated that the number of poor women attended by midwives in villages ranged from 30 to 90 per cent. In market towns, midwives attended at most 10 per cent, but in the large manufacturing towns they undertook between 75 and 90 per cent of all deliveries amongst the poor; in the West End of London, the proportion plummeted to 2 per cent.[102]

By the third quarter of the century, medical practitioners of midwifery were no longer intent on driving midwives out of business, but on keeping them out of the better-paid practice. Midwives, argued James Aveling in 1874, were 'desirable and necessary' because they were 'capable of relieving the general practitioner of an unremunerative, uninteresting, and physically exhausting class of cases'; medical men would have done no good to their profession if they had succeeded in turning all midwives out of every village and into the workhouse.[103] At the time Aveling was writing, general practitioners could expect to earn a guinea or more for attending a case in one of the best practices, but in poor areas the fee was likely to be 10s. 6d.;[104] the fee usually charged by midwives for attending a poor woman was 4s.[105] [In order to shed the unremunerative cases, accoucheurs needed to restrict the role of midwives, so as to create an inferior grade of midwifery practitioners for the poor who would never be equal to the medical man. The registration scheme set up by the Obstetrical Society in 1872 aimed to do just that. As James Aveling said two years later in support of the scheme, the relationship of the midwife to the obstetrician must be 'as a soldier to a general'. Midwives must be trained and competent, but 'under command when a battle has to be fought':[106] they must be no more than midwifery assistants, responsible for natural labours only and happy to undertake household chores as part of their duties.[107]]

[Restrictive as it was, the Obstetrical Society's scheme was opposed by some medical men, who feared the competition of qualified midwives. The feminists' counterblast was to put forward schemes that would have created highly trained, high-status midwives. In 1873 the Female Medical Society proposed that suitably qualified women should be allowed to be admitted to the Medical Register as 'Licentiates in Midwifery'. At the same time, a group of London midwives began to campaign in favour of the establishment of a licence in midwifery for women. First the Royal College of Surgeons, then the GMC were approached with a request that they set up such a licence; neither body however considered that this was their responsibility.[108] James Aveling for one objected that such women would have attracted a better class of patients at the expense of the poor, who most needed skilled care in childbirth, and of the general practitioner, who would lose practice to the licensed midwife: because, he claimed, obstetrics was an integral part of medicine, there could be no intermediate grade between the low-status midwife and the fully qualified medical man.[109] ⌐

Another aspect of midwifery dragged obstetricians into the fray of the battle of women for registration as medical practitioners. A loophole in the licensing system allowed women to be admitted to the Medical Register: under the terms of the 1858 Medical Act the Midwifery Licence of the Royal College of Surgeons allowed any *person* holding it to register as a qualified medical practitioner. In 1876 Sophie Jex-Blake and two of her colleagues at Edinburgh University, who were being prevented from continuing their studies there, decided to take advantage of this expedient in order to qualify for medical practice, and applied to be examined for the licence.[110]

The Council of the College of Surgeons was keen to allow the women's claim, as they were already under some pressure to remove the legal obstacles that prevented women from registering as medical practitioners. The year before they had tried to get an enabling Bill through Parliament, but they had been informed that James Stansfeld, former President of the Local Government Board and a prominent member of the women's rights movement, would oppose the Bill unless a clause were added admitting women as candidates for the diploma. Thus on 17 February 1876 the Council of the College of Surgeons resolved to admit Miss Jex-Blake and her friends to the examination in midwifery.[111] But the examiners for the licence, William Priestley and Robert Barnes, refused to carry out the examination and resigned from the Examination Board. To some extent their action was justified by the fact that the College for some years had debarred from the midwifery licence examination those who did not already possess a qualification in either medicine or surgery. But as the three candidates were not allowed to enter for the other medical qualifications, the Obstetrical Society's argument that the admission of partially qualified practitioners to the Register would have been 'injurious' to the public was something of a double bind.

From the pages of the *Obstetrical Journal of Great Britain and Ireland*, James Aveling criticised the Surgeons' handling of the Jex-Blake affair for displaying 'not only a disregard but a disdain for Midwifery practice'.[112] The decision to admit the three women to the exam for registration lost obstetricians ground in their struggle for supremacy over midwives and opened the floodgates to partly qualified practitioners.(Worse still, the Surgeons' resolution introduced women into obstetrics – and women, Aveling maintained, were not fitted to practise this branch of medicine, since they were 'deficient in the nerve and strength necessary for the successful treatment of Obstetric emergencies'.[113] Aveling had used the same argument two years earlier, when he had successfully resisted the admission of Dr Elizabeth Garrett Anderson to the Obstetrical Society.[114] Opposition to female practitioners was greatest amongst obstetricians and gynaecologists: they had most to fear from the competition of medical women, for the major argument in favour of lady doctors centred on women's need for medical care which did not violate women's modesty. This danger of competition from female obstetricians and gynaecologists had become all the more serious since Elizabeth Garrett Anderson had opened her women-only New Hospital for Women in 1873.

How then could obstetricians defend their 'threatened honour'? Aveling reiterated that the establishment of special qualifications in obstetrics was the only solution: 'Above all', he said,

let us insist upon a higher Obstetric qualification, either by obtaining from universities a special Obstetric degree, or by the establishment of Royal Colleges of Obstetricians.[115]

When the College of Obstetricians envisaged by Aveling finally became a reality in 1929, however, it was not intended to protect obstetricians from the competition of midwives and medical women, but to fight off the grip of the surgeons on gynaecological surgery.[116]

It is probable that the resignation of the midwifery examiners involved in the Jex-Blake affair hastened parliamentary action, for in 1876 the Russell Gurney Act empowered all licensing bodies to examine women for medical qualifications. In the same year the GMC resolved to accept women for registration, and in 1877 the students of the London School of Medicine for Women were allowed to attend clinical instruction at the Royal Free Hospital. The question of the registration of midwives remained a separate issue. It was ambiguously settled much later, in 1902, when the newly established Midwives Board was taken from under the control of the GMC, and yet remained regulated by the medical profession through the Board's governing body.[117]

The campaign for the integration of obstetrics into the medical curriculum began to yield some results in 1881, when obstetrics became an integral part of the examination for the diplomas of Fellow and Member of the College of Surgeons. In 1884, with the establishment of the Conjoint Board Examinations, proficiency in obstetrics, medicine and surgery was required of all the candidates for medical registration, thus debarring partly qualified practitioners from the profession; two years later the Medical Act Amendment Act put the legal seal on the first complete examination for general practice.[118] It took another two years to overcome the opposition of the physicians and surgeons on the GMC to the proposed regulation requiring all candidates to have attended twelve confinements, and to have conducted three personally under the supervision of a registered medical practitioner. But as Dr Robert Rentoul, a Liverpool man who was fighting midwife registration on behalf of the less affluent medical practitioner, complained in 1891, in practice 'being present' at a confinement covered a multitude of sins: it could mean that a student had looked at a case and left, or that he had been taught by a midwife – which was like 'obtaining his training in surgery from a bone-setter, or his medical education from a herbalist'.[119]

The last quarter of the nineteenth century saw the beginnings of a further evolution in the professional organisation of obstetrics and gynaecology. As the women's hospitals became a central locus of gynaecological practice, a class of hospital-based specialists began to emerge out of general practice: before long general practitioners, who had founded and staffed the first women's hospitals in the early Victorian years, would be excluded from these institutions. To a large extent the history of this development is the history of the success of the gynaecological hospitals.

3

The rise of the women's hospitals

As Dr Acland indicated in his evidence to the Select Committee on the Medical Act (Amendment) Act in 1879, the medical establishment did not approve of specialists. Some of the reluctance of the older generation to accept specialties was due to the association of these fields with quackery: this was especially true of urology, orthopaedics and ophthalmology. But the public thought otherwise and patronised specialists with enthusiasm. The proliferation of specialist institutions during the nineteenth century provides a measure of their success: between 1800 and 1890, eighty-eight specialist hospitals, dispensaries and infirmaries were founded in London alone, reaching a peak in the 1860s, when twenty-two institutions were founded.[1]

The first specialist institutions began to appear at the end of the eighteenth century, when a number of dispensaries and infirmaries were set up to care for those charity patients who were excluded from the voluntary hospital – for example, women in childbirth, lunatics, the incurables, fever and venereal disease cases. The most important difference between these establishments and the voluntary hospitals created earlier in the century was that they were founded by medical men rather than by lay philanthropists. During the nineteenth century the range of conditions that were treated at specialist institutions was greatly extended to include the diseases of the eyes, ears, throat, skin and nervous system, to name but a few.

From the 1840s onwards, special hospitals were set up also for the care of women's diseases. The rise of these institutions occupies a central place in the development of gynaecology as a specialist practice. The gynaecological hospitals embodied moral and social views about the 'special' nature of femininity; they were the place where gynaecologists gained their experience of women's diseases and served as vehicles of professional advancement for many individuals who lacked the necessary social connections. Interest in a single locale helped forge professional links between practitioners of gynaecology, favouring the separation of gynaecology from general practice and the creation of specialist gynaecological societies.[2]

The two women's hospitals that are discussed in this chapter exemplify this pattern: they are the Hospital for Women in Soho Square, London (1842), the first hospital of its kind in Britain, and the Chelsea Hospital for Women, founded by James Aveling in 1871. These institutions are of particular historical interest also because they were established for the benefit of different social classes; they thus provide a focus through which the interrelation of class and gender issues in gynaecology may be fruitfully explored.

Hospitals, specialists and nineteenth-century medicine

In founding special hospitals, nineteenth-century medical practitioners were following an accepted pattern of reputation-building. Hospital posts generally carried no remuneration, but they were valuable to medical men as the place where they gained experience and, most importantly, social visibility. Members of the honorary medical staff of a hospital stood a good chance of becoming medical advisers to the wealthy businessmen, merchants and aristocrats who formed the governors' board. Younger practitioners who managed to get a foothold on the bottom of the hospital ladder could be confident that their seniors would help them further their careers and build up their private practice.[3]

During the course of the nineteenth century, hospitals came to play an increasingly important role in the training of the profession and the treatment of the sick. From the beginning of the century, the requirements for the licences of the College of Surgeons and the Society of Apothecaries began to include one year's and six months' hospital practice respectively. In order to cope with the influx of students, medical institutions were induced to set up schools of medicine, and new hospitals were founded to fulfil the needs of medical teaching: this was the case with University College Hospital (1834) and St Mary's (1852).[4]

Between 1861 and 1891, hospital facilities rapidly expanded in response to the growing demand for in-patient care. In the eighteenth and nineteenth centuries, the upper and middle classes were treated at home; hospitals were intended for the 'deserving poor'. The reform of hospital nursing and management in the second half of the nineteenth century led to higher standards of care and hygiene, making hospital treatment attractive to a wider social group. With the introduction of anaesthesia, the type of surgery that could be attempted was extended; this, too, contributed to the increase in hospital accommodation.[5]

Another factor that played a part in the growth of institutional care was the campaign against outdoor relief. In 1834 the New Poor Law attempted to abolish 'outdoor' (i.e. domiciliary) relief of the able-bodied poor; medical relief, which was hitherto widely supplied to the poor by the parish, was restricted to the destitute and attempts were made to restrict its availability to the workhouse. Working-class men thus began to insure themselves against sickness by joining a friendly society or a sick club, a form of self-help for the poor which was either entirely funded from members' subscriptions or subsidised by private philanthropy. Workers who were not covered by any provident scheme were forced to seek general practitioner services at free or part-pay dispensaries, and increasingly resorted to the general hospitals, which provided the largest system of free care.[6]

Given the increasing emphasis on the hospital as the locus of medical practice, it is not surprising that in the first half of the nineteenth century so many doctors chose to found specialist institutions. The typical founder of special hospitals was a practitioner who could not secure positions at the general hospitals, either because he did not enjoy the protection of prestigious surgeons and physicians, or because he was not rich enough to 'buy' the vote of governors in hospital elections.[7] Often he was able to step on to the first rung of the professional ladder, but could not go any further: entrepreneurship thus had to replace patronage as the means of achieving fame and prosperity.

The Moorfields Eye Hospital, founded by John Cunningham Saunders in 1804, was the example on which later specialist institutions were modelled. Saunders was a provincial surgeon who had come to London to walk the wards and work in the capital. He got a post as house-pupil and dresser to the eminent surgeon Sir Astley Cooper at St Thomas's, but as he had not been articled for six years at the Royal College of Surgeons he had little hope of a hospital appointment. Saunders at first went back to the provinces 'anxious about his future prospects'; a letter from Cooper summoned him back to London with the promise of making him 'comfortable in a pecuniary point of view'. At the suggestion of Cooper, who had a special interest in the anatomy of the ear, Saunders established a specialist dispensary for the treatment of ear and eye disease. The dispensary rapidly grew into a hospital for eye disease only, Saunders having apparently realised that he could do nothing for aural disease.[8]

[It was not very difficult to set up a special hospital. First of all, a house was rented in a district where rents were affordable. A favourite haunt of early nineteenth-century medical entrepreneurs in London was the unfashionable Holborn area; this was the neighbourhood where the Hospital for Women, too, began its existence. Once the house had been fitted up with a few beds, a residential matron was put in charge and patients could then be admitted straightaway under the medical supervision of a surgeon, usually the founder himself.[9]

If the institution was to thrive, it was essential to secure the financial support of wealthy philanthropists, and these were not hard to come by. Medical philanthropy was popular with the upper classes as it fulfilled their social obligations to the poor; it was also a means whereby upwardly mobile individuals could improve their image and social standing. Gifts were not always disinterested. In 1880, for example, the management committee of the Hospital for Women considered a gift of clothing from an anonymous donor, who requested that the gift be acknowledged in the *Daily Telegraph* as the 'contents from the wardrobe of an adulterous wife'.[10] Another benefactor from Sydenham near London offered £100 on condition that the 'non-alcoholic treatment of disease' as practised at the Temperance Hospital be tried out for six months and the results published.[11] On both occasions the committee turned the gift down. In some hospitals, preference was given to tradesmen who were subscribers when purchases were made for the hospital.[12]

A number of factors – medical, political and social – provided the stimulus and the momentum for the establishment of specialist institutions. For example, when St Peter's Hospital for the care of Stone in the Bladder and Urinary Diseases was established in 1860, its founders Armstrong Todd and Thomas Spencer Wells advertised the institution by promising a new technique for the treatment of stone (morbid concretions in the bladder) which, they claimed, would dramatically reduce the high mortality rates of lithotomy.[13] Belief in the miasmatic origin of contagion provided a rationale for accommodating cancer patients in special hospitals, as such cases were thought to render the air of a ward injurious and disagreeable to other patients.[14] The origins (and success) of children's hospitals can scarcely be understood without reference to the Victorian ideal of the 'child' – a social category mediating ideas of dependence, innocence and development.[15]

Specialists claimed that a love of knowledge and humanity animated their hospital-building enterprises. They hailed the process of division of labour by which special hospitals and specialisms were emerging as a happy mark of progress and civilisation. Not all their colleagues, however, took their claims at face value. General hospital consultants in particular regarded specialist medicine as a pernicious influence on the practice of medicine and on the profession. Hostility against special hospitals mounted in the 1850s and finally came to a head in 1860, when the proposed foundation of St Peter's Hospital for Stone provoked nineteen of the most eminent London hospital consultants to draw up a statement of protest against the proliferation of special institutions.[16] It was ironic that some of the signatories of the letter were themselves specialists: Sir Charles Locock (1799–1875), for instance, Physician-Accoucheur to the Queen, was one of the obstetricians who had supported the foundation of the first hospital for women eighteen years earlier. The other signatories of the circular included Thomas Mayo (1790–1871), President of the Royal College of Physicians, John Flint South (1797–1882), President of the Royal College of Surgeons, and Sir Benjamin Brodie (1783–1862), President of the Royal Society. Copies of the statement were sent to hospital consultants throughout England, and by mid-October 1860 at least 415 hospital doctors had signed the document.

A nationwide campaign was launched against the 'monstrous evil' of special hospitals. The leaders of the profession criticised the narrow approach to disease they tended to foster: the splitting up of medicine into specialties encouraged practitioners to see bodily parts and diseases in isolation from the whole organism, destroying 'that unity of disease which the philosophic mind should always keep in view'.[17] Consultants were also acutely concerned about the impact of special hospitals on the reputation, teaching functions and funding of their own hospitals. The establishment of special institutions, it was claimed, would result in the multiplication of expensive facilities which were already supplied in the existing general hospitals; it would divert much needed funds away from the general hospitals and starve them of their patients, who were the foundation of clinical teaching. The *British Medical Journal* for 1860 thus summed up the feelings of the medical establishment:

> What is the cause of the growth of 'charitable' bricks and mortar, and what is its tendency? To read the carefully worded advertisements, it would appear that hospitals, in the metropolis at least, were created solely on behalf of suffering humanity ... Anyone who knows anything of our metropolitan charitable institutions, is fully aware how far this is from the real – and we must add, in too many cases, vulgar – truth ... Founded in the grossest self-seeking on the part of some individual, they are matured only through a system of mendicancy already strained to the uttermost.[18]

It was not long before general practitioners joined the chorus of disapproval. They complained that the special hospitals were robbing them of their better-off patients, the skilled artisans and clerks who were well able to pay for medical advice. Specialist charities bitterly competed for financial support, and this depended on the alleged existence of need as measured in particular by the number of patients relieved by the institution. By 'carefully got up statistics' and by turning a blind eye on the actual socio-economic circumstances of patients, special hospitals inflated numbers and bolstered their reputation: specialists 'got their names spread all over England, but in the meantime the profession was being ruined', grumbled W. O. Markham, later to become the editor of the *British Medical Journal*, at a meeting of the British Medical Association in 1860.[19] Some argued that the special hospitals were to blame if general practitioners were reduced to selling bottles of medicine in a desperate and ungentlemanly attempt at economic survival.

Hospital consultants had a battery of weapons they could use in order to contain the growth of specialism. They could refuse to consult with specialists and refer patients to them; they could exclude them from medical societies, denying specialists the social and professional benefits that could be derived from such associations, and ban them from the governing bodies of the profession.[20] The eminent gynaecologist John Bland-Sutton, who made his reputation at the Chelsea Hospital in the late nineteenth century, resigned his post there when it became apparent that this association was preventing him from going any further: in the late 1910s

Bland-Sutton was seeking election to the Council of the Royal College of Surgeons, but he was repeatedly blackballed because of his connection with a 'Woman's Hospital'.[21] Social pressure from their colleagues forced practitioners with dual appointments to choose between specialist and general hospitals. Thomas Nunn was Assistant Surgeon at the Middlesex Hospital when he was elected to the staff of St Peter's Hospital for Stone in 1866. He resigned a year later, saying that he was leaving 'in order to prevent being forced into open rupture with several of my colleagues at the Middlesex Hospital with whom I have been connected nearly twenty years'.[22]

The first women's hospital

Arrangements for the in-patient treatment of gynaecological cases in London varied widely in the early Victorian period. On the whole, though, obstetric physicians had no access to hospital beds and often had their cases taken out of their hands by the physicians and surgeons. Gynaecological patients at St George's Hospital and at the London were referred to one of the physicians or surgeons; in difficult cases, the lecturer in midwifery was consulted for an opinion. At St Thomas's it was the assistant apothecary who selected gynaecological out-patients for the obstetrician; the obstetric physician had charge of twelve beds, which were set apart for him in the three medical wards. At King's College and at University College Hospitals, obstetricians had no beds and were forced to encroach on those of the physicians and surgeons. St Bartholomew's Hospital had no special obstetric officer, but it was customary for gynaecological out-patients to see the lecturer in midwifery one day a week; in-patients were occasionally entrusted to his care by the physicians and surgeons.[23] Only Guy's Hospital offered separate facilities for gynaecological patients. The ward, which contained ten beds, had been opened in 1831 at the instigation of the obstetric physician Samuel Ashwell.[24] It was important that Ashwell had the support of the hospital Treasurer, Benjamin Harrison Jr. At many of the London hospitals the treasurer was the chief administrator; he could exercise great power in the governors' boardroom as well as the hospital wards, and often became the greatest single influence in the hospital.[25]

Shortly after the opening of the gynaecological ward at Guy's Protheroe Smith, a young practitioner from Bideford in Devon,

put forward proposals for the establishment of a charitable institution for the treatment of women's diseases.[26] Born in 1809, Smith
was the son of a physician. He originally intended to join the army,
where he had been promised a commission, but a hip injury forced
him to change his plans. He decided to take up medicine and be a
military surgeon, but soon he became more interested in medicine
and gave up the idea of a military career. After serving as an
apprentice to his father, who had a successful practice in Bideford,
Smith set his sights on London and in 1830 he came to St Bartholomew's Hospital, where he was awarded first prize in Anatomy,
Physiology and Surgery. He qualified MRCS in 1833 and was then
appointed surgeon to the Farringdon Dispensary and Lying-in
Institution, with which he was associated until his death; he also
began to work with Dr Edward Rigby (1804–61) as co-lecturer in
midwifery and the diseases of women at St Bartholomew's Hospital. A keen innovator, he invented surgical gadgets and instruments, and in 1842 he performed ovariotomy in an operation which
is thought to have been the second of its kind ever carried out in the
capital. He was also the first London accoucheur to use chloroform
in childbirth: in 1848 he wrote a pamphlet giving scriptural evidence in support of Simpson's discovery, which the Edinburgh
obstetrician later quoted in defence of the practice.[27] He was a
careful and successful operator and built up a lucrative private
practice.

   Smith set out the reasons for founding a hospital for women in a
circular addressed to all medical men. His arguments deserve close
scrutiny, for they reveal both the gender and the class dimensions of
female disease. Women's complaints, Smith claimed, were difficult
and accompanied by much suffering and 'nervous sensibility', thus
requiring specially trained attendants and a quiet and restful environment to avoid the dangers of nervous excitement. Further,
they called for a 'delicacy of treatment' which was hardly imagina-
ble in the large teaching hospitals, where the physician or surgeon
'walked the wards' in the company of a large crowd of pupils.[28]
This was a pledge to debar medical students from the wards of the
new hospital which was no doubt intended to secure public support
for the project: ever since men–midwives had entered the lying-in
chamber, the suspicion that obstetricians violated women's
modesty had proved one of the major obstacles to the advance of
the male practitioner of midwifery.[29]

The second line of argument hinged on the failure of domiciliary treatment amongst the poor.[30] Smith associated the gynaecological disorders of the poor with the insalubrious conditions of slum living, a relationship for which the constitutional theory of uterine disease provided the mediating link. Edward Rigby, later to become Professor of Midwifery at St Bartholomew's, was a well-known propounder of this doctrine.[31] In the wealthy, overindulgence in food and drink caused intestinal and hepatic derangements which ultimately led to disorder in the sexual organs;[32] the other side of the coin was the aetiology of gynaecological disease in the poor. Rigby discussed the question in the first of a series of 'Reports on uterine disease', published in the *Medical Times* between 1844 and 1847: 'In a great metropolis like London, where the general health of the population is necessarily more or less below the standard in point of tone and strength', he wrote, there were many factors which caused 'defective assimilation, irregular distribution of the circulation, and local congestions'.[33] Residence in damp, cramped and unhealthy situations, long hours spent in close and ill-ventilated workshops depressed the tone of the general health; local uterine disorders, particularly of a functional kind, were commonly the result in women.[34] Such cases, stressed Protheroe Smith, abounded

in the dark and crowded alleys of London, where the sufferer is often found to be a mother, upon whose constant exertions the cleanliness and comfort of the family depend.[35]

As long as the patient remained exposed to the noxious influences of her miserable dwelling, no treatment could prove efficacious: 'the one close room' the poor woman occupied in common with her family,

her careworn aspect – the filthy and squalid appearance of her children – the impure atmosphere in which such misery is necessarily bred, – prove that no remedies can be effectually applied whilst so many causes are operating to counteract them.[36]

The solution was to remove patients from their wretched abodes to a more salubrious environment, where 'perfect rest, good nursing, a well-regulated diet, and proper ventilation' would assist recovery.[37]

These arguments had a moral and political resonance which Smith's contemporaries would have readily appreciated. Overcrowding did not breed only disease – as the sanitary reformers emphasised, it produced crime and sexual immorality; it destroyed the sanctity of the family; it concentrated the masses in a politically dangerous way and favoured the spread of socialism and nihilism.[38] In contrast to Frederick Engels, who described the condition of the English working class in the context of a critique of bourgeois domination,[39] middle-class sanitarians saw the question of urban health as one of morality: ill-health and poverty were due to the individual's indolence and depravity, physical health arose from states of social and moral order. As the statistician William Farr wrote in 1875, there was

a relation betwixt death and sickness . . . betwixt death, health, and energy of body and mind . . . between death and national primacy . . . betwixt the forms of death and moral excellence of infamy.[40]

This assumption underlay constitutional theories of disease in early Victorian Britain. Advocates of the theory tended to underplay the importance of social and working conditions as causes of disease, emphasising the individual's responsibility for his or her own health: self-discipline and good personal habits, it was argued, were the means by which disease could be prevented.[41]

This displacement of political issues onto a moral plane was noticeable in another area of social concern which directly impinged on Protheroe Smith's project. Since the 1820s, when the struggles of the Lancashire textile mills operatives had revealed the terrible conditions of their employment, there had been growing concern about the lot of working women, particularly if they were wives and mothers.[42] The *Lancet* woke up to the 'system of slavery' to which London milliners and dressmakers were condemned in 1853. Young girls worked for sixteen hours a day without a break in unhealthy and overcrowded workshops: it was impossible to 'trace the slow but certain inroads upon their constitutions – the pitiless and destructive drudgery of these "*death-shops*" – without feelings akin to indignation and horror', wrote the *Lancet*.[43] Scrofula, cachexia, menstrual disorders and derangements of the digestive organs were the necessary consequences of want of air and exercise. The journal appealed to the British public to remove this 'blot on the metropolis', but it fought shy of recommending political action: the improvement of the sanitary condition of milliners would be better achieved by thrusting the 'moral weight' of public opinion upon employers than by resorting to penal codes and enactments.

The *Lancet* was not calling for an end to social inequality, it merely desired humanitarianism to smooth out the rough edges of capitalism. Even so, its views were a great deal more radical than the Evangelical response to the problem. During the early Victorian period, middle-class Evangelical philanthropists identified the labouring woman as one of their causes: improving her lot was one step towards establishing the Kingdom of God on earth. The remedy, however, lay not in bettering exploitative working conditions, but in eliminating the moral degradation that female employment was said to bring about. Philanthropists blamed the domestic squalor of the poor on the negligence of the working-class wife and mother, and stressed the importance of acquainting her with good domestic management, thrift, industry, cleanliness and the Christian virtues.[44]

Seen in this light, Smith's argument for orderliness and sanitation was also a plea for a form of moral and bodily discipline which locked poor women into a socially subordinate position. If health and disease were linked to social and moral order, then no cure could be effected unless patients acquiesced to the structure of power and domination in society.[45] Interestingly, not only gynaecological cases, but also women suffering from chronic ill-health and work-related complaints were treated at Smith's hospital during its early years of activity: gender allowed to categorise patients in such a way that the realities of economic exploitation were obliterated.

It is important to understand that the use of hospital admission for moral education was not new, and neither was it unique to medical institutions where women were treated: it was an aspect of the *relations between classes*. Smith's application of this method to the treatment of gynaecological patients illustrates the importance of both gender *and* class issues in shaping medical perceptions of gynaecological disease. In viewing their patients, it was as if Victorian gynaecologists were 'looking at a picture through a double exposure'.[46]

A moral institution

After some initial difficulty, Protheroe Smith finally succeeded in interesting a number of influential laymen and in August 1842 a provisional committee was formed with the object of establishing the hospital.[47] A year later the first Hospital for the Diseases of Women was founded under the presidency of John Henry Manners, the fifth Duke of Rutland. The declared objects of the institution were twofold: first, to relieve those diseases that were peculiar to the female sex, and secondly, to give 'strength and activity' to those who were either 'disabled from performing the duties of life', or performed them with difficulty.[48] A number of well-known medical men, from Samuel Merriman, a prominent member of the London medical establishment, to Charles Locock, Physician-Accoucheur to the Queen, had expressed their support for the venture; all of them emphasised the sanitary advantages of institutional treatment and the opportunities to learn about gynaecological disease that this would provide.

At a cost of £100 a year, a house was rented in Red Lion Square near High Holborn, a stone's throw from the Farringdon Dispensary where Smith held a post as a surgeon. A matron and servants were engaged, two wards comprising eleven beds were fitted up and patients were first admitted on 25 January 1844. During 1844, twenty-eight in-patients and seventy out-patients from every London district and from the outlying counties were admitted under the care of Protheroe Smith, who acted as surgeon to the institution; the consulting physicians were Robert Ferguson and Edward Rigby, but it is not clear whether they actually saw any patients.[49]

Hospital building was a competitive business and the new hospital at first found it very difficult to attract charitable funding. This was attributed to the fact that the title 'Hospital for the Diseases of Women' suggested venereal disease and prostitution to the public. Venereal disease was widely regarded as the wages of sin and no one was prepared to encourage immorality. In order to dispel any misapprehension about the purpose of the hospital, in 1845 the word 'diseases' was dropped from the title,[50] but the new image of the hospital does not seem to have made an immediate impact on would-be benefactors. A note entitled 'Unprofessional Advertisements' appeared in the *Lancet* for 1853 condemning the hospital's fund-raising efforts:

Our attention has for several weeks past been attracted by the frequency of appeals made for pecuniary aid to certain medical institutions by public and oft-repeated advertisements in the leading newspapers. Such constant demands for institutions appropriated to special diseases (that for example, in Soho Square) savour more of quackery than philanthropy.[51]

Notwithstanding the growing medical opposition to specialisation, by the late 1850s the public was beginning to show some interest in the first women's hospital. Thanks to the co-operation of Lord Chelsea and the Marquis of Westminster, in 1856 a fête held in Grosvenor Square raised £750 to finance the move to new premises in Soho Square.[52] In the meantime, practitioners from foreign countries had begun to visit the institution. One of the results of this interest was the foundation of hospitals for women in Boston, New York, Bristol and Manchester.[53]

It is not possible to say very much about the social background of the first patients, apart from what can be gleaned from the sparse references made in the hospital reports to the 'disabled housewife', the soldier's wife and the 'half-starved needlewoman'. Some information about the occupation of patients for a later period can be gained from Protheroe Smith's book of cases from October 1869 to November 1870. About a third of the seventy-six cases in this book were patients admitted to the new pay block that had opened in 1869. Of the fifty charity patients, just over half were married women, and three were widowed. In twenty-eight cases the occupation is stated: servants, nurses, laundresses, dressmakers and a variety of women employed in manual crafts are to be found in this sample. Nearly half of these women were married, three were widowed (see table 1 in appendix).

Evangelicalism exercised a strong influence on hospital life till the 1870s. As the hospital reports emphasised, it was not only the physical, but also the spiritual needs of patients that were catered for by the institution. Lady visitors undertook to read passages from the Bible and to impart some religious instruction; every morning and evening, a period of time was set aside for prayers.[54] The results could be impressive. In 1846, a young woman suffering from a fatal disease was admitted 'as hopeless of the life eternal as that which was rapidly declining; and altogether ignorant of the way of salvation'. During her stay at the hospital, she was gradually converted to Christianity and finally died 'in the peace of God'.[55] Another patient, a twenty-two-year-old woman, was not only cured, but also got to hear 'of Him whom to know is Life Eternal'.[56] Bodily healing and spiritual redemption went hand in hand.

Patients were subjected to a disciplinary regime that bore a striking resemblance to the training of repenting prostitutes in Magdalen Institutions.[57] They were expected to comply with the hospital regulations and to take an active part in religious and domestic activities. Patients could be discharged for misconduct: two such cases were recorded in 1873 out of a total of 294 admissions, but the reasons unfortunately were not stated.[58] Any reading material had to be vetted by the Matron or by the Ladies' Committee; if found unsuitable for the patients, it could be banned from the wards.[59] Patients who were relatively able-bodied were encouraged to mend or make linen for the hospital, or do other light work – not least with a view at defraying the expenses of the institution.[60]

The maintenance of discipline on the wards was the responsibility of the Ladies' Committee through the direct intervention of their subordinate, the matron, who had the task of supervising the conduct of patients and staff. The introduction of lady visitors into the female wards of hospitals and lunatic asylums had been advocated in 1816 by the social reformer Catherine Cappe. The presence of ladies, she argued, would tend to produce 'general habits of order' and a sense of propriety in conversation and behaviour, especially if patients were made aware that every expectation of future patronage depended on their conduct:[61] upper-class ladies could throw their social superiority behind the effort to check the 'moral disorders' that might arise between male physicians and female patients. The ladies' supervisory role was to be modelled on the type of interaction with lower class women that was already familiar to gentlewomen – the mistress-servant relation. Ladies visitors in a hospital

should be to that institution what the kind judicious Mistress of a family is to her household, – the careful inspector of the economy, the integrity and the good moral conduct of the housekeeper and other inferior servants.[62]

The ideology of femininity may have united females into a single biological and social group; in practice, class divides were of overriding significance in determining the pattern of interaction between women.

The work of improving patients' morality was no doubt facilitated by the great length of a stay in the institution – in 1850 one woman was reported to have been under treatment for thirteen and a half months.[63] This was exceptional by contemporary standards, and three years after the opening of the hospital there was some concern that the nature of the cases and the necessity of keeping them in the hospital for a long time might turn the institution into an invalid asylum.[64] The figures for these early days are not available, but in the late 1860s the length of stay stood at ninety-two days on average.[65] This compares with thirty-two days on the gynaecological ward of a general hospital (the Middlesex) in the mid-1860s,[66] a figure which is consistent with the average length of stay in the London general hospitals in 1861 (33.3 days according to Pinker's *English Hospital Statistics 1861–1938*).[67]

The members of the Ladies' Committee were of a higher social class than the medical men and lay managers who ran the hospital. They were conscious of their social superiority and of being in a position to challenge male control over the institution. Ladies and doctors came to blows in 1872–73 over the hospital's nursing arrangements. At the end of 1872 the medical staff instituted an inquiry into the efficiency of the nursing and the private character of the matron; at the same time, they conferred greater powers to the head nurse. This caused so many difficulties between the head nurse and the matron that the ladies were prompted to intervene. They recommended that the head nurse be dismissed and that the matron be entrusted with the superintendence of the whole institution.[68] Shortly afterwards, a new by-law regulating the appointment of the medical staff was passed, which the medical officers interpreted as an attempt to 'weed their ranks of all such as had in any way rendered themselves conspicuous by their desire for reforming the institutions of Soho-square'. When the Management Committee refused to rescind the by-law, the medical staff tendered their resignation.[69]

The episode revealed to the profession the extent of lay control over the institution. Brian Abel-Smith has argued that 'the distinctive feature of specialist hospitals was the fact that most of them were founded and controlled by doctors'.[70] This did not apply to the Soho Square hospital: 'No long time ago', commented the *Medical Times and Gazette* in April 1874,

we had occasion to remark on the evils inherent in that system of hospital government in which the lay authorities have all the power vested in themselves, without sufficient means of making themselves acquainted with the views of the medical officers; and on the system of snubbing these meritorious workers so persistently carried out in some quarters.[71]

Nowhere was the 'abuse' of lay authority more marked than at the Hospital for Women. Not only did the management committee control the medical appointments in the hospital; they also constantly interfered with the medical aspects of the charity. It was galling that Protheroe Smith, who sat on the management committee and should have represented the medical staff, chose 'almost invariably to cast in his lot with the lay body rather than with his medical colleagues'.[72]

However, the medical officers' revolt did indicate that they were no longer prepared to accept lay control unquestioningly. Their growing desire for a say in the running of the institution found its expression in a struggle for freedom over the selection of cases. As was the practice at most other medical institutions, the lay governors rigidly defined the criteria for the admission of patients: for example, cancer cases were excluded as being 'offensive and incurable'.[73] In the early 1880s, however, the medical staff began to admit cancer patients without the authority of the governors. When the Management Committee objected, the physicians replied that to exclude all cases would deprive the hospital of its utility. First, some patients were sent in as cancer cases which were not; secondly, the amount of relief that could be provided and the extent to which the patient's life may be prolonged depended on the nature of the cancer; and finally, such cases could be treated without detriment to other patients. By emphasising the value of their clinical judgment, the medical staff asserted their independence from the lay managers. The hospital authorities capitulated.[74]

From the 1880s onwards, the increasing concern with the clinical teaching of gynaecology brought the staff of the Soho Square hospital into conflict with the Management Committee. Teaching was very important for the professional advancement of specialties. With students in the wards of a special hospital, knowledge was passed on to the next generation of practitioners and, in the process, specialists gained influence and recognition. In 1882 the Medical

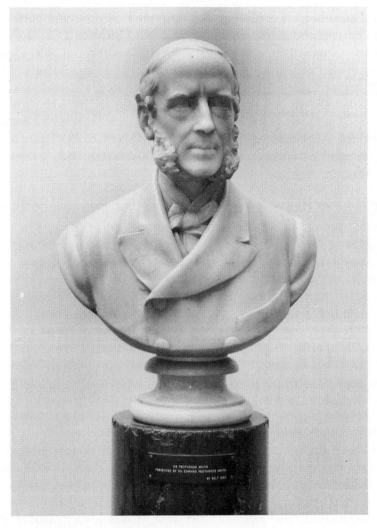

1 Protheroe Smith

Committee moved that medical students be allowed to attend the
in-patient department. They were sharply reminded by the
Management Committee that it had never been decided that the
wards of the hospital should be open to students. Three years later
the medical staff proposed that, in view of the large number of
medical men who came to the hospital to learn, the clinical department should be restyled 'The London School of Gynaecology', but
again their request was turned down.[75]

By the 1880s the Hospital for Women had built for itself a

reputation which could not be questioned. A powerful patroness had been found in the person of Princess Christian of Schleswig-Holstein, one of Queen Victoria's daughters; through her, Queen Victoria herself began to take an interest in the hospital, and in 1885 she demonstrated her appreciation by sending a cheque for five hundred pounds.[76] When Protheroe Smith retired from the hospital in 1884, the management committee honoured him with a marble bust, the accolade reserved for heroes and benefactors of humanity. Smith could certainly look back on his career with pride and satisfaction.

The Chelsea Hospital for Women

As the popularity of specialist institutions grew during the third quarter of the century, the medical establishment became increasingly agitated about the 'rampant evil of over-weening specialism'. The Soho Square hospital had fallen foul of the medical press in 1853, when its loud appeals to philanthropy had offended the professional sensibilities of the *Lancet*; the nursing crisis of 1874 provided yet another pretext for directing attention to its 'disagreeable peculiarities'. 'The Hospital for Women', wrote the *Medical Times and Gazette*,

was one of the first of those special hospitals which have since been sown broadcast over London; and as it was among the first in point of time, so it has been, in professional estimation, one of the first in pre-eminence in working the mischief such institutions are calculated to foster.[77]

One of the most frequent objections levelled at specialist institutions was that they were abused by a class of patients who could well afford to pay for their medical care. It was partly for this reason that in the 1870s medical men began to advocate the establishment of pay beds and hospitals. The system, it was argued, would also benefit middle-class persons of limited means, especially those forming the 'lodger class' – governesses, clerks and students who lived away from their own homes and were left to the 'tender mercies' of their landlady.[78] Finally, pay hospitals would be useful for those who resided outside London and needed the services of a London consultant. The wealthy were treated at home and would pay large sums of money to have a consultant come and visit them in remote areas of the country. Those who were not so rich used to take lodgings in the areas where surgeons and physicians had their consulting rooms; this enabled them to visit the consultant or be visited by him. Private operations were also performed in such lodging-houses. These cases, it was claimed, would be better catered for in a hospital, where patients took advantage of continuous medical and nursing care, easy access to complex and expensive appliances and more cheerful surroundings. Payment of a fee would grant them better treatment than was available in the general hospitals and, above all, they would enjoy greater privacy.[79] Privacy was one of the marks of gentility, so it was important that, within the hospital setting, there should be a way of signalling the distinction between charity patients and their betters.

Women's and children's hospitals were the first to implement these suggestions. In 1864 the Ladies' Committee of the Hospital for Women brought to the attention of the management committee the plight of the

impoverished gentlewoman, the wives, widows, and daughters of professional men, and needy and overworked governesses, who, though unable to incur the expense of protracted medical treatment at home, yet shrink from the want of privacy and repose, common to the wards of the general hospital, and thus are entirely debarred from the advantages which the rich and the destitute poor alike enjoy,[80]

the former because they could afford them, the latter because they received them for free. This middle stratum of society, it was argued, would willingly pay a fee for medical treatment according to their means, thus giving proof of self-reliance and self-respect. This would grant them the right to enjoy superior accommodation, better diet and, most importantly, greater privacy.

These proposals resulted in the opening of the New Wing in July 1869. Housed in premises adjacent to the main building in Soho Square, the New Wing was the first pay block in the British Isles. The facilities on offer ranged from single-bed wards, which were available at a cost of three guineas a week, to five-bed wards, where a bed could be obtained on payment of a minimum of one guinea a week. These charges were in the moderate-to-high bracket. The *Lancet*, for example, recommended payments of one guinea per week, on the grounds that two guinea fees would have excluded many people of the governess and clerk class;[81] however, when in 1879 St Thomas's Hospital considered admitting paying patients for a fee of one guinea per week, it was feared that few people would be willing to pay the sums involved.[82]

Applications for admission to the New Wing had to be accompanied by a certificate from a medical man, who had to testify as to the fitness of the case, both socially and medically; every care was taken to ensure that candidates could not afford to be treated at home. As Protheroe Smith's case-book shows, those who were granted admission to the New Wing were mostly single women engaged in 'genteel' occupations – a governess, a schoolmistress and a lace-worker are to be found amongst the twenty-two paying patients. Other patients were unmarried women of no stated occupation from lower- to middle-class backgrounds, such as a draper's and a clergyman's daughter; only one married woman was stated as being employed (see table 1 in the appendix). Besides offering greater privacy (for example, beds in the shared wards had curtains round them), the New Wing also featured an elegant drawing-room for convalescent patients and a lift, which attracted a great deal of interest as it was a rarity in hospitals in those days.[83]

The economic depression caused by the Franco-Prussian war in 1870 forced the managers of the Soho Square hospital to cut down on expenditure and increase the number of pay beds. A ward of ten beds was opened for patients who could afford to pay 10s.6d. a week – the cost of their food and laundry. The scheme proved so popular with the wives and daughters of artisans and small tradesmen that it was then agreed to retain the arrangement as a permanent feature of the hospital.[84] In 1871, measures designed to check the abuse of charity were extended to the out-patient department. After seeing the physician or surgeon, patients were required to obtain a dispensary ticket from the hospital secretary, without which no medicine could be supplied; patients who could afford to pay were charged 1s. for the ticket.[85]

The establishment of the New Wing was followed two years later by the foundation of a similar institution, the Chelsea Hospital for Women. The founder was the obstetrician James Hobson Aveling, chief advocate of midwife registration and founding member of the British Gynaecological Society. Aveling was not new to that kind of enterprise: in 1865 he had set up a hospital for women in Sheffield, where he was a highly esteemed obstetrician. The son of a Cambridgeshire landowner, Aveling was born in 1828. He qualified MRCS in 1851 and a year later he entered practice at Ecclesfield, near Sheffield, on the recommendation of a friend of Sir James Young Simpson. By the early 1860s he was established in practice in Sheffield and was beginning to specialise in obstetrics and gynaecology. He quickly managed to secure a prominent place within the profession locally, but in 1868 he decided to leave the town, much to the regret of the local notables. The reasons for his departure are unclear: in resigning his post at the Sheffield Hospital for Women, Aveling stressed that his decision was motivated by his wife's ill-health, but his obituary in the *British Medical Journal* suggests that he was seeking a wider professional field. After a spell in the country, the Avelings settled in London. James decided that he needed to get a hospital appointment, but he failed to get a senior post. Thus, like many other provincial practitioners had done in similar circumstances, he resolved to set up his own hospital and became one of its physicians.[86]

The Chelsea Hospital for Women was intended for much the same social mix of patients which the Hospital for Women by then accommodated: on the one hand, there were the respectable female poor, who were admitted free of charge on production of a sub-scriber's letter; on the other hand, there were the 'gentlewomen of limited means', who could afford to pay one guinea a week. The latter class of patients comprised

the wives, daughters, and widows of clergymen, naval, military, and professional men – as well as ... those of business-men, clerks, and others, having but moderate means[87]

but who could still 'help themselves' financially. This arrangement, it was maintained, would stamp out illegitimate claims to free medical relief and enable the 'genteel poor' to enjoy some of the privacy of treatment to which they felt entitled, but which they could not afford: for such patients, whom an 'inherent refinement' prevented from seeking admission to charitable medical insti-tutions, pay wards would provide a welcome compromise between home and hospital.

Concern about the medical needs of the 'impoverished gentle-woman' reflected widespread anxiety about the social condition of 'redundant' or 'surplus' women – 'redundant' in the sense that they had failed to fulfil their 'natural' role in relation to men. Middle-class women were brought up in the expectation of marriage, yet the increasing numerical preponderance of women over men during the nineteenth century put marriage beyond the reach of thousands of women. The result was that large numbers of single, well-to-do women were forced to take up ill-paid jobs for which they had no training; they often had to live away from their own homes, alone and friendless, and resign themselves to the loss of class and status that was consequent upon having to work for a livelihood.[88]

Best known to us of all the Victorian 'surplus' women is the governess, a figure who was uppermost in the concerns of the founders of the first pay systems for gynaecological patients. Jeanne Peterson has described the social position of the Victorian governess as one of 'status incongruence': the governess was brought up in the cultivation of gentility, but as a paid employee she came closer to the servant, thus occupying an indeterminate place within the middle-class home.[89] This invariably created difficulties at times of illness, one of the most 'untoward events' which could befall the middle-class family. As a *Times* editorial entitled 'The hospital for ladies' commented in 1865, the illness of the governess, with its concomitant of professional visits, was never agreeable – last but not the least because her employers had to foot the bill; worse, servants continually refused to wait upon invalids who were not members of the household. If the governess had returned home, she would have lacked the necessary care; removal to a hospital on the other hand would have sounded unfeeling. However, pay-beds would have put an end to 'all indelicacy in mentioning the matter'.[90]

The other category of women who were expected to benefit from pay-beds were middle-class wives of limited means. Henry Burdett, the layman who led the voluntary hospital world until his death in 1920, thought that pay hospitals would be a boon to this class of patient because their family circumstances were not conducive to the cure of disease: noisy children, inadequate nursing care and anxiety about domestic matters hampered recovery.[91] Pay hospitals had none of these disadvantages, yet they offered the privacy and comfort that were central to the ethos of the middle-classes. It never occurred to Burdett that the removal of a mother to hospital was both impractical and counterproductive, for the disruption of family life it was bound to cause could only add to a mother's anxiety.   .

Like the Hospital for Women, the Chelsea Hospital began its life in a rented house. It was situated in the King's Road, a 'healthy locality' in the western district of the capital. The rooms were large, well ventilated and furnished comfortably.[92] Thirty-two patients were admitted in 1873, the first year of activity of the institution, under the care of the physicians Thomas Chambers and James Aveling. Robert Barnes, who had been working as Obstetric Physician at St George's Hospital since 1865, and T. B. Curling, author of the standard Victorian textbook on the physiology and the pathology of the testis, acted as consulting physician and surgeon respectively. The number of out-patients exceeded 6,000.[93]

It is not possible to say what was the proportion of free to paying patients at this hospital, and very little can be gleaned about their social background, as patients' case notes seldom state their occupation. Since virtually all the nineteenth-century case-records of the Chelsea Hospital have been carefully preserved, sampling at five-yearly intervals has been used here, from 1873–4 to 1890, with a total of 932 cases. Between 1873 and 1874, we find a servant, a housekeeper and a teacher of gymnastics. In 1879, a lady's maid, a dairy maid, a servant, a housemaid, a housekeeper and a needle-woman were admitted. In 1889, a sick-nurse, a cigarette-maker, a shopkeeper, a nun, a dressmaker, a servant, a showroom assistant and a hospital ward maid were treated at the hospital. The majority of patients were married or widowed women: in the 861 cases in which the marital status was recorded, 559 patients (64.9 per cent) were married, 227 (26.3 per cent) were single and 15 (1.7 per cent) were widowed.

By 1883, the hospital had outgrown its accommodation and moved to purpose-built premises in the Fulham Road. The new hospital comprised six storeys, and the greatest attention had been paid to its sanitary arrangements. These were deemed to be of the utmost importance in the prevention of post-operative sepsis, one of the problems which had beset the development of ovariotomy. As the women's hospitals began to take a leading role in the expansion of surgical gynaecology, their environment became a central concern of the gynaecological profession. At the Chelsea, a corridor communicating with a balcony ran through the building from north to south on each floor, allowing a current of fresh air to pass through the centre of the building. The wards were arranged along the corridor: there were seventeen on each floor, containing from one to nine beds. The latest building technology had been incorporated: speaking tubes, electric bells, passenger and dinner lifts being provided throughout. The charges for pay beds were set at 10s.6d., 21s. and 42s. per week; extra payments were required for operations.[94]

The teaching functions of the hospital expanded dramatically during the 1880s, in line with similar developments at the Hospital for Women. In 1885 a series of post-graduate lectures was launched; the new venture proved so popular amongst the local practitioners that teaching was resumed during the winter of 1885. Clinical assistant posts were also instituted on a fee-paying basis, thus giving medical practitioners an opportunity to further their training in gynaecology.[95]

When James Aveling died in 1892, the Chelsea Hospital was a flourishing and highly esteemed institution; no one could have foreseen the scandal which two years later threatened the hospital with closure. In January 1894 Dr Louis Parkes, Medical Officer of Health for Chelsea, examined the hospital mortality rate after operations during 1893. It was 6.1 per cent (58 per cent of all deaths) and Parkes thought it was unjustifiably high. Out of the 373 patients operated upon, twenty-six had died; twenty of the deaths were apparently due to septicaemia. A number of theories could be advanced to explain these figures (which were in any case too small to be of any statistical value), but Parkes attributed the deaths to the unsatisfactory state of the drains and ordered the closure of the hospital.[96]

Dr Parkes' charges were serious, for the main argument in favour of gynaecological hospitals at the time was that ovariotomy could not be performed with safety except under the special sanitary conditions they provided.[97] The committee appointed to inquire into the administration of the Chelsea Hospital would later disclose that the mortality after ovariotomy had been 19.3 per cent, nearly double the average mortality from this operation at London hospitals.[98] Dr Parkes further questioned the necessity for major surgery in cases which, he claimed, were not fatal conditions requiring risky operations: for example, uterine fibroids and prolapse of the womb. The *Lancet* took the view that the mortality rate of an operation like hysteropexy (fixing the uterus to the abdominal wall to remedy displacements or prolapse) needed to be nil in order to make the procedure justifiable; at the Chelsea Hospital, however, the death rate after hysteropexy was 22 per cent.[99]

The onus of defending the tarnished reputation of the hospital fell upon its Treasurer, Mr Henry Wright. In an indignant letter to the *Lancet*, Mr Wright pointed out that every appliance that was 'sanitarily perfect' had been adopted regardless of cost when the hospital

had been built fourteen years earlier; he added that Parkes' recommendations as to the way in which the drains should be improved were by no means endorsed by other sanitary experts. Most
of the septic cases, he argued, were infected before entering the
wards. There was no doubt that they had exerted a 'malign influence' on some of the other cases, but that risk had to be taken: it
would have been inhumane to turn out poor creatures 'merely to
keep our statistics in a condition favourable to the medical staff'.[100]
As might be expected, the medical officers violently denied the
truth of Dr Parkes' charges and signified their protest by resigning
in a body.

As the crisis unfolded, the consultants to the Chelsea Hospital
identified another source of evil: Sir Thomas Spencer Wells and Dr
Robert Barnes, former champion of the general practitioner–obstetrician, contended that the general practitioners who worked at the
hospital conveyed the germs of disease into the building and should
therefore be disqualified from serving on the staff.[101] This astonishing conclusion is interesting in view of the subsequent development
of the obstetrical and gynaecological profession: from the 1920s
onwards, obstetricians were to devote much of their time and
energy to excluding general practitioners from gynaecological
surgery.[102]

The controversy at the Chelsea happened to coincide with the
construction of a new temple to medical science in the district, the
Institute for Preventive Medicine. Anti-vivisectionists rose up in
arms against this development and many demonstrations were held
in protest. The high mortality rates at the Chelsea confirmed their
worst suspicions that vivisection encouraged doctors to undertake
cruel 'experiments' on their patients. The women who had died
were mourned as martyrs and the resignation of staff at the hospital
was claimed as a victory for the movement.[103] In a desperate attempt to restore public confidence in the institution, the hospital
authorities resolved to implement the sanitary improvements
suggested by Dr Parkes. A special commission was formed with
the brief of appointing the new medical officers; those members of
staff who were engaged in general practice were not re-elected.

The closing years of the century saw an upsurge in the fortunes of
the hospital. With the appointment of John Bland-Sutton, Comyns
Berkeley and Victor Bonney to the staff, the Chelsea Hospital
gained three of the rising stars of gynaecological surgery. Their

pioneering work put the Chelsea in the avant-garde of Edwardian gynaecology, giving the hospital an international sphere of surgical repute. It was at the Chelsea Hospital that Bland-Sutton developed his remarkable dexterity in abdominal surgery and devised daring and controversial operations; he later became President of the Royal College of Surgeons and received many honours, including a baronetcy.[104] Berkeley and Bonney collaborated in the treatment of cancer of the cervix by Wertheim's hysterectomy. During the 1920s they played a prominent part – though in rival camps – in the events that led to the foundation of the British College of Obstetricians and Gynaecologists. Bonney and Berkeley found that their link with a special hospital was no impediment to their professional advancement and, unlike Bland-Sutton, they never gave up their posts at the Chelsea after joining the staff of the Middlesex Hospital.

The biographies of Bonney and Berkeley illustrate the increasing importance of special hospitals to the careers of late nineteenth-century medical practitioners. During the mid-Victorian period, those who held posts at special hospitals had been ostracised by the medical establishment; by the end of the 1880s, only 31 out of the estimated 195 medical staff in London general hospitals did not hold some post in a special hospital as well, although some of them were not proud of their special hospital connections and did not mention them in the *Medical Directory*.[105] In 1889 the *British Medical Journal*, which had led the campaign against special hospitals thirty years earlier, adopted a more conciliatory tone towards them:

How many men are there waiting outside the hospital, doing dreary drudgery at the dispensaries; or, who, having at length been received within the coveted circle, are exhausting their best energies in the out-patients' departments, waiting anxiously for promotion and release from the thraldom of seniors! What these men, and many more who are not aspirants to the general hospitals, want is opportunity for independent work. And they want it while they are young, with energies unimpaired, still burning with the fresh spirit of original research. Those who by good fortune or merit – the two qualifications are not always united – have achieved hospital rank are apt to lament the multiplication of special hospitals. To some extent they themselves are responsible for this evil, if evil it be. Enjoying what approaches to a monopoly they should not be surprised if young men seek independent outlets.[106]

Medical practitioners were more cautious about what they had to say on the subject of special hospitals: in the 1850s the surgeon

Jonathan Hutchinson had been opposed to the establishment of a special hospital for the treatment of stones and diseases of the bladder; in 1881 he stated that he no longer held this view.[107]

Specialisation was growing within the medical profession and by the end of the century most general hospitals had opened special departments. Ophthalmic departments were established first among the specialties. Guy's Hospital created facilities for skin diseases in 1851 and for aural diseases in 1863. St Thomas's opened the throat department in 1882, the skin and ear department in 1884, and a gynaecology clinic in 1888; in the 1890s, departments for electrotherapy, x-ray and dentistry were established. St Bartholomew's had a full department of ophthalmology by 1869, and by 1880 it had special clinics for throat and skin diseases, for orthopaedics and for obstetrics and gynaecology.[108]

The concentration of similar cases under the same roof provided a most important stimulus for the clinical development of gynaecology. Dr Charles Routh, consulting physician at the Samaritan Free Hospital and founding member of the British Gynaecological Society, thought that this was indeed the greatest merit of specialist institutions: 'In special hospitals there were large numbers of the same kinds of disease', he was reported as saying at a meeting of the British Medical Association in 1860.

Instead of three, four, five, or six, there were fifty, a hundred, or two hundred patients. The medical attendant could, therefore, reason on all of them. This was the way to come to general conclusions. No man could come to any positive conclusion as to the treatment of special diseases till he had many examples.[109]

By comparing and contrasting cases, the gynaecologist learnt to differentiate diseases and assess the value of different treatments. Furthermore, the gynaecological hospital was a gallery of female types as well as a living museum of pathology: it thus afforded the gynaecologist a unique opportunity to refine and expand his knowledge of woman and her diseases.

4

Woman and her diseases

Woman was, by definition, disease or disorder, a deviation from the standard of health represented by the male. As Robert Barnes wrote in 1882, gynaecology bore 'the most instructive testimony to the law which declares that there is no proper boundary between physiology and pathology; that pathology is but a chapter in the history of physiology'.[1] He was echoed by his colleague William Tyler Smith, for whom parturition, like menstruation, stood 'at the boundary between physiology and pathology, being attended by more pain, and being liable to a greater number of accidents, than any other act of the economy'.[2] Not only did woman's biological functions blur into disease; they were also the source of a host of psychological disorders, from strange moods and feelings, to hysteria and insanity.[3] The mid-nineteenth-century physician Thomas Laycock (1812–76), a prominent writer on mental pathology, termed this psychological imbalance 'affectability', and argued that in woman it may be

compatible with a general good health; but in man it is a morbid state, the source of hypochondriasis, and the result of causes which depress the assimilating powers, or excite unequally the nervous system.[4]

These assumptions – that woman's physical and mental peculiarities derive from her reproductive function and that pathology defines the norm of the female body – legitimated the medical supervision of women and demarcated the field of gynaecology, the science of woman.

The pathology of femininity

It was during the period from puberty to the menopause – the peak of sexual activity in the female – that women were most vulnerable to gynaecological complaints. The approximation to the masculine characters after the menopause acted as a natural 'cure' for much female disease. Losing both the physical and the emotional aspects of her sexuality – her childbearing capacity and her sexual feelings – woman tended to 'revert to the neutral man-woman state' and became 'more capable of rendering herself useful'.[5] Once the change was well established, she passed

on to old age better than man, because free from sexual activity and its many demands on the powers of the system at this later period of life; and, as a rule, suffering less from disease and more secure against external battles and exposure to the elements; more cared for, she more frequently outlives her male comrade in the battle for life.[6]

Gynaecology was the study of the 'whole woman'; it thus fused the physical, the psychological and the moral aspects of femininity. This synthetic approach was sustained by an organicist conception of bodily functioning. As the body was a purposeful, integrated totality, functions could not be understood in isolation from the complex structure of which they were a part, nor could local disease be studied without regard to general pathological principles.[7] It was therefore 'impossible to draw an arbitrary line that shall clearly separate what are commonly regarded as the special diseases of women from the domain of general pathology', explained Robert Barnes in 1882.

The study of the diseases centred in the sexual system of women is no more than the application of general pathology to this particular system. Any disease occurring in a woman will almost certainly involve some modifications in the work of her sexual system. On the other hand, the ordinary or disturbed work of her sexual system will influence the course of any disease which may assail her, however independent this disease may seem in its origin.[8]

Thus no reputable gynaecologist practised as a pure specialist, but rather considered female disease in the light of his general pathological and physiological knowledge. This approach became especially important to the obstetrical profession as the general surgeons began to colonise the burgeoning field of pelvic surgery in the last quarter of the nineteenth century.[9] Banned from performing ovariotomy within the walls of the teaching hospitals, obstetricians fought back by arguing that medicine, 'like the body which is its subject, is one and indivisible'. The surgical treatment of women's diseases could not be separated from the study of female physiology and pathology, hence the obstetrician must be a surgeon as well as a physician.[10]

As part of an integrated whole, the sexual organs constantly interacted with the rest of the female organism. Both the vascular and the nervous systems were emphasised as the elements which mediated the relationship between organs, bridging the physical and the mental aspects of the female organisation. Blood, women's life force, was implicated in the processes of menstruation and in gestation, during which period it conveyed vital nutrients to the foetus; it was thus of great biological and metaphorical significance. The nervous system in women was deemed to be extremely susceptible to a wide range of physical, moral and environmental stimuli; hence it played an especially important part in unifying the female body into a single organic base.[11]

Gynaecologists used two main models of nervous organisation in order to explain the mechanisms whereby woman's sexual system interacted with other parts of her body, most notably the brain. The first of these may be termed 'economic'. According to this theory, the body was a closed system in which organs and mental faculties competed for a finite supply of physical or mental energy; thus stimulation or depletion in one organ resulted in exhaustion or excitation in another part of the body. The Harvard professor Edward Clarke, for example, opposed women's entry to higher education on the grounds that intellectual work would reduce the supply of nerve-energy to the female reproductive system, producing 'monstrous brains and puny bodies; abnormally active cerebration and abnormally weak digestion; flowing thought and constipated bowels'.[12] The English psychiatrist Henry Maudsley argued that the overexpenditure of vital energy in mental activity would cause menstrual derangements which might never be corrected; in some cases, he claimed, hysteria, epilepsy and chorea might ensue.[13]

Reflex theories of nervous organisation also played an important role in gynaecology. Victorian neurophysiologists drew a distinction within the nervous system between higher brain levels which were the locus of mind, and lower levels which functioned automatically by reflex action. The higher levels controlled the lower levels by means of an inhibitory mechanism, whereby nervous impulses repressed as well as excited organ activity. While volition, voluntary motion and judgment were believed to be functions of

the central nervous system, the bodily functions, including reproduction, were thought to be regulated by the reflex nervous
system.[14]

Reflex theories of nervous organisation contained allusions to
ideological distinctions between male and female. Gender differences were represented in terms of a different weighting between
the controlling and automatic sectors of the nervous system; while
the higher intellectual faculties played the dominant role in men, an
imbalance of physical over mental events was posited in women.
Thus mental derangements such as puerperal mania, epileptic con-
vulsions and hysterical phenomena were thought to be common at
times of intensified sexual activity such as childbirth. Gynaecological disorders, it was claimed, were usually attended by nervous
excitability and sometimes they were the direct cause of insanity –
for example, uterine 'irritation' could induce nymphomania, 'con-
gestion' of the ovaries could bring about attacks of mania, melanch-
olia and hysteria.[15]

Given the sexual etiology of much female insanity, it is not
surprising to find that, over the century, a number of gynaecological treatments were devised for the purpose of managing women's
minds. Mr Isaac Baker Brown, a member of the Obstetrical Society
of London, believed that masturbation led to madness and that the
surgical removal of the clitoris could cure it. He carried out this
work in his private clinic in London between 1859 and 1866,
claiming a high success rate, but he was accused of coercing patients
into the treatment and eventually expelled from the Obstetrical
Society on these grounds.[16] In the 1880s, especially in the United
States but also in Britain, a number of gynaecologists began to
advocate the removal of healthy ovaries for the cure of a range of
conditions, from dysmenorrhoea and uterine fibroids, to incipient
insanity and epilepsy.[17] By the end of the century, medical practitioners were advocating the appointment of gynaecologists to the
staff of insane asylums and recommending routine gynaecological
examinations in the diagnosis of women's mental disorders.[18]

Nineteenth-century psychiatrists were eager to propound the
view that mental illness was a disease of the brain, not a spiritual
state, yet scientific theories about insanity remained deeply imbued
with Christian notions of sin. The mid-Victorian alienists Bucknill
and Tuke, authors of a best-selling manual of psychological medicine, confidently stated that every physician would repudiate the

'Pope's slander' that women were rakes at heart; yet it had to be acknowledged that 'religious and moral principles alone give strength to the female mind, and that, when these are weakened or removed by disease, the subterranean fires become active, and the crater gives forth smoke and flame'.[19] Insane women excelled over men in sexual depravity and immorality. 'To many people the most striking difference between the sexes in asylums is the language, and here the women hold the palm for volubility, abuse and foul-mouthedness', wrote T. Claye Shaw, physician at St Bartholomew's Hospital, in 1888: 'Certain it is', he continued,

that noise, filthy conduct, and sexual depravity, both by speech and act, are much more common on the female than on the male side of an asylum ... Women in acute states of insanity are abusive, indiscriminately violent, impulsive, obscene, and wayward out of all proportion to what men are.[20]

As Roger Smith has noted, madness in women 'exemplified the manner in which disease released evil by eliminating mental control'.[21]

In their efforts to understand the nature of gynaecological disease, physicians did not overlook its social dimensions and addressed themselves to the influence of habits, environment and social activities on women's physiology. Both men and women were deemed to be affected by their physical *milieu* and life-style, but while man's confrontation with the external environment, the strife of public life and of the market-place explained his pathology, the nature of female disease became intelligible in the light of woman's social role within marriage and the family: 'The integration of man with surrounding nature', wrote Robert Barnes in 1880,

is more essential to the understanding of his physiology and pathology than in the case of woman. To the woman the integration with man and with offspring assumes predominant importance. Man's ambition and daily work is the contest with the surrounding world, physical and moral; the ambition of the work of woman, more restricted, is the study and conquest of man. This relation governs her being, and is the secret of a great part of her physiology and pathology.[22]

Man's greater exposure to physical dangers and the stresses of waged employment rendered him more vulnerable to the influence of climate and to the wear and tear of life: thus sudden death, traumatism, fractures and dislocations were deemed to be more common in men than in women.[23] Because of their alleged social and physiological characteristics, men and women differed also in the way they responded to the same external stimuli: for example, intemperance in men led to gout, in women it caused amenor-rhoea.[24] However, both sexes were advised to take the same measures in order to keep disease at bay: physicians stressed the importance of prevention and argued that the observance of regular habits was the key to ensuring the optimum adjustment between individual and environment.

The attempt to construct a science that could explain woman's nature in its various physiological, moral and social aspects can be seen in the development of a special branch of obstetrics called 'obstetric jurisprudence'. This field was the interface between gynaecology and the law: it was where knowledge about women's physiology and pathology was applied to the regulation of social life.[25] 'Is it not true that the gravest issues, even those of life and death, liberty, loss of character and reputation . . . frequently hang upon the evidence of the gynaecologist?' asked the late nineteenth-century obstetrician Henry Macnaughton-Jones (1845–1918) in a discussion of medico-legal issues in gynaecology. And he went on to bemoan 'that confident self-assurance which occasionally in the witness-box asserts itself in matters that require considerable and special pathological experience to decide.'[26] Jones's claims to ex-pertise in medico-legal questions involving marriage, divorce, il-legitimacy, rape, infanticide and abortion, implied that the maintenance of the public order depended on the medical surveil-lance of women's sexual functions. Thus from the medico-legal point of view it was necessary to recognise, for example, the disorders of the sexual apparatus that mimicked the signs of parturi-tion, the abnormalities of the hymen which might be mistaken for rape, the malformations of the female sexual organs that consti-tuted a bar to marriage, the length of gestation and the development of the foetus.

As the debate on women's rights to education, work and political participation reached a crescendo in the last quarter of the century, physicians focussed on female emancipation as a cause of gynaeco-logical disease. This thesis was strongly challenged by British and American feminists: it was not higher education, but boredom and idleness that led to disease in upper middle-class women, argued Elizabeth Garrett Anderson in her rejoinder to Henry Maudsley's 'Sex in mind and education'.[27] The anti-vivisectionist campaigner

Frances Power Cobbe for her part blamed the 'little health' of the lady of leisure on women's social relations and on the medical profession. Cobbe found it hard to believe that the Creator could have planned 'a whole sex of Patients'; not even the 'holy claims of Motherhood' ought to have involved a state of invalidism for the larger part of married life. The primary cause of female valetudinarianism lay in society's 'false ideals of womanhood', which put a premium on delicacy and self-sacrifice; but the 'great Medical Order' was also to blame. Doctors were interested in making work for themselves, not in preventing disease; furthermore, they resisted the admission of women to the profession. Women were often reluctant to disclose their symptoms to a male physician, with the result that much female disease went untreated. There was only one remedy to the evil: male doctors must sacrifice their pride and their trade unionism and allow women to enter the profession. Thus despite the radical potential of her critique, Cobbe was unable to transcend the medical terms in which the discourse on femininity had been set.[28]

Surgical analysis

From about 1860 onwards the organicist approach to women's diseases was challenged by the rapid expansion of surgical gynaecology: surgery fostered an anatomical outlook which tended to reduce gynaecology to the study of women's pelvic organs, shifting the emphasis from the study of the 'whole woman' to the treatment of a localised pathology. Until the mid-1800s, gynaecological surgery was limited to the removal of polyps, the excision of a hypertrophied clitoris, the incision of an imperforated hymen and rare attempts to repair severe perineal lacerations. The second half of the nineteenth century brought the development of daring abdominal operations such as ovariotomy (the surgical removal of cystic ovaries), hysterectomy and the removal of the gravid uterus. Operations were also devised for the repair of vesico-vaginal fistula and for the relief of uterine and vaginal prolapse.[29]

The evolution of surgical techniques in gynaecology reflected the growing relevance of surgery to medicine. Traditionally, surgeons had relied on physical signs in their diagnosis, and correlated the clinical picture to structural changes, while physicians had drawn their evidence of disease from the existence of symptoms which indicated a departure from good health. From the end of the eighteenth century onwards, physicians gradually began to accept the clinical-anatomical orientation of surgery in the diagnosis and treatment of internal disease. The surgeon's external diseases, such as tumours, abscesses, ulcers and inflammations, came to provide the model for understanding the anatomical changes wrought by disease on the inner fabric of the body. Efforts were made in order to render internal disease accessible to the senses, as was the practice in surgery, and increasing emphasis was placed on instrumental and surgical interference in diagnosis and treatment.[30]

During the course of the nineteenth century, surgery also came to play a very important role as a method of research into questions of health and disease. Beginning with Georges Cuvier, professor at the Paris Museum of Natural History, and the physiologist François Magendie at the turn of the century, physiologists questioned the scientific status of the vital properties of organisms, on the grounds that they were the result of speculation unsupported by scientific evidence. Prompted by a rising technological attitude which encouraged intervention and manipulation as the foundation of knowledge, they increasingly argued that the goal of their discipline was to establish knowledge on a strict programme of experimentation. Complex organisms had to be broken down into constituent parts and simpler actions, so as to determine the conditions under which living phenomena appeared: knowledge was control, and its test was the certainty that the imposition of the same conditions would always produce the same limited succession of events. These analytical and interventionist currents culminated in experimentation based on vivisection. Experiments on living animals were extensively carried out at the French veterinary schools in the early nineteenth century. By the second half of the century, physiologists had adopted vivisection as the means of raising their discipline to the status of a fully developed experimental science, on a par with physics and chemistry. For the French physiologist Claude Bernard, one of the chief advocates of vivisection, only the experimental sciences like physics or chemistry could give man power over natural phenomena; as far as he was concerned, the practice of vivisection was the one and only way for the life sciences to become experimental.[31]

Bernard's faith in the methods of surgery as the means by which man could master nature was echoed by one of the late-Victorian champions of surgical gynaecology, the gynaecologist James Murphy. Speaking at the first Congress of the British Gynaecological Society in 1891, Murphy argued that at the beginning of the century the gynaecologist had been a physician, not a surgeon,

for then the female genital organs were regarded as so mysterious and so sacred that no matter how serious the disease that afflicted them might be, it was no justification for an examination either by sight or touch, and as long as that state of affairs continued there naturally was no work for the hand of the surgeon.[32]

Gradually, though, a rising interventionist approach to women's diseases had eroded the quasi-sacred status accorded to the female genitalia. The tumours and malformations of the female sexual system were no different from those occurring elsewhere, and likewise they had to be treated by surgery: thus 'the modern gynaecologist', said Murphy in triumphant tones, 'has shorn the female genitalia of their mystery, and examined by sight and touch every portion of them, and has successfully attacked their disease with the scalpel and scissors'.[33]

In describing gynaecological surgery as the 'shearing' of the female genitals, Murphy wrapped up the idea of surgical progress in sexual metaphor. The medical unveiling of woman's mystery was analogous to another situation in which the female body was unclothed by and for the male gaze, namely, the pictorial representation of the female nude. In the European tradition, the naked female body was depicted in an attitude of passive abandonment that was intended to appeal to the beholder; the 'ideal' spectator was always assumed to be a male, and the image of the woman was designed to flatter him. The convention of not depicting the woman's body hair was an integral part of the relationship between male actor and female object, for hair was associated with sexual power and passion, which in their turn were related to the idea of nature as a wild, dangerous and unknown entity. Thus, the absence of body hair conveyed the idea that the woman's passion had been tamed for the exclusive benefit of the owner of the painting.[34] Through these sets of metaphorical associations, the 'shearing' of the female genitalia also alluded to the domination of nature by man: in this way, to the image of the gynaecologist's eyes and hands unveiling the secrets of femininity, there was juxtaposed that of woman as subjugated nature, the castrated object of male science.

Not all obstetricians shared Murphy's enthusiasm for operative gynaecology. Some, like the Professor of Gynaecology at Chicago Medical School, Henry Park Newman, feared that surgical interventionism might lead physicians to lose sight of the 'whole woman' and treat their patients as if they were hardly more than objects to act upon. In 1896 Newman, when urging his colleagues to pay more attention to prevention in gynaecology, stressed that

in our devotion to the experimental and purely scientific side of our art, we must not forget that we are dealing not with cold facts and interesting phenomena, but with the highest of human interests ... We should remember that the 'ology' is not the whole of our speciality. We know all about the pelvic organs of women; we can teach our students how to cope with serious conditions, to treat grave lesions, and to do brilliant operations; but woman must be more than the material upon which to exploit skill in perfecting radical and often mutilating operations.[35]

It was important that the gynaecologist should not neglect the study of physiology, of diagnostic techniques, and of socio-environmental conditions, Newman argued, because

the surgeon and the diagnostician must be one and the same, so often the diagnosis cannot be complete or procedure fully determined until the operation is under way. And to be a good diagnostician in the diseases of women one must know as much about women as about disease; as much about environmental and social and domestic conditions as about pelvic lesions; as much about causes as results.[36]

Across the Atlantic, Newman's sentiments were echoed not only by a section of the British obstetrical and gynaecological profession, but also by feminist and anti-vivisectionist campaigners. [Their criticisms were chiefly directed at two practices: the performance of ovariotomy, an operation which was said to 'mutilate' and 'castrate' women, and the use of the speculum, which earned widespread condemnation as the 'instrumental rape' of women.] This controversy occupies an important place not only in the history of gynaecology, but also in the development of scientific medicine, for as well as being a vehicle through which ideological views about femininity and female sexuality were articulated, it provided an outlet for a wider debate about the morality of experimentation based on vivisection. In the next section, we shall examine these interlocking themes as they were developed during the debate on the use and abuse of the speculum in the mid-Victorian period.

Penetrating private parts: the 'speculum question'

The *speculum matricis* is an ancient instrument. It was known and used in the Greco-Roman period, but it lapsed into disuse during the Middle Ages and the Renaissance.[37] It was not until the beginning of the nineteenth century that the speculum was rediscovered and popularised by Joseph Récamier (1774–1852), Professor of Medicine at the Collège de France in Paris. In 1801 Récamier had a patient with a purulent vaginal discharge which failed to clear up despite irrigations of various sorts. He examined her by the finger, but failed to gain any information as to the source of the complaint. He then constructed a slender tin tube through which he inspected the uterine neck and vagina. This revealed a marked ulceration of the cervix, which Récamier treated with topical applications of syrup of carrots and a preparation consisting of honey and rose petals, on analogy with the treatment of ulcers and inflammations in the throat. Récamier subsequently applied the speculum to the treatment of ulcerated carcinoma of the cervix by means of caustics such as fused potash and nitrate of silver. This therapy became very popular in Paris, although there was some disagreement as to its value.[38]

When the Parisian authorities implemented the regulation of prostitution in 1810, the speculum became an instrument of the police. Every prostitute had to be registered; in return, she had to submit to an examination by the speculum and, if found to be suffering from venereal disease, she was compulsorily detained for treatment within the prison hospital.[39] These examinations were publicly witnessed by medical students and visitors from foreign countries, some of them British. Men like William Acton, the renowned writer on genito-urinary diseases and prostitution; James Henry Bennet, physician-accoucheur first to the Western General Dispensary and then to the Royal Free Hospital, and William Jones, founder of the Gynepathic Institute Free Hospital (later the Samaritan Free Hospital for Women), became familiar with the use of the speculum while studying medicine in Paris and, upon their return from the continent in the 1830s and 1840s, they began to use the instrument on their patients.

The most cogent argument in favour of the speculum was supplied by William Jones, one of the first to recommend the systematic use of the instrument in Britain, in his *Practical Observations on*

Diseases of Women, published in 1839. Disease, he argued, could be efficaciously treated only once it had been properly diagnosed, and this had to be done not in the light of external symptoms, but after ascertaining the alterations of structure on which these were dependent. A vaginal discharge generally termed as leucorrhoea, for instance, was at times common to every form of uterine disease, from polypi to syphilis: hence, to attempt to relieve the discharge without any knowledge of its underlying pathological condition was in his view 'unscientific, empirical and inhuman'.[40]

Jones's arguments seem almost banal in the light of modern approaches to diagnosis, but in the early Victorian period few practitioners found them acceptable. In May 1850 the Professor of Midwifery at St George's Hospital, Robert Lee (1793–1877), one of the first to criticise surgical and instrumental interference in gynaecology, opened fire against the speculum at an unusually crowded meeting of the Royal Medical and Chirurgical Society, the established forum where all the important medical controversies of the time were discussed. Dr Lee did not condemn the use of the instrument in all cases, but he was anxious to define its 'legitimate use and real value' in gynaecological practice.

In his paper Dr Lee claimed that the incidence of ulcerations in the neck of the womb did not justify the extensive employment of the speculum. To prove this, he cited the results of two investigations that had been carried out at his request. In 1832 he had asked his colleagues at the St Marylebone Infirmary to conduct the post-mortem examination of the uteri of over seven hundred women; this had shown cervical ulcerations to be very rare. More recent statistical data, which Lee had obtained from the resident medical officer at the St Marylebone Infirmary and from the curator of the pathological museum at St George's Hospital, pointed to the same conclusion. Dr Lee concluded his paper with a particularly horrific account of the evils perpetrated by the 'apostles of the speculum'. A middle-aged woman affected by paraplegic symptoms had consulted a physician who believed that her disease arose from uterine inflammation. He wanted to demonstrate this by an examination with the speculum, despite the fact that the woman had never suffered from gynaecological disease. According to her general practitioner, who was in attendance at the time of the examination, the proceedings were shocking: the woman's hymen was unbroken, and all the doors had to be closed in order to prevent the

FIGURE 8.

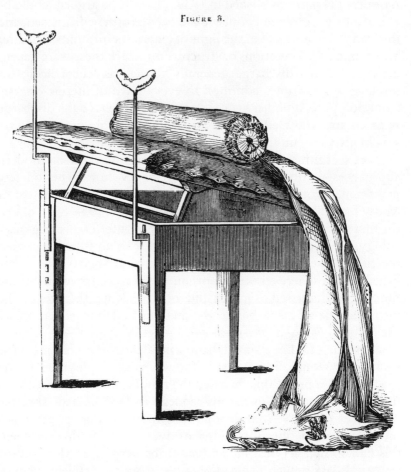

SPECULUM TABLE.—JONES

2 The first illustration of a table for gynaecological examinations

people in the house from hearing her screams and being alarmed. A week after the examination, the woman's paraplegic symptoms recommenced and she died. It was found after her death that she had an inflammation at the base of the brain; the uterus however was perfectly healthy.[41]

These examples gave a medical veneer to arguments that had little to do with science, and everything with morals. An examination by the speculum, involving as it did the exposure and instrumental penetration of parts that were defined as 'private',

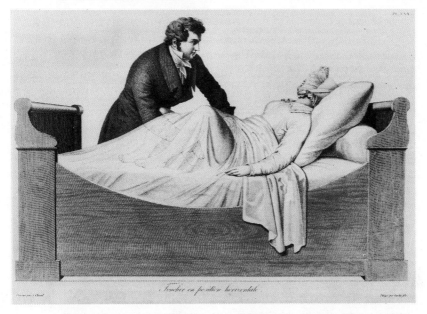

3 Vaginal examination by the 'touch'; note the avoidance of eye
contact

'wounded' and, if repeated daily, eventually 'blunted' women's
modesty; thus for Dr Lee it was 'unjustifiable on the grounds of
propriety and morality', unless the diagnosis proved impossible on
the basis of the symptoms alone. In unmarried women especially,
Lee argued, 'the integrity of their structures should not be destroyed with the speculum, nor their modesty wounded by an
examination of any kind without a necessity for such a proceeding
being clearly shown'.[42] It was not so much anxiety about preserving
the *physical* virginity of the patient that troubled Dr Lee and his
supporters: as the Queen's accoucheur Charles Locock pointed out,
it was sometimes necessary to break down the hymen during an
examination by the finger, but obstetricians were never condemned
for such a practice.[43] For the participants in the speculum debate, a
woman's virginity was less physical than moral and mental. As the
experimental physiologist Marshall Hall argued, it was not exposure, but the 'dulling of the edge of virgin modesty, and the
degradation of the pure minds, of the daughters of England', which
had to be avoided. Even if there was no exposure of the person, 'the
female who has been subjected to such treatment is not the same
person in delicacy and purity as she was before'.[44]

Once introduced to the pleasures of instrumental sex, young girls lost their innocence and turned into lustful temptresses. Robert Brudenell Carter, author of an influential study on hysteria published in 1853, was convinced that the use of the speculum in cases of hysteria aggravated by uterine disease could do nothing but harm:

I have, more than once, seen young unmarried women, of the middle classes of society, reduced, by the constant use of the speculum, to the mental and moral condition of prostitutes; seeking to give themselves the same indulgence by the practice of solitary vice; and asking every medical practitioner, under whose care they fell, to institute an examination of the sexual organs.[45]

For the physiologist Marshall Hall, the speculum induced a kind of 'mental poisoning' in the guise of a 'new and lamentable form of hysteria ... of *furor uterinus*'. Patients became 'reserved, and moody, and perverse'; they spoke 'unintelligibly in broken sentences' and directed all their thoughts to the uterine organs. 'I have known cases of the most revolting attachment, on the part of such patients, to the practice and to the practitioner', Hall noted. 'I have known them to speak of "the womb" and of "the uterine organs" with a familiarity which was formerly unknown, and which, I trust, will ere long be obsolete.'[46] The child as evil incarnate and the child as innocent flower – the dual image of childhood which dominated Victorian art and fiction – was much in evidence in the mid-century speculum debate, as indeed it would be during the agitation against child prostitution three decades later.

Dr Lee's paper sparked off a lively discussion during which three practitioners rose to speak in defence of the speculum. William Acton said that, if the speculum had been abused in the treatment of uterine disease, so had drugs and washes, yet nobody dreamed of denouncing the latter. He further contended that the speculum was of the greatest value in the detection of venereal disease: in consequence of the speculum not being in general use in British hospitals, he claimed, many women were only partially treated and discharged supposedly 'well', who then went on to infect 'fresh men'.[47] William Jones candidly stated that 'he saw no more harm in the use of the speculum than in the use of a spoon to ascertain the condition of the throat. (*Laughter.*)'[48] Henry Bennet, author of a treatise on uterine ulcerations, congratulated himself on having been the first to point out to the profession the existence of inflammatory ulceration in the virgin and challenged the Society to nominate an independent committee for the purpose of investigating their frequency. It was a 'conscientious feeling of imperative duty', he argued, which had led him to overcome his own scruples about examining unmarried women in cases of severe ulceration.[49] But Acton, Jones and Bennet were in a minority. In his final rejoinder to his critics, Dr Lee denounced Bennet's 'ulcers' as having 'neither centre nor circumference, beginning nor end', and declared the speculum to be 'wholly useless' to the enthusiastic cheering of the entire assembly.[50]

Correspondents in the medical papers were divided over the benefits of speculum examinations. In a letter to the *Medical Times* for 1850, 'Pudor' gave short shrift to Henry Bennet's 'speculum committee'. The writer shrank back from such an 'indecent proceeding', and claimed that no respectable medical practitioner would belong to such an 'obscene association'. He thought, however, that a few 'speculumizers' (a word which perhaps all too easily rhymed with 'womaniser') would have no objection, and suggested that the Opera House might be the most appropriate sphere for the proposed 'operations' of the Committee:

A box might be engaged at the top of the house for a moderate price, which would hold the whole fraternity. Between the acts there would be abundance of time, and no lack of ladies, who would be delighted with the exhibition. At the close of the season the Committee would be expected to furnish a report, for the satisfaction of the public. It would be invidious to mention names for the office of president and secretary of this Committee; but the appointment of Dr. Locock, and his friend Dr. Bennet would, I have no doubt, be satisfactory to all concerned.[51]

By conjuring up this picture, 'Pudor' brought together the image of a place where men and women publicly displayed themselves and of the womanising speculum doctor. In the theatre box, which enabled the spectator to enjoy a private view of a public performance, the inspecting practitioner might witness a public exhibition of private parts.

Those who favoured the 'judicious' use of the speculum suggested ways of defusing the sexual tensions engendered by vaginal examinations – a futile effort, since it was not the technique of gynaecological examinations, but its interpretation that was at the root of the problem. In a letter to the *Lancet* for 1845, 'Censor' proposed that the speculum be '*fixed* in the centre of a large handkerchief or shawl, that it be inserted in the vagina under the bed-clothes, whilst the shawl is spread over the patient's person, and that the patient be then placed in the proper position for examination. *Not the slightest exposure need be made'*.[52] The *Lancet*, however, did not think this plan was advisable, first because every mean which rendered diagnosis more difficult reduced its usefulness, secondly, and most importantly, because 'we should shew so plainly to our patients that we consider the operation indecent, that we much doubt whether they would submit to it under any circumstance'.[53]

Historians of obstetrics will have no difficulty in recognising an affinity between this debate and the controversy over the employment of male attendants in childbirth. From the middle of the eighteenth century to the last quarter of the nineteenth, the rise of the man-midwife was accompanied by the publication of pamphlets, mostly by pro-midwife physicians and alternative practitioners, which vehemently condemned the practice as a cover for adultery.[54] In the view of the mid-eighteenth-century accoucheur Frank Nicholls, men-midwives were allowed

to treat our wives in such a manner, as frequently ends in their destruction, and to have such intercourse with our women, as easily shifts into indecency, from indecency into obscenity, and from obscenity into debauchery.[55]

The accoucheur insinuated himself into the home of the pregnant woman; by sight and by touch – a term which was used technically to describe the method of gynaecological examination, but which was also slang for 'sexual intercourse' – he became acquainted with every charm a woman possessed. Once the woman's erotic feelings had been aroused by his manipulations, it was not difficult for the accoucheur to seduce his patient into an illicit sexual relationship. Women were 'invaded *by the presence, and violated by the actual contact* of the *man*-midwife', thundered the author George Morant in 1857 in his *Hints to Husbands*, a book which, turning the metaphor of 'man-unveiling-woman-as-nature' on its head, was significantly subtitled *A Revelation of the Man-Midwife's Mysteries*.[56] Man-midwifery, Morant alleged, was just a piece of '"scientific" rascaldom' which led the unaware public to permit 'unspeakable and hideous mysteries . . . under the hypocritical guise of scientific discovery'.[57] It was no wonder that the practice had first become fashionable at the corrupt Parisian Court before the revolution, in an age of luxury and lewdness when 'adultery was the fashion, and marriage but a cloak for vice'.[58] Man-midwifery, in other words, created the possibility of a dangerous alliance between a woman and her physician, posing a serious threat to marriage and usurping a husband's rights over his wife; thus ultimately it was less a violation of female modesty than an insidious challenge to male authority.

This is where the similarities between the speculum controversy and the debate on man-midwifery end. The discussion on the use of the speculum in fact brought to the fore not the cuckolded husband, but the question of *consent*, which separated lawful from unlawful sex, seduction from rape, therapy from assault, and in particular the *age* at which a young person could be considered to be able to consent to sexual intercourse. Medical disquiet about the propriety of the speculum in young unmarried women must be examined in the light of mounting public anxiety about prostitution, and particularly about the 'trade' of young girls for sexual purposes. The existence of juvenile prostitution in London and of a traffic of English girls to state-regulated brothels on the Continent was well known at the time of the Royal Medico-Chirurgical Society debate. By the 1880s, it had become a prominent concern of moral reformers. Organised protest against child prostitution was an offshoot of the social purity movement, whose primary goal was to achieve a single standard of sexual morality for both men and women. It took its origins from the campaign of the 1860s and 1870s against the Contagious Diseases Acts (1864 and 1866), which instituted a form of state regulation of prostitution in garrison towns. Anti-regulationists saw the traffic as an inevitable result of state regulation, and in the early 1880s they began to put pressure on the government to introduce legislation to control this trade and raise the age of consent.[59]

The crusade against the 'dark and cruel wrong' of child prostitution culminated in a series of sensational articles entitled 'The Maiden Tribute of Modern Babylon', published in the *Pall Mall Gazette* in 1885. In the 'Maiden Tribute' series the author, William Stead, exposed the rape of children who had been ensnared and trapped by wicked men. Stead described the evils of the 'white slave trade' in highly emotional and inflammatory tones, emphasising the corrupting effects of sexual intercourse upon innocent children. These revelations made a deep impression on a broad spectrum of

public opinion: during the appearance of the articles, a wide variety
of reform groups and individuals, from socialists and feminists to
Anglican Bishops, found themselves united in vocal protest against
the sexual abuse of children. Finally, in August 1885 the government bowed to pressure and passed the Criminal Law Amendment
Act, which raised the age of consent from thirteen to sixteen as well
as making provisions for the suppression of brothels and the repres-
sion of male homosexual behaviour.

Age of consent legislation must be understood in the context of
other laws aimed at defining the social boundaries between childhood and maturity, for example those which forbade the employment of children. In middle-class Victorian ideology, childhood
had great symbolic importance as a world apart from adult society.
Children were excluded from the public market-place where everything, including sex and human labour, were treated as commodi-
ties; they were seen to be sexually innocent and economically
dependent – hence the concern with child prostitution, which violated the social, economic and sexual dimensions of childhood. Yet
the need for legal definitions of the age at which children may work
or become sexually active revealed profound ambiguities about the
nature of childhood and the relationship of children to the family
and society. On the one hand, it was intimated that children were
not objects which could be bought and sold either for economic or
sexual purposes; on the other hand, it was suggested that they *were*
sexual and economic beings – why else would they need to be
placed under surveillance?[60] It was precisely this ambivalence that
was at the root of anxiety about the use of the speculum in young
unmarried girls.

Unlike labour laws, age of consent legislation applied only to
girls, not to boys, and many of its provisions were in fact intended
to protect a guardian's right to control a girl's sexuality rather than
to safeguard the defenceless from danger. The underlying principle
was that a father had rights to the services of his children, thus if a
girl under sixteen entered into a sexual relationship with a man, her
father could bring an action for the loss of services of his daughter.
The Offences Against the Person Act of 1861 even gave parents
power to prevent a girl's marriage up to the age of twenty-one if she
had property, provided that they could prove that her suitor had
used 'false allurements'.[61] The coercive implications of age of consent legislation were not lost on those social purity reformers who

were also civil libertarians and supporters of women's rights. They argued that such measures would subject girls 'to an amount of espionage and control ... damaging to their self respect and strength of character'[62] and vigorously opposed successive versions of the Criminal Law Amendment Act in the name of personal freedom.

The contentious issues of personal liberty and parental authority that were raised by age of consent legislation had direct relevance to the speculum debate. There was a danger that by using a 'corrupting' instrument such as the speculum, gynaecologists might infringe fathers' rights to control the sexuality of their daughters. 'What father amongst us, after the details which I have given, would allow his virgin daughter to be subjected to this "pollution"?', asked Marshall Hall at the height of the controversy.[63] The speculum might have engendered a conflict between the interests of fathers and those of doctors – a most undesirable prospect at a time when gynaecologists were seeking to consolidate their position as the 'true guardians' of women's interests and the 'custodians of their honour'.[64]

Issues of personal liberty and authority were at stake also in the relationship between a gynaecologist and his patient. As the Secretary of the Obstetrical Society of London, Seymour Haden, stated during the debate over Baker Brown's clitoridectomy operations in 1867, patients

are obliged to believe all that we tell them, they are not in a position to dispute anything that we say to them. We, therefore, may be said to have ... our patients, who are women, we being men, at our mercy.

It was thus essential that the gynaecologist should not abuse the power he possessed by virtue of his sex and his profession: 'If we should depart from the strictest principles of honour', Haden concluded to applause, 'if we should cheat and victimise ... [our patients] in any shape or way, we should be unworthy of the profession of which we are members.'[65]

Strict rules of professional conduct were required not only to safeguard the patient's interests, but also to protect the gynaecologist from legal liability. For the law, medical power was neither absolute nor automatic: it was based on a contract between doctor and patient which legitimated the doctor's right to intrude into the living body. The patient had to agree to place herself in the hands of the doctor, while the doctor undertook to do only what he believed good for the patient. In order for a person's consent to medical treatment to be legally effective, it was necessary for the therapy to be fully justified, and for the patient to understand its implications. If these criteria were not fulfilled, a doctor became liable to the crime, as well as the tort, of battery (commonly known as 'assault'), the category under which all medical procedures involving bodily touchings are subsumed by the law. With minors, it was generally assumed that a child's parent or guardian had the power of authorising medical procedures on the child.[66]

It is in the light of the rules governing individual capacity to consent to medical procedures that Dr Lee's opposition to the 'abuse' of the speculum must now be viewed. In claiming that the speculum was being used *without proven necessity*, Dr Lee suggested that speculum practitioners betrayed the trust of their patients and were not far from committing a form of rape for their own vicarious sexual gratification: the 'abuse' of the speculum, the sexual abuse of the patient and the abuse of medical authority were inextricably bound up together.[67] And indeed in 1852, the Jackson and Wife versus Roe case showed that the patient's consent may not be legally effective in protecting a medical practitioner from liability, if he used the speculum for no good reason. Two years after the debate at the Royal Medico-Chirurgical Society, Mr and Mrs Jackson of Plymouth brought legal proceedings against a Dr Roe on grounds of maltreatment. Roe was accused of using the speculum unnecessarily. He countered the accusation by arguing that Mrs Jackson had syphilis, and that he had therefore been justified in giving her a course of treatment by speculum and caustics. The evidence of the case was contradictory, and a verdict of not guilty was returned.[68]

Another important professional dimension of the speculum debate was hinted at in 'Pudor's' letter, which was quoted earlier. At a time when Queen Adelaide had given the royal seal of approval to 'quackery', anti-speculum practitioners intimated that the speculum had become fashionable amongst the aristocratic 'ladies of leisure', who always took the lead in quackery and easily became prey to speculating practitioners. Setting medical men in opposition to the fashionable lady and her speculum practitioner, they reminded their colleagues that the success of the medical profession depended on respecting the moral codes of its predominantly middle-class clientele: using the speculum might have cost obstetricians ground in their struggle for professional advancement. The physician Thomas Litchfield explained the professional issues raised by the speculum in a letter to the *Lancet* for June 1850:

The fast hold our noble science yet has of [sic] the middle and thoughtful classes renders it highly necessary that we practise our art with decent propriety, and never have recourse to such instruments unless the urgent necessity of the case renders such an examination unavoidable. Without that urgent necessity it is highly indecorous; and, depend upon it, the virtuous and delicate sensibilities once shocked by the medical attendant, he may find his position as the medical adviser of the family circle not so firm as previously.[69]

Speculum examinations did become technically 'instrumental rape' with the passage of the Contagious Diseases Acts. In these Acts, provision was made for the forcible examination of prostitutes: the 1864 Act, which was designed 'to Prevent the Spreading of Contagious Diseases to certain Naval and Military Stations', gave JPs, inspectors, magistrates and medical practitioners the power to apprehend a woman and 'convey her with all practical Speed to the Hospital' for an examination; the 1866 Act gave the police greater power to detain and examine any prostitute they suspected of carrying venereal disease. Women could be issued with a notice requiring them to be examined, and detained in hospital against their will and without their consent; if they refused to be medically examined they could be imprisoned.[70]

These regulations provoked an outcry on behalf of the principle of individual liberty, and a campaign for the repeal of the Acts rapidly gained momentum. Anti-regulationists violently opposed the examination of prostitutes by the speculum, which they depicted at best as a voyeuristic intrusion in the womb, and at worst as the 'instrumental rape' of women. Women were forced to submit to brutal and degrading inspections to 'make vice safe for men', while the men who consorted with them were allowed to go unpunished. This asymmetry made the speculum a prime target for the campaign against the 'double standard' of sexual morality. Both 'White Slavery' and prostitution were deemed to be the result of the two great vices of which men were culpable, cruelty and sensuality. Male control over women had to be combatted at all levels: sexual, social and economic, for it was women's social dependence that made them liable to become instruments of male pleasure. Demands for the vote and for male chastity went together.[71]

The attack on male depravity provided a key link between the campaign against the CD Acts and the antivivisection movement. For many Victorians, scientific medicine based on vivisection posed a major threat to traditional assumptions about the connections among individual responsibility, behaviour and disease. Science was driving vitalist doctrines out of physiology, thus undermining belief in the sacredness and inviolability of the organism; it was also introducing the idea that disease was due to the attack of invading germs, a morally random event.[72] Woman, the quintessence of life, a symbol for nature, and the custodian of natural morality, became the vehicle for these concerns.

A disturbing parallel was drawn between women as the actual or potential victims of sadistic monsters, and the animals tortured by male scientists in vivisectionist experiments. Frances Newman, a leading social reformer active in the feminist and temperance movements, equated the subject of an inspection for venereal disease to a carcass laid out for dissection and claimed that, with the CD Acts, doctors had been empowered to torture women, children and animals.[73] The speculum exemplified the manner in which the new science was devaluing and degrading life: it was as if women were reduced to inanimate status in the hands of the inspecting doctor.

For the feminist and anti-vivisectionist physician Elizabeth Blackwell (1821–1910), one of the most outspoken critics of surgical gynaecology, exposure to cruel vivisectionist experiments could only encourage doctors to treat their patients with callousness and brutality, as if they were nothing more than 'clinical material' devoid of life and feelings. It was to the corruption of the moral sense resulting from 'unrestrained experiment on the lower animals' that Blackwell attributed the gynaecologists' willingness to submit women to 'degrading' vaginal examinations.[74] As Elston has noted, the metaphor of medical science as rape became a dominant theme in late-Victorian anti-vivisectionist literature: women and animals shared the same fate as the victims of materialist medical men.[75]

It was not only feminists, but also working-class radicals that found anti-vivisection appealing. In the last quarter of the nineteenth century, anti-vivisectionist novels like Edward Berdoe's

Dying Scientifically: A Key to St. Bernard's popularised the belief that the interests of charity patients were subordinated to the research objectives of their doctors. There was a widespread fear among the working classes that charity patients were used for experimentation, and hospitals were shunned by the poor as promising a fate worse than death. As Coral Lansbury comments, 'it was not only Robert Louis Stevenson who felt that the soul of a ravening, amoral monster could be found in the breast of a kindly man of medicine like Dr Jekyll'.[76] The view that women and the working classes shared the same social oppression led to the identification of feminist demands for female emancipation with radical politics, and a curious alliance between middle-class feminists and working-class men was forged in the campaign against the CD Acts.[77] It was in this context that doctors, the people who had to work the Acts in conjunction with the police, were described by repealers as the 'oligarchy', although they belonged to the same class as the feminists who were fighting against male vice and state-sanctioned prostitution.

The complex metaphors that drew male vice, vivisection, gynaecology and class oppression together found their expression in the image of the horse as a symbol for social and sexual exploitation. Equine metaphors were much in evidence both in pornographic fiction and in gynaecological practice. Victorian pornographic novels typically portrayed women as horses which were 'broken to the bit' by the riding master: straps, ropes and whips were the standard equipment of the fictional libertine. In gynaecology, women were strapped to saddles and tables and indecently exposed for the purposes of examination and surgery; footrests, which were widely used after 1860, were referred to as 'stirrups', thus evoking the language of the stable which was so prominent in pornographic fiction.[78]

The language of horses and the dialogue of the stable were also accepted modes for speaking about the working classes. Horses, the beasts of burden, were held up to the working man as a model of patience and forbearance, and equine parables were used in religious tracts and fictional works as means of inculcating docility in recalcitrant workers. Drawing upon this fund of shared metaphors, social reformers represented the exploited worker as a horse being beaten and flogged to death. Workers and horses shared the same fate: when they became too old and sick to work, the horse went to the knacker's yard, the worker to the workhouse.[79] Interestingly, in the early part of the nineteenth century old and diseased horses were widely used in the vivisectionist experiments carried out at the French veterinary schools. These institutions, especially the Ecole Vétérinaire in Alfort, were strongly opposed by the English Society for the Protection of Animals, and it was in consequence of pressures from the Society that a commission was nominated by Napoleon to investigate the utility of vivisection.[80]

By the last quarter of the nineteenth century, the medical opposition to the speculum had waned: the clinical records of the Chelsea Hospital for Women in London, for example, show that the procedure was carried out routinely at this hospital, even on young single women. A number of reasons for this change of heart can be suggested. The experience of examining prostitutes may have diminished the gynaecologists' sensitivity to the speculum; the need to woo the middle class market may have been less pressing. But perhaps the most likely explanation lies in the acceptance of anaesthesia after 1850. As is well known, the introduction of anaesthesia in obstetrics and gynaecology was the subject of keen debate. One of the arguments in its favour was that it overcame women's moral sensitivities and subdued their resistance to medical authority.[81] It is interesting that gynaecological patients at the Chelsea were usually examined under chloroform: one wonders whether they were ever fully informed of what would be done to them once 'under the influence'. In contemporary gynaecological practice, patients anaesthetised for gynaecological operations are often used to teach medical students the technique of vaginal examinations.

It is therefore relevant to consider the objections that were levelled against the employment of chloroform in the early Victorian period. The medical and lay opponents of anaesthesia contended that it gave doctors unchecked power over their patients; popular caricatures of the practice in the early Victorian period significantly rendered this domination in sexual terms by portraying the administration of chloroform as the taming of the shrew.[82] Charges of improper conduct towards anaesthetised patients became rife from 1870 onwards, as anaesthesia came to be extensively employed in gynaecology and dentistry. There is no doubt that some practitioners did take advantage of the patient's unconsciousness, but medical men did not see it that way. Anaesthesia, they argued, produced sexual fantasies in the patient; in some cases it even induced displays of sexual excitation.[83] Rape in other words was only in the patient's mind and doctors must be protected from false allegations of sexual assault.

Precept and practice

During the second half of the nineteenth century hospitals became a central locus of gynaecological practice: studying their activities must thus be a priority for any historian interested in charting the medical management of woman and her diseases. The information drawn from clinical records, hospital reports and management committee minutes serves to illustrate routine treatments and changing patterns of medical care; it allows for comparisons with similar establishments and offers some useful insight into the relationship between gynaecologists and their patients.

Recent historical work on nineteenth-century gynaecological therapeutics has argued that treatment was shaped by cultural prejudice against women. At times of social upheaval and feminist agitation, doctors used harsh therapies to punish women and induce conformity to the prescribed feminine role.[84] It has also been claimed that women physicians rebelled against male definitions of female pathology and appropriate treatments by shunning heroic therapies and developing a feminist approach to women's diseases: 'The women doctors who began to appear on the American scene in the 1850s', writes Ann Douglas, 'saw women's diseases as a *result* of submission, and promoted independence from masculine domination, whether professional or sexual, as their cure for feminine ailments.'[85]

Evidence about the practice of nineteenth-century gynaecology does not support these views. Harsh therapies were used to control male as well as female sexuality: Regina Markell Morantz-Sanchez, for example, relates a case of male masturbation in late nineteenth-century America that was treated with doses of quinine, strychnine, calomel and podophyllin, and strong quantities of faradic shock to the penis and scrotum.[86] Medical men were as divided over gynaecological surgery as were medical women. Elizabeth Garrett Anderson, for instance, was the first female physician to practise ovariotomy, but her assistant Frances Hoggan criticised the decision and resigned from the New Hospital for Women, London.[87] In our effort to understand the relationship between gender and medicine, it is important to realise that there are no simple patterns, no easy explanations. Morantz-Sanchez's comparative study of obstetric practice at a female-run and a male-run Boston hospital during the last quarter of the nineteenth century has shown only minor variations in the use of heroic therapies.[88] Marked differences in the surgical practice of *male* gynaecologists have been revealed in my analysis of cases treated in the 1860s at the Hospital for Women and at the Middlesex Hospital in London.

For the purposes of this study, I have examined the cases admitted to the Hospital for Women under the care of Protheroe Smith between October 1869 and November 1870. This appears to be the only surviving evidence about the practice of gynaecology at the Hospital for Women in the Victorian period. For the Chelsea Hospital, where virtually all nineteenth-century case-records have been preserved, sampling at five-yearly intervals has been used, from 1873, the year in which the first patients were admitted, to 1890. The records of gynaecological patients admitted to the Prudhoe Ward at the Middlesex Hospital between June 1863 and October 1866 have provided some comparative material on gynaecological practice at a London general hospital.

Although there are no clinical records relating to the early years of activity of the Hospital for Women, we know from the Hospital Reports that in those days admissions were not confined to gynaecological cases. The 1850 Report stated that the aims of the hospital were, first, to cure the ailments peculiar to women, and secondly, to give 'strength and activity to those who are either disabled from performing the duties of life, or perform them with difficulty.'[89] This suggests that some of the patients suffered from occupational diseases or chronic ill-health rather than from gynaecological complaints.

Protheroe Smith's book of cases reveals that by 1869 admissions were restricted to cases of gynaecological disease. Women sought treatment for ovarian cysts, uterine fibroids and inflammations, menstrual derangements such as amenorrhoea (absence of menstruation) and dysmenorrhoea (painful menstruation), displacements of the uterus and perineal lacerations following parturition. Diseases of the urinary apparatus were also treated. The usual therapy for fibroids was by means of fused potash injections into the uterus at frequent intervals. Pessaries were used for the treatment of displacements, leeches and blisters for pelvic inflammation; oper-

ations were done for perineal tears. Two cases of hysteria were
admitted under Smith's care between November 1869 and January
1870. Hysteria had been associated with the afflictions of the female
sexual system since Greek times, but in the second half of the
nineteenth century it became central to definitions of femininity
and female sexuality, encapsulating cultural views about feminine
waywardness and irrationality.[90] The first patient was a young
married woman; she complained of pain in the back, restlessness
and leucorrhoea (white discharge from the vagina). The second
patient, an unmarried woman of twenty-six, had suffered from
hysterical fits at the menstrual period ever since puberty.[91]

The range of conditions treated at the Middlesex was very similar
to the Protheroe Smith series. There was a large number of cases of
cervical ulceration – a controversial disease, as we have just seen –
and of pelvic cellulitis; the latter diagnosis was much in vogue at the
time. Most of the patients were married women. Compared with
the married charity patients in Smith's case-book, it is curious that
most of the patients gave 'housewife' as their occupation (see tables
2 and 3). This may have reflected either the patient's or the practitioner's expectations of the female role; it is more probable,
though, that the admitting officers at the Soho Square hospital
exercised greater care in investigating patients' socio-economic
circumstances, since the introduction of a system of payments
required them to differentiate more subtly between levels of
poverty.

One of the most interesting differences between the Hospital for
Women and the Middlesex concerns the figures for ovariotomy.
Protheroe Smith had six cases of ovarian disease and performed
ovariotomy in four, with two deaths. Of the remaining two
patients, one was tapped and the other died before she could receive
any treatment.[92] At the Middlesex Hospital, on the other hand,
surgeons were more conservative and preferred tapping the cyst.
There were sixteen cases of ovarian disease between June 1863 and
October 1866, and ovariotomy was performed on two occasions,
both of them ending in death.[93] One of these patients was later
found to have a tumour of the kidney; the other appears to have
suffered not from an ovarian cyst, but from a pregnancy, as the
presence of a 'tawney areola round nipple, enlarged follicles, milk
in breast' indicates. It seems extraordinary that this particular case
should have been so grossly misdiagnosed, but such errors were not

uncommon at the time. In another case, which was also fatal, it was attempted to remove the tumour through an incision in the uterus. Environmental conditions were believed to affect the outcome of an operation, thus in 1865 the 'unsettled state of the weather' was deemed to be a sufficient reason for not performing ovariotomy; the patient, a servant who had been ill for ten years, was discharged *in status quo.*[94] Gynaecological practice at the Middlesex remained very conservative right up to the late 1880s: when John Bland-Sutton was appointed Assistant Surgeon in 1886, he soon incurred the displeasure of his colleagues by his zeal for abdominal surgery, especially in regard to pelvic operations on women.[95]

The Chelsea Hospital was founded in 1871, and the first patient was admitted at the beginning of 1873. According to the Report for 1871–3, the case was one of paralysis subsequent to a fall, which had injured the lower part of the patient's spine and displaced the womb to such an extent as to induce progressive paralysis of the left side.[96] The physician Thomas Chambers was in charge of in-patients, and two books of cases under his care are still available, covering the period 1873–81. The cases admitted between April 1873 and December 1874 included tumours of the womb, ovarian cysts, urinary complaints and diseases of the bowel (piles in particular), menstrual derangements and uterine displacements and inflammations. Cases of dysmenorrhoea were usually attributed to atresia of the os (narrowing of the opening into the womb) and were treated by dividing the cervix. Operations were done for ovarian cysts and cancer of the rectum; leeches were applied to relieve uterine inflammation. The average length of stay was seven weeks.

The range of cases treated at the hospital in 1879 was much the same as during the previous period. An interesting case of utero-vaginitis was admitted that year. The patient, a twenty-year-old single girl, was suffering from irregular menstruation; she had been unable to use one foot and one leg on account of 'paralysis', and had lost her speech for eighteen months. She was also suffering from a great deal of 'irritation'. Iron and strychnine were administered, and the clitoris and the labia minora were excised; the girl was discharged 'cured' after one month.[97] Another case of clitoridectomy had occurred at the Chelsea Hospital in 1877. The patient was a nineteen-year-old unmarried girl, but no further notes were made about her case.[98]

During the 1880s, the number of admissions increased dramatically, not only because of the greater capacity of the hospital (which had by then moved to new premises in the Fulham Road), but also thanks to the quicker patient turnover. The average length of stay decreased from 30 days in 1886 to 20.6 in 1894;[99] over the same period, the number of patients rose from 306 to 664.[100] Uterine cases form the largest class of disease in the sample: they comprise tumours, displacements, inflammations and malformations ('conical cervix' accounts for twenty-two out of twenty-eight cases of uterine malformation). Other cases include the complications of pregnancy and childbirth, such as abortion and subinvolution, diseases of the ovaries and tubes (such as salpingitis, ovarian prolapses and cysts), perineal tears, piles, anal fissures and fistulae, breast tumours and diseases of the urinary system. Cases of dyspareunia and vaginismus were also treated.

The breakdown of cases by diagnosis provided in the hospital reports shows that a small number of cases of hysteria were admitted each year. Three such cases were found in our sample. The first patient, a twenty-four-year-old single woman, was admitted in 1884 under the care of James Aveling. She suffered from irritability of the bladder, pain at the end of micturition, constant pain in the left iliac region and leucorrhoea. She was treated by means of infusions of gentian and pills of zinc valerianate. The latter (a sedative) was a favourite remedy for hysteria.[101] The other cases occurred in 1889 and were treated by Fancourt Barnes and William Travers respectively. Barnes' patient was a thirty-three-year-old single woman who was afflicted with sick headaches, a white discharge and pains that got worse on menstruation; upon examination, the cervix was found to be soft and the uterus anteflexed.[102] The patient treated by Travers was a thirty-year-old woman who had been unwell since her first confinement and was suffering from pain in the left iliac fossa and dysmenorrhoea. An examination revealed that the uterus was anteflexed and a thickening was discovered in the right broad ligament. It is not clear what was done in these two cases, but the application of blisters to relieve pain was recorded in the latter.[103]

One striking feature of the 1880s and early '90s is the high percentage of operations performed at the hospital (see table 5). Some of these were carried out for uterine fibroids, malignant tumours and polypi, others for the relief of uterine prolapse; ovaries also began to be removed more frequently, not only for the cure of cysts, but also for that of ovarian prolapse. It was often the case that, after removing one diseased ovary, the other was found to be 'cyrrhosed' or 'atrophied' and was removed for good measure. Exploratory incisions for suspected ovarian disease also began to be performed in this period. Patients did not always take surgery lying down: a number of women refused to give their consent to a proposed abdominal operation.

From 1888 onwards, patients who dreaded surgical intervention were able to benefit from a new treatment by electricity, based on the work of the Frenchman George Apostoli (1847–1900), which was carried out for the cure of uterine fibroids and scirrhus (hard carcinoma) of the breast.[104] The treatment unfortunately proved fatal in one case. In 1889, a thirty-nine-year-old woman was admitted for scirrhus of the breast. Punctures were made round the growth, and a current was passed through them. When the current was passed in a puncture made to the left of the median line, the patient's pulse stopped. Attempts at resuscitation, which included artificial respiration, brandy and ether injections, hot water bottles and a mustard leaf over the cardiac region alas proved of no avail.[105]

Case-notes and minutes of hospital committee meetings, if read from the standpoint of the patient, can reveal precious information about the relations between gynaecological patients and their medical attendants. Charity patients were at the mercy of the practitioner's goodwill and the calls of his private practice. In 1885, a patient discharged herself from the Hospital for Women to protest against her treatment by one of the surgeons. She alleged that Mr Reeves had abandoned an operation he was about to perform on her because of an urgent private call. When the incident was discussed at a meeting of the management committee, Mr Reeves declared he was very surprised the woman had left so suddenly, since he had given 'every attention to her gratuitously' prior to admission. At the Soho Square hospital, the practice of calling out the hospital's nurses to attend private cases seems to have been widespread. Not until 1885, when a patient in one of the paying wards complained that wards were left understaffed, did the management committee take steps to reduce the extent of the practice.[106]

Paying for one's treatment increased patients' expectations of medical care and gave them the right to criticise if the treatment fell short of the desired standard. Nine years after the establishment of a pay system at the Hospital for Women, the management committee was receiving so many complaints from patients that a complaints book was introduced in each ward: some paying patients expected the same comforts and privacy of their own homes and were disgruntled when they discovered that neither could be easily provided in a public institution.[107] Unfortunately none of the complaints books has survived, but it is possible to capture some of their flavour from the complaints reported to the hospital management committee.

The quality of the food seems to have been a common source of dissatisfaction. In 1884, a GP from Taunton wrote that one of his patients, while under treatment at the hospital, had found 'the butter always bad, fish rarely eatable'. In reply, the hospital committee said that the patient was at fault for failing to enter her complaint in the book provided. In the early 1880s, there were complaints about the noise caused by revellers on Saturday and Sunday nights and the long waiting times in the out-patient department.[108]

Sometimes the nurses were the butt of criticism. In 1885 a patient reported that surgical appliances were being used for more than one patient without cleaning; on one occasion after receiving a 'hot air bath', she had had to wait for her bed to be made, uncovered, while the doors and windows of the ward were wide open; on another occasion, she had been left on a couch for several hours without proper nourishment, uncovered, and again with the windows and doors open. All charges were firmly denied by the matron and nursing staff. In 1886 the conduct of two nurses was reported to the management committee. The nurses had apparently been sacked following the reorganisation of nursing at the hospital, and they were taking out their anger on the poor patients under their care.[109]

Thus, while the definition of femininity propounded by gynaecological science clustered round ideas of disease, frailty and instability, the clinical records of the patients admitted to the Soho Square and the Chelsea hospitals reveal that women were not always the passive recipients of medical care. Nor did practitioners necessarily agree as to the best way of treating their patients, as can be seen from the debates on gynaecological surgery.

5

The 'Unsexing' of women

Of all the therapeutic innovations introduced in gynaecology during the nineteenth century, ovariotomy was undoubtedly the one which met with the greatest opposition from medical practitioners and the lay public.[1] This is as might be expected, for the ovaries were the 'grand organs' of sexual activity in women, the source and symbol of femininity itself; their removal 'unsexed' woman, thus threatening deeply held beliefs about woman's nature, her social role and moral responsibilities.

In the early Victorian period the surgical removal of cystic ovaries by abdominal section was a very dangerous operation, carrying a mortality rate comparable to that for amputations. By 1870, ovariotomy had become established as an accepted procedure and was hailed as the triumph of gynaecology and the beginning of abdominal surgery. Ovariotomy, said the gynaecological surgeon James Murphy at the first conference of the British Gynaecological Society in 1891, had

opened up the whole field of abdominal surgery, so that many men who started as gynaecologists are now our most brilliant surgeons, successfully attacking the uterus, the spleen, the liver, and all the organs contained in the abdomen.[2]

This was a dazzling apotheosis for a practice which was initially regarded as little short of murder. What is particularly intriguing about the development of ovariotomy is the asymmetry it reveals in the treatment of similar conditions in man and woman. Surgeons do not remove testicles for the cure of hydrocele, they resort to the palliative drainage of the cyst by tapping. This procedure was also used in the treatment of ovarian cysts before the first trials of ovariotomy; it was the preferred method for some time afterwards, in the belief that it carried fewer dangers to life than ovariotomy.

The rise of this operation cannot be seen simply in terms of scientific progress, nor can it be regarded as an expression of medical mysogyny and male oppression. In this chapter I shall argue that the rise of ovariotomy must be seen as an integral part of the social construction of femininity in the last century; I shall also suggest that ovariotomy might have been used as an abortion and contraception procedure. Gynaecological texts, iconographic material, literary evidence and hospital records form the basis of my analysis.

Early controversies

Ovariotomy, or the removal of one or both ovaries as a radical cure for ovarian disease (cysts in particular), was suggested by several British and continental surgeons during the course of the eighteenth century. One of the earliest advocates of the operation in England was the famous surgeon John Hunter (1728–93), who thought that there was no reason why women should not bear 'spaying' as well as other animals did.[3] There seems little doubt that ovariotomy was attempted in a few isolated cases from 1700 onwards, but at the time it was not an elective procedure. The standard treatment for ovarian tumours was then by tapping, injections of sclerosing fluids such as iodine solutions, incision and drainage; sometimes, a permanent fistula through which the tumour could discharge its secretion was created.[4] An instance of unintended ovariotomy is provided by the well-known case reported by Percival Pott in his *Chirurgical Works*, published in 1775. In an attempt at removing an abdominal hernia in a young woman by laparotomy, Pott discovered that the hernia was in fact a tumour affecting both ovaries, which he successfully removed.[5] Pott's patient survived, but other sporadic operations in the eighteenth century generally had such dire consequences that any deliberate attempt at ovariotomy was held to be too hazardous and cruel to be justified.

The first ovariotomy was performed in 1809 by the American surgeon Ephraim McDowell (1771–1830). While studying medicine at Edinburgh during the 1793–4 session, McDowell had heard the surgeon John Bell lecture about the dangers of ovarian disease and argue in favour of the surgical removal of ovarian cysts by abdominal section. It is said that McDowell resolved to put his teacher's suggestion into practice, and in 1809 the opportunity finally presented itself while he was practising medicine in the backwoods village of Danville, Kentucky. McDowell's patient suffered from a condition which had at first been diagnosed as an advanced state of pregnancy, but labour had not commenced at the expected time. Upon examination, McDowell found nothing in the uterus; this led him to think that the 'pregnancy' must be an enlarged ovary. He proposed its removal, and the patient consented notwithstanding the enormous hazards of the operation. During her ordeal, which lasted twenty-five minutes, the patient apparently supported herself by singing hymns. At some point in the proceedings, loops of intestine gushed onto the abdominal wall and were eventually replaced with great difficulty. The tumour however was successfully removed, and five days later McDowell found his patient on her feet, busy making her bed. She fully recovered and lived for thirty-one years.[6]

McDowell's report of the operation, which he published only eight years after the event, was generally received with hostility and incredulity in Britain. James Johnson, editor of the *Medico-Chirurgical Review*, disbelieved the seemingly miraculous recovery of 'Dr. Mac's' patient and doubted that his example would encourage British surgeons to open the abdomen of their patients: 'Craedat Judaeus, non ego', was his lapidary comment.[7] In the meantime, however, the news of McDowell's operation had also reached a more receptive practitioner, John Lizars (1787–1860), who had been a pupil of John Bell and was a surgeon and lecturer in Anatomy and Physiology at Edinburgh University. Lizars became convinced that elective laparotomy (i.e. the cutting of the abdominal wall) and the removal of diseased ovaries could be carried out successfully, and in 1824 he performed the first British ovariotomy on a twenty-seven-year-old woman whose abdomen had reached the size of a nine months' pregnancy.

The patient's case-history is of interest, as it indicates some of the reasons why women might have consented to submit to such a fearful surgical practice. The woman, a shoe-binder, had come to Lizars after consulting several practitioners, all of whom had diagnosed a pregnancy and poured scorn on her when she had maintained that this could not be the case. She was in fact separated from her husband, and on her part she attributed the abdominal enlargement to several blows and kicks she had received from him. Being without means of support, she had applied to the county hospital, but had been turned away on the grounds that she was pregnant. Her neighbours had then started to abuse her for the same reason and had made such complaints to her employers that they had dismissed her. At that point she chanced to consult Lizars who, upon examination, diagnosed a tumour occupying the abdominal cavity. Against his colleagues' advice, but with the full consent of his patient, Lizars performed ovariotomy. It is harrowing to think that the woman need not have submitted to such an ordeal, as the Edinburgh surgeon found that he had misdiagnosed the disease: he had been deceived by the woman's great obesity, and no tumour was found. Luckily the patient survived, but three further attempts by Lizars ended in death.[8]

Between 1825 and 1833, two attempts at ovariotomy were made by the obstetrician Dr Augustus Granville, President of the first Obstetrical Society. In the first case, the adhesions were so strong that the operation had to be abandoned; in the second case, no tumour was found on opening the abdomen.[9] These problems hardly encouraged the adoption of drastic operative measures, and no attempts at ovariotomy were reported until 1838, when a successful operation by William Jeaffreson (1790–1865), a provincial general practitioner who was also a successful lithotomist, revived interest in the practice.[10]

From that epoch, the number of operations carried out in Britain increased steadily: according to the statistics published by the obstetrician Robert Lee in 1851, ovariotomy had been performed over 130 times in Britain since Jeaffreson's operation.[11] These figures most likely represent only the tip of the iceberg, as operators at the time did not often report their cases, nor were they forthcoming with data about their results. Those which were available were far from reassuring: according to the statistics of all published ovariotomy cases gathered by Charles West in 1855, the death rate after ovariotomy was 44.5 per cent, the number of operations to which this applied being 200.[12] These dire results were a matter of grave concern to the medical establishment, and in the 1840s and 1850s a controversy broke out over the justifiability of the procedure. Medical opinion became split into a conservative and an interventionist camp, the first led by the obstetrician Robert Lee, the second vaunting men such as the Edinburgh obstetrician James Young Simpson, the Manchester general practitioner Charles Clay and, later, the surgeon Thomas Spencer Wells.

The advocates of ovariotomy claimed that ovarian disease was so grave and dangerous to the life of the sufferer as to warrant surgical interference. Simpson, for example, maintained in 1846 that in nine out of ten cases of ovarian cysts, the disease pursued a regular progress towards enlargement, insufferable distension, local irritation, constitutional exhaustion and death.[13] Patients became weak and emaciated, developing a peculiar appearance which Spencer Wells was later to dub *facies ovariana*.[14] Drainage, it was claimed, was a mere palliative, and in most cases patients died within four years of the first tapping.

Ovariotomists did not deny that the death-rate of the operation was high. However, they pointed out that tapping was nearly as dangerous as ovariotomy, and further, that other capital operations (i.e., those likely to involve loss of life) had comparably high mortality rates, yet nobody ever questioned their propriety.[15] Thomas Inman's tables of the mortality rates after capital operations, collated in 1844, show that the death-rate after ovariotomy was 33.3 per cent, approximately the same as after tying the large arteries and after amputations (see table 4).

The relative benefits of ovariotomy compared to palliative treatment had to be assessed also in relation to women's life expectancy. This was estimated in Mr Finlaison's tables at nearly forty-four years for a woman aged twenty-four, and at thirty-one years at age forty.[16] If these figures were contrasted with the average expectation of life after drainage, the balance was clearly tipped in favour of ovariotomy: at twenty years of age, claimed an advocate of the operation in 1851, the sufferer 'perils four years of wretched life', while a radical operation, if successful, promised 'forty years of existence and renewed powers of social and domestic enjoyment'.[17]

For the critics of ovariotomy, these arguments were so much medical mumbo-jumbo and their proponents hardly more than sow-gelders and butchers in frock-coats. They claimed that the risks of ovariotomy far outweighed those of ovarian disease and argued in favour of tapping and medicinal treatment. First, the disease could never be diagnosed with absolute certainty, since the symptoms of ovarian cysts mimicked those of pregnancy and of a host of other abdominal conditions. Secondly, there was the danger of exposing the abdominal cavity to the air, which was thought to cause peritonitis and lead to death. Thirdly, there was a risk of injuring the intestines and of causing internal haemorrhages; last, but not the least, it was feared that the presence of adhesions or of a thick pedicle, neither of which could be established prior to operation, might prevent the removal of the cyst, thus putting the patient unnecessarily at risk.[18]

The opponents of ovariotomy maintained that it was inadmissible to justify ovariotomy by comparing its high mortality rate with the death-rates of other capital operations. In the first place, the conditions were not the same. Capital operations were usually carried out under the worst possible circumstances in crowded and comfortless hospitals, on patients who suffered from other conditions, often aggravated by intemperance, and who had not one chance of life; ovariotomy on the contrary was performed on selected patients, often in the favourable surroundings of a private home.[19] Secondly, the justification for capital operations rested solely on the grounds that their performance was essential to the preservation of life; this point was by no means established in the case of ovarian cysts, as the disease was hardly ever fatal.[20]

The suggestion that the ovariotomists outraged the Hippocratic oath was made in 1843 by the reviewer of Charles Clay's *Extirpation of Diseased Ovaria* in the *British and Foreign Medical Review*. Having considered each of the cases reported by Clay and denied that they were legitimate cases for operation, the writer thus concluded:

We have merely sought to establish the real amount of danger which attends *one* of the operations which have been practised for the cure of ovarian dropsy . . . We earnestly hope that they will prevent the younger members of the profession from being dazzled by the alleged success of an operation, which though it may excite the astonishment of the vulgar, calls neither for the knowledge of an anatomist nor the skill of a surgeon . . . A fundamental principle of medical morality . . . is outraged whenever an operation so fearful in its nature, often so immediately fatal in its results, as gastrotomy, is performed for the removal of a disease, of the very existence of which the surgeon is not always sure; of the curability of which, by his interference, he must be in the highest degree uncertain. There are unfortunately no means of gaining notoriety in the practice of medicine as by the performance of some bold operation, which the aged and the timorous are reluctant to attempt, and we can fully sympathise with those who, just setting out in their medical career, are unwilling to let slip an opportunity of advancing their reputation. We would, however, entreat all such to ponder well before they jeopardy [sic] the lives of their patients by operations such as that the claims of which we have been investigating.[21]

Criticism of Clay's pioneering work was coloured by personal prejudice and parochialism. Clay was a provincial, and the members of the London surgical élite could not bring themselves to recognise the merits of colleagues practising in remote places such as Manchester. One of Clay's most outspoken critics was the renowned surgeon Robert Liston (1794–1847), who would quote from Spenser's *Fairie Queene*: 'As if a man should be dissected / To see what part should be disaffected'. Liston did not mince words when he discussed the activities of the ovariotomists. As Dr Lee recalled at a meeting of the Royal Medico-Chirurgical Society in 1862, he was in the habit of referring to the ovariotomists as '"belly rippers" with a B before and a B after'; the meaning of those two Bs Lee refrained from stating plainly to the Society.[22]

By the mid-1800s ovariotomy was in disrepute. The operation was generally condemned at a meeting of the Royal Medico-Chirurgical Society in November 1850, when Dr Robert Lee analysed 162 operations for ovarian tumours done in Great Britain. Lee estimated that a third of the cases had been found to be inoperable or to have no tumour. Of 102 completed operations, 42 had ended with the death of the patient. At this meeting even the famous surgeon Caesar Hawkins, who had performed ovariotomy with some success, denounced the operation as too dangerous. William Lawrence, twice President of the College of Surgeons, stated that he had never performed the operation and never would, unless his view of the matter was 'essentially altered'.[23]

This polarisation of attitudes towards ovariotomy was of no help to those surgeons who needed practical advice about individual cases: 'If I turn to one side', complained the surgeon Benjamin Phillips (1805–61) in 1850, 'I am assured that the operation is little short of murder; if I turn to the other side, I am told that it is comparatively harmless.'[24] The arguments were persuasive enough on both sides because the data were open to interpretation: ultimately, the decision to opt for palliative treatment or for a radical operation was, as Clay's reviewer put it, a matter of 'medical morality' rather than of hard statistical facts. Views about the extent to which surgical interference should be allowed to govern treatment were shaped by beliefs about the value of human life. As a comparative analysis of attitudes to ovariotomy and to the caesarean section in both France and Britain can show, it was this evaluation that provided the basis on which the costs and benefits of palliative versus radical treatment were assessed.

A question of values

Mid-nineteenth-century obstetricians in Britain and France agreed that there was a striking analogy between ovariotomy and the caesarean section. The methods of closing and opening the abdomen were the same (see plates 4–7); the danger of post-operative peritonitis was thought to be as grave in ovariotomy as it was in the caesarean section; the risk of internal haemorrhages was also comparable.[25] The mortality of the caesarean section was only marginally higher than that of ovariotomy: according to the data collected by the French historian Pundel, the maternal mortality in Britain and France was about 50 per cent in the first half of the nineteenth century, while the foetal mortality was approximately 40 per cent.[26]

These similarities present a stark contrast to the prevailing attitude towards the caesarean section and ovariotomy in Britain and France. It was apparent to contemporary medical observers that practitioners in these countries took diametrically opposed views about the propriety of abdominal section in cases of difficult labour or ovarian disease. In his lectures on obstetrics, published in 1847, Tyler Smith noted that obstetricians could be divided into two camps with regard to the caesarean section, the 'maternal sect' and the 'foetal sect': one was British and Protestant, the other was French and Catholic.[27]

Compared with their British colleagues, French obstetricians were much readier to resort to the caesarean section in cases in which the contraction of the maternal pelvis did not permit of a natural delivery. Their criteria for performing the operation were broader than in England: the caesarean section was recommended if the smallest diameter of the pelvis was 2 inches or less, and it was still the preferred method of delivery if the contracted pelvis measured from $2^{1}/_{4}$ to 3 inches and the child was alive. In Britain, on the other hand, the propriety of performing the operation only began when the short diameter of the pelvis measured $1^{1}/_{2}$ inches or less; with measurements exceeding this figure, British obstetricians preferred to extract the foetus by craniotomy.[28] This was a brutal and crude procedure: a hook was passed into the uterus and fixed into the foetus, which was then extracted bit by bit. As well as being obviously fatal for the baby, the operation also carried some risk for the mother: in 1859 Tyler Smith for instance estimated that craniotomy was performed in Britain twice as often as in France and four times as often as in Germany, with a maternal mortality of one in five.[29]

In choosing between a caesarean section and craniotomy, French obstetricians took into account first of all the duty to preserve the life of the child: this was partly because, according to the precepts of the Catholic religion, failure to baptise the (live) foetus would result in its losing the promise of eternal life. Secondly, they considered the danger likely to ensue to the mother from a protracted delivery by craniotomy.[30] This, as Tyler Smith's figures show, was not inconsiderable: in Britain, cases in which the child could not be extracted and the mother was abandoned to die were often exposed by the critics of craniotomy.[31] Such a risk, however, was regarded as acceptable by the majority of British obstetricians, who gave little or no weight to the duty to preserve the child. The life of the mother, they argued, was far more valuable than that of the foetus because her social relations and moral and religious responsibilities were greater and more important; it was therefore unwarrantable to put the mother's life to certain risk for what was no more than a small chance of saving the foetus.[32] This desire to prevent the loss of maternal, rather than foetal, life is borne out by the treatment of abortionists in Britain until about 1870. There was strong public sympathy for abortionists, and the penalties that existed against them were motivated not by concern about the lives of the unborn children, but by fear for the safety of women.[33]

British obstetricians looked upon their French colleagues' willingness to jeopardise the life of the mother with horror and indignation: 'Every principle of humanity and religion is opposed to such a practice; nay, even the cold dictates of mere science and physiology must condemn it', stated the reviewer of Lee's *Clinical Midwifery* in 1843. 'Why, then, it may be asked, should practitioners abroad have recourse to it with such little hesitation? The answer', he claimed,

is simple, and will at once be surmised by those who are all acquainted with medical practice on the Continent, and more especially in France. Patients, at least those amongst the poorer classes, seem to be regarded, not so much as fellow-creatures that have the same hopes and fears and the same feelings and destinies as ourselves, but rather as objects, so to speak, of natural history, which the learned doctor has to speculate and experiment upon.[34]

The view that French practitioners regarded human life as a valueless object for experimentation was shared by the obstetrician William Campbell, who argued in 1833 that the caesarean section was never delayed in France because 'there is neither that dread of operating so generally entertained by British practitioners, nor that high estimate of human life'.[35]

Amazingly, though, the allegedly brutal and insensitive French made the same allegations against the British with regard to ovariotomy. In France, medical practitioners considered ovariotomy to be an entirely Anglo-American creation and claimed that the prudent French surgeons would never resort to such a practice. The question of ovariotomy was discussed by the Académie de Médecine at a series of meetings which extended over a period of four months, from October 1856 to February 1857. In this debate the obstetrician Pierre Cazeaux (1808–62) stood practically alone in defence of that procedure, while the highest medical and surgical authorities of the country hurled anathema against the extirpation of the ovaries.[36] It was not until 1862, when the surgeon Koeberlé began to operate successfully, that the Académie de Médecine reconsidered its views.[37] The reason for this strenuous opposition was explained in 1875 by Jules Rochard, a physician and historian of French surgery:

Une opération qui consiste à ouvrir l'abdomen d'une femme pour en éxtirper une enorme tumeur . . . ressemble trop à une autopsie, elle heurte trop les idées reçues au sujet de la gravité des plaies pénétrantes de l'abdomen et de la lésion du péritoine, pour qu'elle ait pu se faire accepter sans résistance dans un pays où les chirurgiens se sont toujours fait remarquer pour leur prudence.[38]

The likening of ovariotomy to dissection recalled another aspect of medical endeavour which, since the beginning of the century and in France in particular, had been characterised by an increasing reliance on the methods of surgery – namely, the use of vivisectionist experiments in the study of bio-medical questions. This was a method which the experimental physiologist Claude Bernard thus defined in his *Introduction à l'étude de la médecine expérimentale* (1865):

La vivisection est la dislocation de l'organisme vivant à l'aide d'instruments et de procedés qui peuvent en isoler les differentes parties. Il est facile de comprendre que cette dissection sur le vivant suppose la dissection préalable sur le mort.[39]

Bernard further maintained that surgery was an extension of the experimental and vivisectionist approach on which scientific medicine was founded. Every time the surgeon performed an operation he could be said to be performing a vivisectionist experiment: here, however, the interests of the patient and those of science coincided, because a surgical procedure carried out for therapeutic purposes could at the same time throw light on physiological and pathological questions.[40] It was in these terms that Barnes saw ovariotomy when, at the end of the century, he wrote that the surgery of the abdominal and pelvic cavities was at once 'experimental and therapeutical. It is vivisection of the noblest kind. It teaches physiology, the rational basis of the healing art; it demonstrates pathology at the same time as it heals'.[41] Claude Bernard could not have agreed more, and it is no coincidence that he was the only one to support Cazeaux at the time of the Académie de Médecine debate on ovariotomy.

As a method of research, however, vivisection was extremely controversial in Britain. There were tensions in the medical profession between those who saw progress in medicine as being inextricably linked up with scientific research, which involved vivisection, and those who preferred to see the practice of medicine as an art to which any method of research overlooking the patient must be inconsequential.[42] Medical opposition to vivisection first flared up, interestingly enough, shortly before the ovariotomy controversy got in full swing. In the 1830s, during the celebrated Bell-Magendie priority dispute over spinal nerve root function, the vivisectionist experiments carried out by the French physiologist Magendie were strongly condemned in Britain as an expression of materialist philosophical doctrines which the pious English abhorred.[43]

Underneath these nationalistic disputes, one can thus identify a deeper convergence in the methods of studying and treating problems of life and disease. Ovariotomy and vivisection were unified by the same analytical methodology, by the same activist and empiricist approach, and the suggestion was made that ovariotomists, like the vivisectionist experimenters, were devaluing life to the point of treating human beings like objects. Within a perspective in which belief in the sacredness and inviolability of life were becoming progressively undermined, ovariotomists could feel justified in jeopardising the life of their patients during the course of a dangerous operation, while the rationale for medical intervention became a question of assessing the *relative* value of the patient's life. It could be argued, as the physician Thomas Radford did in defence of the caesarean section, that the value of women's lives derived from their reproductive function;[44] thus if a woman was unfit to fulfil her domestic duties because of disease in the generative organs, it was no great loss if her life was sacrificed, either for the sake of the foetus, or in the hope of a cure.

Pathological pregnancies

The proponents of ovariotomy emphasised the dangers of ovarian disease and argued that women stood a far greater chance of dying from this malady than from ovariotomy. What grounds were there for this assertion, in the face of counterclaims that ovarian disease was never fatal? From the beginning of the nineteenth century, the view had gradually emerged that cysts were more likely to occur in the ovary than in any other organ of the female body. Cysts developed from an unnatural accumulation of fluid in the Graafian follicles: they were vesicles that failed to rupture and became pathologically enlarged. The period from puberty to the menopause, when the ovaries were at the peak of their activity, carried the greatest danger of ovarian disease.[45] 'In proceeding to estimate the frequency and importance of the diseases of the ovaries', wrote the famous surgeon and ovariotomist Thomas Spencer Wells in Quain's *Dictionary of Medicine*,

we have to consider the wonderful series of periodical processes which go on in women every month for some thirty-five years ... We have to remember that at each menstrual period one or other of the ovaries becomes swollen ... We must consider, further, how these periodical processes are associated with much that is of supreme importance in the state of the nervous centres, and in the mental condition of women ... When we bear in mind these highly complex conditions, processes, and relations, the wonder is, not that ovarian disease should be so frequent, but that so many women pass through life without suffering from them.[46]

The alleged incidence and seriousness of ovarian disease legitimated the view that sex and reproduction dominated women's body and mind. Ovarian cysts were the pathological analogue of ovulation and pregnancy; ovariotomy, with its likeness to a caesarean section, became the method for their delivery.

The perceived similarity between ovarian disease and pregnancy was often the source of diagnostic errors: it was not uncommon to mistake an ovarian cyst for a pregnancy, and vice-versa. Hospital records provide evidence of what was a recognised hazard of ovariotomy. In 1864, for instance, two of the patients on the gynaecological ward of the Middlesex Hospital were mistakenly diagnosed as suffering from an ovarian tumour. In one case, the patient was examined on admission and found to be pregnant.[47] The other is a little more perplexing. The patient, a twenty-two-year-old servant, presented an 'obscure fluctuation in right side ... Tawney areola round nipple, enlarged follicles, milk in breast'. No medical practitioner should have failed to make a diagnosis of pregnancy on the basis of these signs, yet the patient underwent an operation for ovariotomy which ended in her death.[48]

We cannot surmise what prompted the surgeons at the Middlesex to perform ovariotomy in this case, but it is possible that the diagnosis of ovarian disease may occasionally have served to conceal a pregnancy. In the 1907 edition of his *Medical Ethics*, the physician Robert Saundby maintained that an eminent gynaecologist had once been asked to take a young unmarried woman to his Surgical Home as a case of ovarian tumour in order that the child might be born there.[49] In Saundby's example, the gynaecologist refused to be a party to the plan, but less scrupulous practitioners may well have acted otherwise. Some may sometimes have colluded with wealthy patients in abortion and sterilisation under the guise of ovariotomy. Abortion and birth control were officially condemned by the Victorian medical profession, hence we should not expect to find evidence for these practices in textbooks of obstetrics and gynaecology.[50] Fiction writers were not so constrained by ethical considerations and were thus able to treat these sensitive issues without reticence. In his novel entitled *Fécondité* and published in 1899, Emile Zola devoted a lot of space to investigating the contraceptive uses of ovariotomy. Medical practitioners were familiar with this work and agreed that it was well researched.[51]

Fécondité is a novel about fertility, written at a time of internal political turmoil in France, when the Dreyfus affair, fears about population decline, concerns over national security and class conflicts divided the nation.[52] The novel was the first of a planned series of four *Evangiles*, in which the French author intended to set out his social religion of the future. Zola believed that social reconciliation could be accomplished through fertility, work and justice, and in

Fécondité he elaborated his dream of a prosperous France secured through the victory of fruitfulness and maternity over selfishness and sterility. The novel is the epic tale of a family, the Froments, who abandon the town and settle in the country where they struggle to raise a large family and make a living out of the land. While everyone derides their efforts and their wondrous fecundity, the Froments continue to procreate and reclaim sterile land. The novel ends happily with the celebration of the new peasant dynasty they have succeeded in creating after 70 years of marriage – an army of 158 children, grandchildren and great-grandchildren. This is in sharp contrast to the tragic lot of their selfish friends and acquaintances, who have been led to death, financial ruin, disease and lunacy by the pursuit of worldly pleasures. The female characters in particular, unlike Madame Froment, have rejected the sacred calling of motherhood in favour of sterility and licentiousness; none of them however escapes the dire fate which Zola thinks they deserve.

Perhaps the most tragic of these figures is Reine Morange, the only daughter of an honest and law-abiding couple. The Moranges have high hopes for Reine, but alas they are destined to remain unfulfilled, for the young girl is fatally led astray by the beautiful Baroness Sérafine de Lowicz. Sérafine's depravation is legend among the Parisian beau monde: people claim that she roams the streets of Paris at night, driven by her insatiable passion, and dressed up as a servant she searches for brutal males whose violence she relishes. Sérafine becomes Reine's mentor and introduces her to a life of vice and illicit pleasures. After a secret holiday in the country in the company of the Baroness and her friends, Reine discovers that she is pregnant. Sérafine resolves to help her by seeking out the services of an ovariotomist of dubious reputation. Deeming it expedient not to draw the surgeon into open complicity, Sérafine explains to him that the girl is suffering from some obscure ailment, probably of ovarian origin, but hints that Reine's disease is pregnancy: after all, muses Sérafine, ovariotomists often diagnose an ovarian cyst only to find a foetus when they open the abdomen. Upon payment of a large fee, the surgeon obligingly colludes: he diagnoses a tumour and advises an operation. This is secretly carried out, but Reine subsequently has a haemorrhage and dies.[53] Only a few pages earlier, her mother had preceded her into the grave after an illegal abortion, which she had sought as a means of limiting her family.[54]

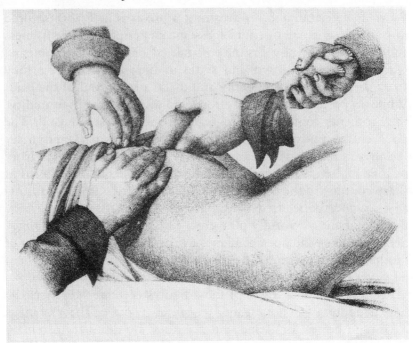

4 Extraction of foetus by caesarean section

Another episode suggests that the removal of ovaries may have been carried out for contraceptive purposes. In Book 4 the hyper-sexed Sérafine confides in Mathieu Froment and tells him that a 'miscarriage' has deranged her whole system. For this reason she has sought the advice of a local practitioner, the evocatively named Dr Mainfroy, who is trying to build up a gynaecological practice in the neighbourhood. Mainfroy has realised that Sérafine is suffering from a procured abortion, but he says nothing. He claims instead that the alleged miscarriage has displaced something in her repro-ductive system, greatly enhancing her chances of becoming preg-nant. Sérafine shudders at the thought; during the consultation, Mainfroy speaks of a 'certain operation' which, he intimates, would at a stroke cure her disease and render her incapable of having children. Thus from the time of the abortion there takes place a 'slow comedy' between Sérafine and Mainfroy, 'in which they could mutually believe themselves the victims of good faith'. Séra-fine gradually exaggerates the gravity of her sufferings; Mainfroy for his part emphasises the chronicity of her complaint, as he does

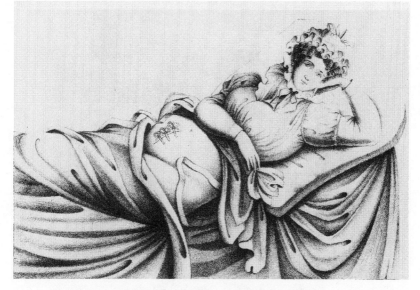

5 Closure of the wound after caesarean section

not want to lose his wealthy patient too soon. Finally, one day he diagnoses an ovarian cyst and arranges for Sérafine to have an ovariotomy.[55] Sérafine cannot wait to be freed from the fear of pregnancy, but she too will receive her just deserts: with the loss of her ovaries, Sérafine not only loses her sexual passion, but also her peculiarly female attractions and her youthfulness, which contemporary medical opinion held to be dependent on healthy ovarian functioning. Sérafine will end her existence a frigid spectre of her former self, yet another victim sacrificed on the altar of selfish pleasures and lust.[56]

In England the removal of healthy ovaries was suggested by the obstetrician Alfred Meadows as a sterilisation procedure in cases in which childbirth might endanger the mother's life: 'It may be a question for consideration', he wrote in 1886,

whether, in women who are the subjects of such pelvic distortions, that the birth of a living child *per vias naturales* is an impossibility, the removal of the ovaries, and with them the Fallopian tubes, as being both useless and, possibly, troublesome, ought not to be performed.

In Meadows' view, the removal of both ovaries as a preventive measure was preferable both to the caesarean section once the pregnancy had occurred, and to mechanical means of birth-control:

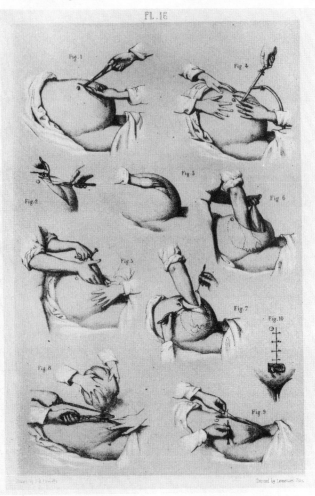

6 Extraction of an ovarian cyst

I contend that, on moral grounds, too, it is far better that, in these special cases, this operation should be performed rather than those so-called safeguards should be practised to prevent impregnation, which are, too often, not only disgusting and revolting to the female mind, but are absolutely demoralising, and tend to destroy that proper modesty which should exist between married people.[57]

Whether the removal of healthy ovaries as a safeguard against pregnancy was in the best interest of the patient as well as of morality, though, was a question which Meadows did not care to elaborate. By the time he was writing, ovariotomy patients still had approximately a 10 per cent chance of death in the hands of the more

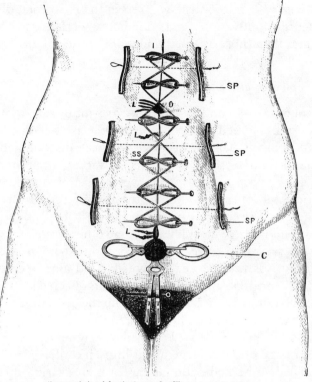

Closure of the abdominal wound. (Wieland and Dubrisay.)

7 Closure of the wound after ovariotomy

skilled operators. Medical men regarded this figure as acceptable, but patients thought otherwise and, as we saw in the last chapter, often refused to consent to the operation. This took place against a background of increasing surgical interventionism, as illustrated by the number of operations performed at the Chelsea Hospital for Women in the last quarter of the nineteenth century. Until 1884, ovariotomy was performed in half of the cases of ovarian disease; by 1889, the proportion had risen to over two-thirds (see table 5).

What factors led to the acceptance of ovariotomy? Much has been made of a presumed reduction in the mortality of the operation during the 1850s, yet it seems clear that ovariotomy became accepted long before there had been any significant diminution in its mortality rates.[58] Doubts must also be cast over the role of anti-sepsis in reducing the mortality of ovariotomy: many late nineteenth-century ovariotomists worked in the most total distrust of such scientific innovations, and nonetheless were able to boast even lower rates than those attained under antiseptic conditions.

The triumph of ovariotomy

After Robert Lee's condemnation of ovariotomy in 1850, it had been generally agreed that the operation was unacceptable. Surgeons and obstetricians in London had been discouraged by this denunciation and most had given up any further attempts at ovariotomy. In the provinces surgeons were undeterred and continued to perform the operation despite the risk of censure from their colleagues, but it seems clear that in the early 1850s ovariotomies were few and far between. The only one other surgeon apart from Clay who seems to have performed more than the occasional ovariotomy was Isaac Baker Brown. He did nine operations between 1854 and 1856 and only two patients survived.[59]

In 1857 Thomas Spencer Wells took up the operation, and over a period of twenty-one years he managed to reduce the mortality of ovariotomy from over 50 to 11 per cent.[60] Few could have predicted such a dramatic improvement. Wells himself confessed in 1884 that when he had embarked upon his career as an ovariotomist everything was against the venture. His first attempt in 1857 had been a complete failure and had strengthened the conviction in his mind that he 'might be entering upon a path which would lead rather to an unenviable notoriety than to a sound professional reputation'.[61] Wells claimed that the suffering of increasing numbers of poor women, who were anxious for relief at any risk, had spurred him onto the dreaded path of surgical intervention. There is no reason to doubt the genuineness of Wells' claims, but for critics of ovariotomy like Robert Lee ovariotomy was largely a 'money question and not one of science or humanity'. Ovariotomies were lucrative, Dr Lee alleged in 1862, and the reason why operators were rushing into the field was greed, not altruism.[62]

In 1862 Dr Lee once more attacked the ovariotomists at a meeting of the Royal Medico-Chirurgical Society. He repeated much the same arguments he had used in 1850, stressing that the published results of ovariotomy did not truthfully represent its statistics. Wells protested that his own pre-operative diagnoses had been remarkably accurate and that he never failed to record his results.

His mortality rate, however, was appalling. He had performed fifty operations by the end of 1862 and lost thirty-three patients – well over half. These results compared unfavourably with those of Charles Clay, who had been so harshly criticised by the London medical establishment in 1850, yet Dr Lee found that few practitioners were now prepared to endorse his condemnation of ovariotomy. Dr Savage, of the Samaritan Free Hospital, accused Lee of never having seen the operation. Dr William Tyler Smith, one of the founders of the Obstetrical Society of London, declared himself a convert.[63] Shortly before Dr Lee was due to deliver his paper, a leader in the *British Medical Journal* warned the profession that Dr Lee would, 'we doubt not, blow a counterblast to the proceedings but one as unavailing as was the trumpet of King James against tobacco smoking'.[64] After Dr Lee's onslaught against all 'belly rippers', the journal admonished the eminent obstetrician that he should 'moderate his tone and his language at these discussions'.[65] Although the mortality of ovariotomy had not changed since 1850, the tide had turned in favour of the operation.

This dramatic change of opinion was largely due to the introduction of anaesthesia in the late 1840s. Anaesthesia had slowly revolutionised the social relations between surgeon and patient, removing some of the moral and psychological barriers to the performance of excruciating operations. Surgeons, who had been accustomed to inflicting torturing pain, now found themselves operating on an unconscious patient in place of a writhing, screaming creature. The result was that surgeons began to operate on a greater proportion of cases, while patients, who in pre-anaesthesia days were not unknown to flee from the operating table, started to request surgery more frequently. By the late 1850s, surgeons were operating far more often and covering a wider field, and operations for hernia, vaginal fistula and diseased joints had been devised.[66] Anaesthesia also removed one of the main moral objections against vivisection, which is why Claude Bernard started to use anaesthetic agents in his experiments as soon as they were introduced.[67]

The attempts at ovariotomy made by men like Wells, Charles Clay and Baker Brown in the 1850s were carried out without any knowledge of antisepsis; later, in the 1870s and 1880s, after Lister had publicised his antiseptic method, they were continued in an atmosphere of widespread scepticism about 'Listerism'. This was commonly understood as the 'carbolic acid treatment' of wounds

and was variously interpreted by Lister's contemporaries. Some
surgeons applied the acid freely to the wound, others took it to
mean the continuous irrigation of the wound with carbolic acid for
five weeks; some had come to regard the acid as a panacea that
would prevent suppuration even in the most appalling septic conditions.[68] On the whole, however, British surgeons were notori-
ously slow in accepting Lister's antiseptic methods and grasping the
rationale for it, and ovariotomists were no exception – indeed many
obstetricians must have carried the germs of infection from septic
ovariotomy patients to their maternity cases. Even Spencer Wells,
who in 1878 adopted antiseptic techniques in his practice, argued
that the environment in which the operation was performed was far
more important than carbolic acid. He attached great weight to
comfort and clean air, special nursing care and the isolation of the
patient in a single room: 'For my part', he maintained at the end of
1878,

I would rather operate in a clean, quiet, well-warmed, and well-ventilated
building, be it large or small, without any antiseptic precautions, than run
the risk of trusting to the neutralising or destructive power of chlorine or
iodine, sulphur or tar, borax or the permanganates, salicylic or any other
acid, in a place tainted by the presence of sewer-gas, or the seeds of some
infectious or contagious disease.[69]

His ideal was to operate in a private home or in the country, and
long after the introduction of antisepsis he believed that ovariotomy should not be performed in a large hospital, where patients
were exposed to foul odours and exhalations.

While Wells was at least disposed to give Listerism a fair trial,
other ovariotomists were strongly opposed to it and argued their
case on the strength of operative results that were even better than
those produced by the Listerian ovariotomists. An interesting
example of this was provided by the gynaecologist Granville Bantock, who was a colleague of Wells at the Samaritan Free Hospital.
Both practised under the same environmental conditions, but while
Wells had adopted antiseptic precautions, Bantock used the soap
and water method, and claimed that this yielded better operative
results than Spencer Wells'. At a meeting of the British Gynaecological Society in 1889, Bantock stated that he had until then
performed 400 ovariotomies. In his first one hundred cases, carried
out under antiseptic conditions, he had lost nineteen patients; in the
second series of one hundred cases, while he was abandoning that

method, he had lost fourteen. Since then, the mortality rate in his practice had fallen to four only in the last series of one hundred operations. Between April 1885 and October 1888, Bantock had had ninety cases and no deaths; in the same period at the Samaritan Hospital the mortality rate under the Listerian method exceeded 12 per cent.[70] Bantock had abandoned the spray devised by Lister to kill the airborne germs around the operating table. He believed that the spray had come to be used like a fetish by the Listerian surgeons, without any understanding of its rationale and purpose. 'For the most part', Bantock remarked,

it is seen to be put to a purpose for which it was never intended by its inventor, i.e. playing upon the ceiling, or against a wall, or anywhere but on the field of operation. This is at best a most illogical proceeding, and I am quite at a loss to understand the process of reasoning – if there be any – which leads to such a practice.[71]

The reason why the spray was pointed away from the operating table was that often both surgeon and patient became drenched with carbolic acid: the chemical badly affected the operator, turning his fingers white and numb and causing severe skin irritation. This is also why the spray was eventually discarded by surgeons. Bantock's reasons for abandoning it, however, were theoretical rather than practical: he totally disbelieved in the harmfulness of germs, thus in his view cold water from the tap was just as good as antiseptic solutions when washing out the peritoneum during ovariotomy.[72] Similar views were shared by Lawson Tait, who had begun to perform ovariotomy in 1872 in spite of having seen thirty ovariotomies in Edinburgh without a single recovery. In 1871 Tait reported ten ovariotomies with three deaths. At this stage he used what he called 'Listerian precautions', but without much conviction:

My opinion of the antiseptic treatment is that its merits have been greatly over-rated, and its good results, which are quite as uncertain as those of other means, are due more to the greater care taken of the cases, and to the exclusion of air.[73]

By 1882 Tait had become a strong opponent of Listerism, which he later defined as a 'strange phase of surgical eccentricity'.[74] He had performed one hundred ovariotomies without antisepsis, with only three deaths in the series.[75] Antisepsis, he argued, did not prevent suppuration, and the good results depended not on the exclusion of germs, but on the 'power of vital resistance' of the tissues and on the condition of the patient.[76] Tait attributed his success to increased personal experience, the disciplinary regime to which he subjected both the nursing staff and the patient and the improvement of some of the techniques of ovariotomy, in particular the treatment of the pedicle to which the ovary was attached.[77] This was a question to which ovariotomists paid a lot of attention, as a haemorrhaging pedicle was a frequent cause of death. Tait preferred to tie the pedicle and drop it into the abdomen;[78] his colleague Thomas Keith instead cauterised it, and claimed that this alone gave a mortality rate of 8 per cent without using antisepsis.[79]

Many reasons thus accounted for the improvement in the mortality rates after ovariotomy. Attention to hygiene and pre- and post-operative care played a part; so did the general conditions of the patient, and these had greatly improved. Encouraged by the prospect of painless surgery, ovariotomists now intervened more frequently and at the early stages of ovarian disease; they had also begun to remove ovaries that were 'prolapsed' but otherwise healthy, and to perform ovariotomy for the treatment of nebulous conditions which are not nowadays regarded as pathological states, for example 'ovarian cyrrhosis'.

A triumphant mood now accompanied the operative exploits of the ovariotomists, which Zola admirably captured in his fictional portrayal of the celebrated Parisian ovariotomist Gaude. Here the conquest of ovarian disease by surgery became subtly blended with the domination of the passive female patient by the brutal male surgeon:

À l'hôpital, Gaude regnait sur les trois salles de femmes, en maître tout-puissant et glorifié. C'était un praticien de premier ordre, une admirable intelligence, gaie et brutale, servie par une main d'une décision, d'une adresse sans pareilles ... Il pratiquait au plain jour de la publicité, il aurait convié tout Paris autour de sa table d'opération. Des peintures, des gravures, des dessins l'avaient popularisé, au travail, le grand tablier blanc noué sur la poitrine, les poignet nus, beau comme un dieu qui tranche et dispose de la vie. Il était seul à ouvrir un ventre, à régarder, puis à recoudre, avec cette ampleur magistrale. Parfois, il le rouvrait, pour mieux voir ... S'il y avait erreur de diagnostic, s'il se trouvait en présence d'un organe sain, il enlevait tout de même quelque chose, ne voulant pas recoudre sans avoir coupé. Et, d'un bout de Paris à l'autre, ses succès opératoires répandaient, célébraient cette maîtrise prodigieuse qu'il avait acquise, en s'exerçant la main sur des milliers de pauvres diablesses.[80]

Ovaries also began to be removed in the 1870s and 1880s for the cure of uterine fibromata, dysmenorrhoea and 'menstrual epilepsy', a condition which was believed to originate from continued ovarian pain during the menstrual period. This controversial procedure was popularised by the American Robert Battey, who called it 'normal ovariotomy' to denote the fact that it involved the removal of non-cystic ovaries. Battey at first removed only one ovary, but when he found that the operation did not always produce the hoped-for results, he began to extirpate both ovaries. Normal ovariotomy was renamed 'Battey's operation' by the American gynaecologist J. M. Sims, one of the most enthusiastic advocates of that procedure; in Britain, the term 'oöphorectomy' was generally used.[81] There was considerable debate as to whether the ovaries thus removed were diseased or not: Battey himself insisted that he was excising diseased ovaries, reflecting a general lack of consensus on what constituted ovarian disease. The German gynaecologist Hegar (1830–1914), for instance, gave examples of surgeons who assumed the existence of anatomical disease in the ovaries if nervous symptoms appeared, in spite of the negative results of the examinations.[82] As Thomas Savage (1839–1907), one of the British proponents of Battey's operation, acknowledged, the exact line of demarcation between ovariotomy proper and Battey's operation could not be clearly made out.[83]

Oöphorectomy was not as prevalent in Britain as it was in America. Most gynaecologists objected to the operation because they believed that it induced not only sterility, but also the loss of sexual feelings and the assumption of the masculine characteristics. At a time of fears about the decline of the race, labour unrest and feminist agitation, the 'unsexing' of women was focussed on as a threat to marriage and the sexual division of labour, the two pillars on which the stability of society and the supremacy of the British nation rested.[84] As the *British Medical Journal* argued in 1887, there was a widespread feeling that the ovaries should be respected because they were 'the organs of sexual life, making a woman what she is, fitting for the duties of womanhood, including childbearing'.[85] The *Lancet* took the view that there was a field for Battey's operation, but it pointed out that a field was such by virtue of hedges or other limits, and reminded oöphorectomists in America that a field was 'not a *prairie*'.[86]

Uncertainty about the nature of ovarian disease gave many British gynaecologists reason to believe that too many ovaries were being removed unnecessarily, either for what they regarded as trivial diseases or notwithstanding the fact that, they claimed, the ovaries thus removed were perfectly healthy. Foremost critic of the operation in Britain was the surgeon Thomas Spencer Wells. In 1891 Wells launched a scathing attack against oöphorectomy:

The meshes of the physical, mental, and moral network of reasons why the operation should be done are so closely woven that few cases of a perplexing nature, that can anyhow be connected with the generative organs or functions, have a chance of escaping laparotomy or something more ... We might at least require some evidence of the ovaries being diseased before consenting to their extirpation in the hope of curing any of those vague disorders to which women are so subject, which are often dispelled by moral treatment or social changes ... [and which] often return after cure in any way, and leave the hopeless being the prey of unscrupulous or illogically enthusiastic experimenters. The danger is now increasing as the operation is becoming world-wide. The oöphorecto-mists of civilization touch hands with the aboriginal spayers of New Zealand. The ovary is, in fact, the nucleus of gynaecological science and the source of gynaecological practice. Its products give occupation to the obstetrical art. The disturbances it sets up in the system at large are the prairie of gynaecological proletarians. The morbid structural changes, displacements, and accidents of it and its appendages are the arena of its operators. Wonderful, indeed, is woman's hydra-like tolerance of sections and mutilations under their hands![87]

Wells also led the campaign against salpingo-oöphorectomy, or 'Tait's operation', a procedure involving the removal of the ovary and Fallopian tube, which Tait had devised as a cure for pelvic haematocele. Wells made it sound more barbarous than ovari-otomy and denounced it as a 'spaying' operation; Tait retorted that the removal of the uterine 'appendages' and the spaying of animals could not be compared because they were done for entirely differ-ent purposes.[88] The controversy, which was fuelled by the rivalry between Wells and the flamboyant Birmingham gynaecologist, divided the profession for many years, culminating in a rumpus over the surgical work of the Liverpool obstetrician Francis Imlach in 1886.

Oöphorectomy was also opposed by feminists and anti-vivisec-tionists: 'The great increase in ovariotomy, and its extension to the insane is a notable result of this *prurigo secandi* [itch to cut]', wrote Elizabeth Blackwell in *Essays in Medical Sociology*.[89] For Blackwell, who was committed to a vision of social progress through the 'spiritual power of maternity', the removal of ovaries was a heinous crime. Oöphorectomy deprived women of their true essence and prevented them from fulfilling their proper destiny in society as mothers and moral leaders; indeed the operation, like the practice of vivisection, outraged morality and violated life itself. The idea that gynaecological surgery was an extension of vivisection can be seen in the belief, current in 1888, that the gruesome series of murders of women attributed to 'Jack the Ripper' was the work of a vivisecting surgeon from London University.[90] The high mortality rates at the Chelsea Hospital in 1894 did very little to allay these fears.

The view that the removal of ovaries was a crime against society was forcefully expressed by terms such as 'maim' and 'mutilation', which came to be widely used as synonyms for oöphorectomy during the last quarter of the nineteenth century. In common law, 'maim' or 'mayhem' defined any act which permanently disabled and weakened a man, rendering him less able to fight. Breaking the incisors, blinding an eye, cutting off an arm, hand, foot or finger and, significantly, castration, were maiming injuries because they reduced the value of the victim as a soldier. As the sovereign was deemed to have a right to the services of those who owed him allegiance, maim was classed as a crime and it was punishable with life imprisonment under Section 18 of the Offences Against the Person Act (1861). The offence of maim did not apply to maiming injuries inflicted upon women: this was probably because women were not required to engage in military service, and because castration was regarded as a standard example of maim.[91] By defining the removal of the ovaries as a 'castrating' or 'spaying' operation, the critics of oöphorectomy exposed the sexual asymmetry which underlay the crime of maim and suggested that oöphorectomy, too, was unlawful and contrary to the public interest. An implicit parallel was drawn between the military value of men and that of women: men were useful as the backbone of fleets and armies, women as the suppliers of the future fighters for the nation. In the last quarter of the nineteenth century, as Britain embarked upon its most ambitious programme of colonial expansion, imperialism stood little chance of success without motherhood.

The sexual imagery which suffused gynaecological surgery took on disturbing connotations for feminists and anti-vivisectionists: oöphorectomists violated life and, by metaphorical association, they raped women, who were the quintessence of life. This theme was clearly articulated in *The Beth Book* (1897), a loosely auto-biographical novel written by the anti-vivisectionist and purity reform campaigner Sarah Grand. In this novel the heroine Beth is married off to Dr Daniel Maclure, medical superintendent of a Lock Hospital. Beth finds it very difficult to tolerate her husband's interest in venereal disease, but what finally induces her to leave him is the discovery that he is a vivisector. Beth's rebellion against her husband's scientific activities is at one and the same time a refusal to submit to his authority:

Look here, sir, I am not going to have any of your *damnable* cruelties going on under the same roof with me. I have endured your sensuality and your corrupt conversation weakly . . . but I know better now. I know that every woman who submits in such matters is not only a party to her own degradation, but connives at the degradation of her whole sex . . . I cannot understand any but unsexed women associating with vivisectors.[92]

Only a woman who had herself lost the capacity to engender life could contemplate marriage to a sexual sadist who negated life in cruel and violent experiments. The meaning of the *Beth Book* was symbolic, but it is uncanny how close it came to describing the marital vicissitudes of none other than Claude Bernard. Bernard, as we have seen, was an avowed vivisector, whereas his wife supported the French equivalent of the Society for the Protection of Cruelty to Animals. It did not make for a happy marriage, and a decree of separation was granted in 1870.[93]

The Imlach affair

The controversy over the 'unsexing' of women reached a peak in 1886, when a scandal broke out in Liverpool over the surgical work carried out by Dr Francis Imlach (1851–1920) at the Hospital for Women in Shaw Street. The son of a doctor, Imlach had qualified as an MD at Edinburgh University. He was instrumental in establishing the Women's Hospital and, when the hospital opened in 1882, he joined its staff as a gynaecological surgeon. Imlach was deeply influenced by Tait's teaching. Between 1884 and 1885 he presented a number of papers at the Liverpool Medical Institution, in which he described many operations for the removal of the uterine appendages. At these meetings the senior surgeon at the Women's Hospital, Dr Thomas Grimsdale (1823–1902), and the Professor of Midwifery, John Wallace (1839–98), strongly criticised Imlach's tendency to perform radical surgery in cases previously managed by medical means. Wallace and Grimsdale were renowned for their conservative approach to operative intervention in gynaecology; there may also have been professional rivalries, since young Imlach claimed success in about 94 per cent of cases, against Professor Wallace's statistics of twelve operations with a 50 per cent mortality.[94]

In December 1885 Imlach read a paper at the Liverpool Medical Institution, relating forty-one operations in which he had removed both ovaries and tubes for the cure of pyosalpinx (accumulation of pus in the Fallopian tubes), hydrosalpinx (accumulation of serous fluid in the Fallopian tubes) and haematosalpinx (accumulation of blood in the Fallopian tubes). Imlach had only had three deaths, but his colleagues were not impressed. The discussion revealed deep concern about the number and nature of the abdominal operations Imlach was performing at the Women's Hospital. It later transpired that he had been practising salpingo-oöphorectomy in cases of 'menstrual epilepsy', prolapsed and atrophied ovaries and ovarian pain. The number of abdominal operations performed at the Shaw Street hospital had doubled from 86 in 1884 to 176 in 1885 with a mortality rate of 9 per cent. Nearly half of all the patients admitted had undergone abdominal section, and 64 per cent of these had had ovaries and tubes removed. Imlach had performed 80 per cent of the total number of operations for the removal of the uterine append-ages.[95] Dr Wallace condemned the procedure as 'unsexing women' and claimed that its consequences were not properly explained to the patient. In the discussion a member argued that the function of the ovaries was already destroyed by disease, but the vast majority of speakers supported Dr Wallace.[96]

In February 1886 Dr William Carter reported the case of a woman who had been successfully operated on by Mr Frank Paul (1851–1941) for urinary calculi. He observed that a year before the patient had had her ovaries removed by Dr Imlach on the suppo-sition that she was suffering from ovarian disease. Carter alleged that the woman had been unsexed and that Liverpool was gaining a 'most unenviable notoriety' in consequence of the frequency with which ovaries were removed at the Shaw Street hospital. Imlach, who was in attendance, refuted the charges of over-operating and argued that the ovaries he removed were diseased. Without warn-ing, Dr Grimsdale proposed a motion to set up an inquiry into the 'grave question of practice and ethics' of these operations at the Women's Hospital. The motion was carried and a Committee of Inquiry was elected, with Grimsdale himself nominating the members.[97]

The publication of the report was delayed by a civil action for damages brought against Imlach by a patient called Casey. In August 1886 Imlach was accused of improperly removing the ovaries and Fallopian tubes of Mrs Casey after diagnosing her condition as a case of haematosalpinx and haematocele. Imlach was charged of performing the operation without any proven necessity and without the patient's consent. It was also claimed that the operation had been performed without prior consultation with one of the medical officers for in-patients, as required by rule 39 of the hospital. During the trial Mrs Casey stated that as a result of the operation the menopause had set in, and there had been 'a change not only in her own life, but in the life of her husband'; she also complained of weakness and giddiness. Summoned as a witness for the plaintiff, Dr Grimsdale stated that Mrs Casey's condition did not justify an operation. He had had many cases like that, and most of them recovered with medical treatment and prolonged rest. Lawson Tait, Thomas Savage, James Aveling and J. Grieg Smith, surgeon to the Bristol Royal Infirmary, supported Imlach and criticised Grimsdale as 'out of date'. Luckily for Imlach, a nurse confirmed that the patient had been informed of the nature of the operation. This cleared Imlach's name and a not-guilty verdict was promptly returned by the jury.[98]

The trial and the inquiry into the practice of gynaecology at the Hospital for Women caused a furore in Liverpool. Letters from the public and from medical practitioners questioned the ethics of oöphorectomy and alleged that the women of Liverpool were being unsexed and subjected to experimentation. This was ironic, since Tait, the eponym of the operation under discussion, was one of the chief medical opponents of vivisection.[99] In a fit of pique Grimsdale leaked to the Liverpool daily papers a letter by Spencer Wells, which indicted Imlach's surgical work. Wells was one of a number of eminent gynaecologists who had been asked by the hospital secretary to comment on the statistics of abdominal operations at the women's hospital. 'I feel bound to say', he had replied,

as the total number of in-patients in the Hospital in 1886 [sic] was only 347, the statement that 111 [sic] of these, or nearly one-third, were subjected to abdominal section, is so shocking as to be almost incredible.[100]

Wells, of course, was one of the arch-critics of 'Tait's operation'; as a surgeon, he was also opposed to the performance of gynaecological operations by obstetric physicians. Imlach, who was an obstetrician practising salpingo-oöphorectomy, gave Wells a golden opportunity to kill two birds with one stone.[101]

Tait at once wrote to the *Liverpool Courier* to protest against the publication of this letter and stated that the percentage of cases submitted to abdominal section at the Samaritan Hospital in London, where Wells worked, was the same as at the Shaw Street hospital. He later accused Grimsdale of having instigated Mrs Casey to bring an action against Imlach.[102] The controversy was eagerly pursued in the chief medical journal. The editor of the *Lancet* claimed that Imlach had removed healthy ovaries for a trivial disease, and emotively described the operation as 'spaying'.[103] The *British Medical Journal*, apparently inspired by Lawson Tait, took the opposite view. Tait believed that Mrs Casey was suffering from an old ruptured tubal pregnancy with recurrent haemorrhage, and claimed that her case was therefore unique.[104]

It was in this heated atmosphere that the Committee of Inquiry instituted by the Liverpool Medical Institution set about its work. The investigation left no stone unturned. The acting medical officers were requested to draw up a full report of all the operations performed during the previous twelve months, stating the circumstances of each case, the subsequent state of the patient, whether the operation had been done after consultation with another member of staff and with the full consent of the patient. The reports were subsequently analysed by the Medical Board of the hospital, and a number of patients were visited in their homes by members of the inquiry committee. Information about the subsequent progress of surgical patients was also sought from medical practitioners in Liverpool. Finally, specimens of ovaries and Fallopian tubes removed by Imlach and voluntarily submitted by him were subjected to pathological investigation.[105]

In November 1886 the report of the Inquiry Committee was published. It was stated that the performance of ovariotomy for the removal of ovarian cysts, and of exploratory incisions into the abdomen had been justified. However, the Committee had reser-

vations about the propriety of oöphorrhaphy (the fixation of prolapsed ovaries) and of salpingo-oöphorectomy, the operation
which had been at the centre of the controversy. No evidence had
been found that ovariotomised women had lost their feminine
characters; several women, however, had reported that they had
suffered a distinct loss of their sexual feelings, causing serious
domestic unhappiness. Commenting on these findings, the Committee stressed that the question under investigation was not purely
surgical, but ethical and moral,

for whether it be regarded as a mere sentimental objection or not, the
removal of the organs which are characteristic of sex is, and always will be,
viewed by the public and the profession with great misgiving. In consequence, such an operation should only be performed after the most careful
consideration.[106]

As a result of the inquiry, the Committee expressed the opinion that
the staff at the Hospital for Women had failed to exercise sufficient
care and discrimination in the selection of cases for operation. The
Committee further stated that operations had been performed
without proper consultation between members of staff, and that
patients had not been fully apprised of the dangers and consequences of salpingo-oöphorectomy. This report wrecked Imlach's
promising career: when he came up for re-election in 1887, he was
turned down after a somewhat suspect organisation of proxy votes.
Imlach had to give up practice as a gynaecologist and was never
reinstated, despite the efforts made by his supporters within the
Medical Institution to have the inquiry overthrown.[107]

   The Imlach affair brought into relief not only beliefs about the
biological basis of femininity, but also profound tensions within the
obstetrical profession over the propriety of radical operations. It
further catalysed a professional dispute between surgeons and obstetric physicians over the performance of gynaecological operations. This conflict underlay the establishment of professional
organisations of gynaecologists between 1884 and 1929.

6

From the British Gynaecological Society to the Royal College of Obstetricians and Gynaecologists

When the three Goddesses met on the Summit of Mount Ida, the envy, hatred, malice, and all uncharitableness with which each regarded the other two, as possible possessors of the apple about to be awarded by the too happy shepherd, were no doubt veiled under the usual compliments about personal appearance of which the sex is so great a mistress. But had these ladies had an idea of the prophetical significance of the scene which they were unconsciously enacting, especially of the apple ... charity forbids us to doubt that they would have resorted to the quickest and most certain means of its destruction. Whether they would have thrown it at the head of PARIS or down the slope of Mount Ida ... we have not time to speculate. But ZEUS or HERMES would have won our eternal gratitude had he whispered in the ear of any one of the three that the apple was an ovarian tumour, and that the three Goddesses were the prophetical types of the general surgeon, abdominal surgeon, and obstetrician respectively.[1]

Thus wrote the *Lancet* in the summer of 1884, on the eve of the foundation of the British Gynaecological Society. The question discussed in the venomous editorial divided the obstetrical profession for many years to come. It provoked a schism within the Obstetrical Society of London which led directly to the establishment of the first association of gynaecologists in Britain; it provided much of the impetus for the foundation of the College of Obstetricians and Gynaecologists in 1929; it was also a focus for other divisions within the profession – between the advocates of radical operations and those who favoured a more conservative approach to women's diseases, between general and special hospital practitioners, between the provinces and London.

The 'handcuffed obstetrician'

A variety of practitioners had contributed to the development of ovariotomy in the first half of the nineteenth century: some were general surgeons, others were obstetricians, others still were sur-

geon-apothecaries. In the last quarter of the century, as ovariotomy
became an accepted surgical procedure, the allocation of cases in
hospital practice emerged as the cause of a fierce dispute between
obstetricians and surgeons. The centre of the controversy was in the
London teaching hospitals, but its ripples also reached some of the
metropolitan women's hospitals and the provinces. At the London
general hospitals, the solution most generally adopted on the
suggestion of the medical staff was to forbid obstetricians to perform ovariotomy. Abdominal cases were concentrated in the hands
of the surgeons: either the surgeon operated each case that was
referred to him, or a surgeon was appointed to perform all ovariotomies for a term of years.[2] This policy was not dictated by
judicious considerations as to the skill and experience which such
operations demanded, but by what the *Lancet* defined as 'the great
principle of "grab" – "that those should take who have the power,
and those should keep who have"'.[3] In the London general hospitals the surgeons outnumbered the obstetricians by four to one on
average; with the physicians remaining almost neutral on the question of abdominal surgery, the surgeons had had no difficulty in
outvoting the obstetricians when the matter had come up for deliberation. Ousted from the operating theatre, obstetricians sometimes tried to get their own back by attempting to dictate to the
surgeon when and how he should operate; sometimes they
managed to circumvent the ban by removing the patient to lodgings near the hospital, where they proceeded to perform
ovariotomy.

The *Lancet* was deeply concerned that discussions about who
should perform ovariotomy regularly overlooked the interests of
patients. Taking up the cudgel on behalf of this silent majority, the
journal argued that the wrangle over ovariotomy should be settled
not by a vote, but on the principle of proven skill and experience.
Generally speaking, the obstetrician knew more about pelvic anatomy and the growth of tumours than the surgeon did, while the
surgeon was more familiar with the treatment of wounds; yet
neither had any special training in abdominal surgery. Thus 'against
the entrance of any person not specially skilled and experienced',
the journal concluded, 'we should feel disposed to keep our own
peritoneal cavity and those of our friends peremptorily closed'.[4]

There was, however, a category of obstetricians who were also
skilful and competent surgeons: they were those who held appoint-

ments at the women's hospitals. Free from any restriction on their practice, the obstetricians on the staff of the special hospitals were playing a leading role in establishing and extending gynaecological surgery. They were the vanguard of a rising generation of dedicated specialists, who would pass through the women's hospitals as an essential part of their training, distinguishing themselves for their bias towards the surgical treatment of women's diseases. This growing band of gynaecologists regarded the surgeons' ban as the usurpation of a right and took a dim view of those among their colleagues who seemed unable or unwilling to fight back. They had a vocal and controversial champion in Robert Barnes, consulting obstetric physician at St George's Hospital and physician at the Chelsea Hospital for Women since 1877. His views on ovariotomy were part of a long-standing commitment to the cause of obstetrics and gynaecology. Since the early 1860s the eminent obstetrician had been fighting to raise the status of the specialism with regard to education, staffing levels and the representation of obstetricians on the GMC.[5] For Barnes the question of ovariotomy, implying as it did that obstetricians were incompetent surgeons, was further evidence of the low regard in which they were held by the physicians and surgeons. He thus took it upon himself to challenge the ban in an open letter to the eminent American gynaecologist Paul Mundé, which was published as a pamphlet in 1884.

In the *Relations Between Medicine, Surgery and Obstetrics in London*, Barnes exposed the 'somewhat peculiar, even anomalous' position of obstetrics in the capital. Only in a few general hospitals were obstetricians able to admit and treat gynaecological cases to the point of operation. At St Mary's Hospital, Tyler Smith, one of the founding Fellows of the Obstetrical Society, had established his right to carry out abdominal surgery when he had been appointed obstetric physician to the hospital in the 1850s. He had initiated the practice of having ovariotomy performed by the obstetric physician, which was afterwards continued by his successors Dr Meadows and Dr Wiltshire and imitated at University College Hospital and at King's College Hospital. At St George's, where he was obstetric physician, Barnes was allowed to perform abdominal surgery; this however rested on a personal concession and was not part of the statutory rights of the obstetric physician.[6]

At all the other London teaching hospitals the 'surgical dynasty' had managed to monopolise ovariotomy. At Guy's, for example, the obstetric physician had been able to perform the operation until the early 1880s, when the surgeons had rebelled against this: bringing their influence to bear on the autocratic treasurer, they had taken ovariotomy away from the obstetricians. Braxton Hicks, who was at the time obstetric physician to the hospital, was near his retirement and did not fight to get the right back; his successor Galabin, 'with his whole career before him, was content to pass under the surgical yoke. In vain protest he held out his hands and – was handcuffed'.[7] This strange spectacle could also be seen at St Thomas's, the Middlesex, Westminster, Charing Cross and at the London. At St Bartholomew's, a law debarring obstetricians from the performance of all operations, including caesareans, had been passed in 1855. There was a curious arrangement regarding perineal operations: obstetricians could repair a ruptured perineum for the relief of uterine prolapse (which can cause incontinence of urine), but not for incontinence of faeces and flatus: 'What a nice distinction' was Barnes' sarcastic comment. 'How ingeniously the line is drawn just between wind and water!'[8]

Surgeons justified their monopoly over abdominal surgery by invoking the ancient legal prerogatives of the Colleges, which established the principle of the division of labour between medical and surgical work. They argued that obstetricians were physicians, thus they may diagnose disease and prescribe treatments, but they may not undertake ovariotomy. The case of Dr Culver James, physician to the Vincent Square Hospital for Women and founding fellow of the British Gynaecological Society, provides an example. In the early 1880s James performed an ovariotomy while temporarily acting for Mr Smythe, who was one of the surgeons at the Vincent Square Hospital. Mr Skene Keith, Smythe's surgical colleague, deemed this to be an invasion of the surgeons' functions. He accused Dr James of performing an operation contrary to the laws of the hospital, and of knowingly and wittingly inducing him, Mr Keith, to take part in a breach of lawful procedure. James took exception to the surgeon's conduct, and in his turn brought a complaint against Keith and Smythe before the Metropolitan Counties Branch of the British Medical Association. His case was dismissed, on the grounds that the incident had arisen 'from the [unlawful] union in one and the same person of two distinct and separate functions'.[9] Obstetricians may have seen some irony in this: earlier in the century the same rule had been invoked when men-midwives had been debarred from the Fellowship of the College of *Physicians*. The rule which forbade Fellows of the Royal Colleges from engaging in mixed practice was, as we saw in chapter 2, purely formal and had never carried any real weight in practice;[10] that it should be enforced on the eve of the establishment of joint qualifications in medicine and surgery for all medical men seems almost unbelievable in retrospect.

For Robert Barnes the splitting up of a case into a medical and a surgical part had disastrous consequences. Firstly, it weakened the practitioner's interest in the welfare of the patient, as it encouraged the surgeon and the physician to shift the blame of error in diagnosis and failure in treatment upon each other. Secondly, it hampered the development of gynaecological science. At the same time therapeutic and experimental, surgical operations were the 'culminating point which brings all the theories hitherto formed as to the nature and complications of the disease to the test': thus, Robert Barnes pleaded, holding out ovarian tumours as an example,

how can a mere man-midwife arrive at a full or accurate knowledge of the manifold varieties in these tumours, in their origin, development, history, complications, and the many accidents they are liable to, unless he enjoys frequent opportunities of seeing and handling these tumours as exposed in operations? How otherwise can he possibly cultivate the diagnostic skill which is necessary for the differentiation of ovarian tumours from the numerous other tumours of pelvic and abdominal origin? As well might he pretend to understand the anatomy of the pelvic and abdominal organs without dissection.[11]

Last but not the least, the surgeons' ban prevented obstetricians from fulfilling their teaching functions, as no one could teach who had not himself learnt through practical experience.

The interests of patients and of gynaecological science were not the only reasons why abdominal surgery was so important to the obstetricians. Economic issues were also at stake in the scramble for ovariotomy cases. Patients had to be reassured as to the number of ovariotomies successfully performed by the proposed operator before putting their lives in his hands; practitioners who could not give that reassurance stood no chance of gaining a foothold in a profitable market: 'We need not further allude to the constant discussion and wrangling on the subject which is heard at our Societies and is to be read in our periodicals, except to remark that the substance of the apple is unmistakably golden, and that the chink of fees seems to us to have repeatedly and effectually drowned the feeble voice of the patient, whose interests have surely *some* claim to our attention', chided the *Lancet* in 1884.[12] Private ovariotomy operations in London commanded fees which in the mid-1870s were believed to be as high as one hundred guineas – a sum equal to the annual income of a young doctor in the first year or two of practice.[13]

Gynaecological surgery was especially valuable to the obstetricians as an alternative to obstetrical practice. Midwifery was unremunerative in proportion to the time and skill employed: in the mid-1870s London consultants might expect to earn an average of five guineas per 'attendance' for midwifery cases (visiting usually ceased on the tenth day after the birth).[14] Besides, the work could be irksome; it often involved calls in the middle of the night and constraints as to holidays. By contrast ovariotomies were more lucrative and could be scheduled to suit the practitioner. The pattern which by the early twentieth century had become typical of the career cycle of obstetricians clearly indicates a decline in the popularity of obstetrics and a corresponding shift towards gynaecological surgery as the preferred occupation: midwifery, still useful as a means of building up a practice, would be discarded by the obstetrician as he grew older and busier, and gynaecological surgery would step in its place. Further, ovariotomy could be an entrée to the wider field of abdominal surgery. By the 1880s, obstetricians at women's hospitals were operating in cases of renal and hepatic tumours; it did not take them long to argue that obstetric physicians at general hospitals, too, should assume the major responsibility of abdominal surgery.[15]

The force with which Barnes put his argument might convey the impression that obstetricians unanimously shared Barnes' discontent. This is far from the truth. Barnes' letter to Mundé was as much a harangue against the surgeons as a manifesto addressed to his own profession: ranked against him were the supporters of an older school, which had grown up in the non-interventionist tradition inaugurated by the late eighteenth-century men-midwives. Their differences came to a head in 1884, when the election of the President of the Obstetrical Society of London sparked off a major confrontation over the obstetricians' right to operate in abdominal cases.

The Meadows incident

On 3 December 1884 the annual nomination of the officers of the Obstetrical Society of London was due. The outgoing President, Dr Gervis, put forward the names of Drs Meadows, Aveling, Potter and Thorburn as candidates for the presidency of the Society. All of them were well known and respected gynaecologists. Alfred Meadows (1833–1913) was a Fellow of the Royal College of Physicians; he had studied medicine at King's College Hospital, London, where he had received many prizes, and was at the time physician-accoucheur to St Mary's Hospital. James Hobson Aveling was the founder of two women's hospitals and the initiator of the *Obstetrical Journal of Great Britain and Ireland*. John Baptiste Potter (1839–1900) was a Fellow of the Royal College of Physicians, and obstetric physician and lecturer in obstetric medicine to Westminster Hospital. John Thorburn (d. 1902) was obstetric physician to the Manchester Royal Infirmary and professor of obstetrics and gynaecology at Owens College, Manchester; he had also taken part in the foundation of the Southern Hospital for Women and Children in 1866.

The dispute began when Alfred Meadows, the candidate proposed by Robert Barnes and James Aveling, failed to be elected. Amidst the dissenting voices of Barnes and Aveling, the Council chose in his stead Dr Potter.[16] Barnes and Aveling were later to claim that the election had rewarded a man who had never been able to make a reputation for himself beyond the Society's council-room. This was probably a fairly accurate evaluation of Potter's talents, but it did not do justice to his contribution to the Obstetrical Society. Potter was undoubtedly more skilled in administrative work than he was versed in clinical questions. His biographer records that in 1869 he and Arthur Edis, one of the future Presidents of the British Gynaecological Society, were candidates for the post of assistant obstetric physician to Westminster Hospital. The two men decided to abide by the result of a spun coin, Potter won the toss and got the job. Potter had made only one contribution as a clinician to the Obstetrical Society, which he had joined in 1864, but he had shown both zeal and ability in its administration. In 1872 he had been elected onto the Society's Council, and in 1882 he had become its treasurer: his election to the presidency in 1884 was thus not wholly undeserved.[17]

Alfred Meadows too felt entitled to this honour on account of his long-standing services to the Society. Seething with resentment and hurt pride, he severed his connection with the Society, while Barnes and Aveling resigned their seats on the Council and on all committees. Ostensibly the Meadows incident smacked of petty rivalries between prima donnas; in fact, far more substantial issues were at stake. Barnes, Aveling and Meadows were challenging not so much Potter's credentials, but the views he represented. They were those of a section of the Council which, Barnes argued, was refusing to uphold the principle on which the Obstetrical Society had been founded, namely:

equality for the obstetric branch with the medical and surgical branches, including the independent right to carry through the clinical study of obstetric and gynaecological cases even to operation.[18]

In order to combat the discouragement met within the Obstetrical Society and throw off the 'dead weight' of the corporations and of the general hospitals, Barnes and his allies joined forces and on 22 December 1884, they founded the British Gynaecological Society. Because of the 'extraordinary neglect of gynaecology in the General Hospitals', argued the founders, special hospitals for women had been established where the most distinguished gynaecologists had gained their experience and 'effected their triumphs'. These practitioners now wished to create a Society 'at which they may record their experiences, exhibit their specimens & surgical improvements, and by so generous interchange of thought gain & give information on all gynaecological matters'.[19]

The thrust of Barnes' polemic provides some clues about his opponents on the Council of the Obstetrical Society: they were those general hospital obstetricians who had no desire to expand the field of gynaecological surgery and preferred to leave ovariotomy to the general surgeons. Chief amongst them was James Matthews Duncan. Born in 1826, Duncan was a leading obstetrician from Edinburgh, where he had been a close associate of James Young Simpson. As his assistant in the late 1840s, Duncan had been a guinea-pig for Simpson's first experiment with ether; he had subsequently become physician to the gynaecological ward of the Edinburgh Royal Infirmary. When Simpson died in 1870, Duncan was widely tipped to be his successor in the Chair of Obstetrics at the University, but he was passed over, and Alexander Russell

Simpson took his uncle's place. Duncan was bitterly disappointed. Thus in 1877 he accepted an invitation to join the staff of St Bartholomew's Hospital and settled in London, where he quickly established his reputation as a leading obstetrician and Robert Barnes' greatest rival.[20]

Competition for patients possibly reinforced an antagonism which stemmed in the first place from different approaches to the treatment of women's diseases: while Barnes' methods were unashamedly surgical, Duncan's were distinctly medical. The Scottish obstetrician persistently set his face against the idea that all pelvic diseases required an operation: when in 1890 John Bland-Sutton, one of the pioneers of gynaecological surgery, began to advocate the partial removal of the uterus for the cure of fibroids, Duncan labelled him a 'criminal mutilator of women'.[21] Duncan simply had no inclination to turn his department into a scene for the surgical triumphs so dear to Barnes' heart and was quite happy to leave gynaecological surgery to the general surgeons. No doubt the governors of St Bartholomew's, where the 'surgical dynasty' ruled supreme, had taken this into account when they had chosen him for the post of obstetric physician.

Matthews Duncan had two supporters on the Council of the Obstetrical Society: one was Francis Champneys (1848–1930), obstetrician at St George's Hospital, who would later step into Duncan's shoes at St Bartholomew's and carry on the medical tradition the Edinburgh obstetrician had brought to London; the other was an influential member of the surgical camp, Thomas Spencer Wells. At the Samaritan Free Hospital in London, where he was consulting surgeon, Wells had successfully fought against the performance of ovariotomy by obstetric physicians.[22] He was also critical of the tendency to over-operate in gynaecology, exemplified by the work of his arch-enemy, Lawson Tait. This goes a long way to explain why Spencer Wells did not follow Barnes in his new venture, whereas Tait, who as an abdominal surgeon had every interest in hindering Barnes, did, and with a vengeance: in 1886, he succeeded Alfred Meadows as the second President of the BGS. For Lawson Tait the Society was a valuable platform from which he could expound his views on gynaecological surgery, express his dislike of Spencer Wells and vent his antipathy toward the London surgical élite of which Wells was a member.

Other Council officers may have opposed Barnes not because they were in principle critical of gynaecological surgery, but because Barnes' views went together with an allegiance to the women's hospitals. It was no secret that specialists and general hospital physicians and surgeons were at loggerheads. The élite in the medical profession deemed specialists responsible for draining resources and stealing patients, and an affiliation with a specialist institution was thought to be a hindrance to practitioners who sought appointments at the general hospitals. All the obstetricians who sat on the Council held positions in the London teaching hospitals; significantly, none of them joined the BGS, despite the fact that it was fighting *their* cause. It may well have been that they did not want to associate themselves with an initiative emanating from their rivals, the gynaecologists at the women's hospitals, with Robert Barnes at their head. Even Peter Horrocks (1850–1902), assistant obstetric physician at Guy's Hospital, chose not to side with Barnes and Aveling, despite the fact that in 1882 he had been forced to join the Chelsea Hospital for Women in order to further his thwarted surgical ambitions.[23] It was preferable to face the vituperations of his colleagues at the Chelsea than the ostracism of the medical establishment at Guy's.

The British Gynaecological Society

Given the many personal, professional and political interests that were vested in the BGS, it was not surprising that, by the end of its first year of activity, the Society could boast 280 members, seventy of them renegades from the Obstetrical Society of London. It was a motley crowd in which the leaders of the gynaecological profession rubbed shoulders with humbler general practitioners, who had a direct interest in the BGS, for midwifery and gynaecology were the bread and butter of their professional life.

Evidence about hospital affiliation, biographical data and the information supplied at the Society's meetings can shed some light on the social and professional identity of its members. Nearly a quarter of the Fellows (sixty men, or 21.4 per cent) held hospital posts in London and in the provinces. In their majority, these practitioners were associated with maternity charities or special hospitals for women. The Chelsea Hospital for Women and the Hospital for Women in Soho Square provided the largest contingent from any single institution with ten and eight members each respectively. Two Fellows were affiliated to the Samaritan Free Hospital for Women and Children in London, an institution which had only just started to specialise in gynaecological work: they were Charles Felix Routh (1822–1909), and George Granville Bantock (1837–1913), Wells' successor in the post of full surgeon. Not all hospital specialists were obstetric physicians. As well as Tait and Bantock, there were practitioners such as William Swain (1834–1916), Henry Reeves (1850–1914), Thomas Jackson (1836–1901) and Thomas Nunn (1825–1909) who were general surgeons with a special interest in gynaecology.

Many of the Fellows were engaged in general practice, but it is difficult to tell what proportion of the Society they formed, as the boundaries between obstetric specialists and general practitioners were to a large extent blurred – very few obstetricians were able to make a living solely by practising midwifery and gynaecology. Several of the leaders of the BGS had started their careers as general practitioners: for example, Barnes, Aveling, David Lloyd Roberts (1836–1920), gynaecological surgeon to the Manchester Royal Infirmary, and John Halliday Croom (1847–1923), physician to the Royal Maternity Hospital in Edinburgh. Thomas Lycett is another instance of this pattern: he joined the Society as a general practitioner, and later became a gynaecological surgeon. Of all the Fellows, only twenty-two, or 7.8 per cent, held the Midwifery Licence of the Royal College of Surgeons. An even smaller number (six men, or 2.1 per cent) were Fellows of the Royal College of Physicians. Members holding the Fellowship of the Royal College of Surgeons were more numerous, possibly because the FRCS could be gained on grounds of seniority: this group reckoned thirty-eight men (13.5 per cent).

From the point of view of social background, too, the members of the BGS did not form a uniform group. The men who filled posts of responsibility in the Society as President, Vice-President, Councillor, Treasurer and Secretary, were those who came from middle-class backgrounds, who had received the highest professional recognition for their work, and who had built up fashionable and lucrative private practices. They provide a contrast to the rank-and-file members of the Society, many of whom struggled to make ends meet as general practitioners to the poor.

There were thirty-two officers of the British Gynaecological

Society in 1885, and biographical data are available for twenty-seven of them. The father's occupation is known in fourteen cases, showing a mixture of physicians, surgeons, clergymen and civil servants. Only David Lloyd Roberts had been born in humble circumstances: he was the son of a Midlands cotton-spinner, and had served in a chemist's shop before starting his medical education. All but four officers had university degrees, and in four cases they held the Fellowship of the Royal College of Physicians as well as a degree. Robert Barnes was unique in being both an honorary Fellow of the Royal College of Surgeons and a Fellow of the Royal College of Physicians: this was indicative of an emerging trend for obstetricians and gynaecologists in London to take the Fellowship of the College of Surgeons. Five other officers were Fellows of the College of Surgeons. In ten known cases, postgraduate study had been pursued abroad: Charles Routh, for instance, had been a pupil of Semmelweis in Vienna, and is remembered as a staunch defender of his theory of the aetiology of puerperal fever. Barnes, Meadows, Lloyd Roberts, Nunn and John Halliday Croom had studied in Paris; others, including A. W. Edis (1840–93), T. M. Madden (1844–1902), C. Routh, A. H. Freeland Barbour (d. 1927) and W. Chapman Grigg (1836–1900), had spent periods of study in various European medical centres, from Montpellier to Vienna and Berlin. Interestingly, one of the gynaecologists who sat on the Council of the BGS, William Travers (1838–1906), had been one of the founders of the Anthropological Society of London in 1863.

Such an international breadth of vision, however, was the privilege of only a handful of specialists: other members of the Society were not so fortunate, and found the going rough in an extremely competitive medical world. Evidence for this is provided by a letter written by A. Shaw Mackenzie to the Secretary of the BGS in 1895. Mackenzie had been on the staff of the Chelsea Hospital, where he had filled the post of pathologist. In 1894, like all the other members of staff, he had resigned during the controversy over the sanitary arrangements at the hospital;[24] he had not been reappointed, however, and from what can be deduced he had then settled in general practice in the Fulham area in West London, where he had a job as general practitioner to a Sick Club. These organisations, which had started in the last quarter of the nineteenth century, contracted doctors to provide medical care for their working-class subscribers.

They were encouraged by local boards of guardians to foster independence amongst the poor and relieve parishes of the cost of their medical care. Doctors were generally willing to engage in contract practice, partly because it was a stable source of income, and partly because they saw it as a means of controlling competition amongst practitioners.

Mackenzie wrote to plead his case after being reprimanded by the Society for advertising by means of medicine bottles and labels. He began his defence by arguing that advertising was an evil caused by competition amongst practitioners, which was rife in his neighbourhood. Advertising was common in his area largely by means of cards, labels and circulars. Sometimes religion was used as a bait for prospective patients. A man in Fulham held prayer meetings at his surgery, and exhibited a board outside with the hours of prayer just underneath; a lady doctor carried out a dispensary at a church mission and charged 2d. for a bottle of medicine. Another source of local competition came from the Holy Cross nursing home which sent women out to attend confinements for only 6s. a case. Mackenzie's Club allowed its doctors to charge what they liked for confinements – usually between 15s. and 21s.

Mackenzie believed that his Club offered reasonably good terms. He was paid 4s. a year per head for the first one hundred members, and 3s. 6d. each afterwards. Other Clubs, like the Fulham Sick Club, were not so generous. In 1894, £923 had been divided between its fifteen doctors: this seemed to allow about 1s. 6d. a year per member, but the amount was reduced by payments for confinements, which stood at 15s. each, and which came out of the total amount so divided. In Mackenzie's view, Sick Clubs were a great evil, in that they kept doctors' incomes unacceptably low, yet in poor districts they were also a necessary one: the alternative was between getting paid too little and not getting paid at all. Only a system of Industrial Insurance, controlled by the medical profession, he thought, could stop all keen competition amongst doctors and stamp out both Sick Clubs and advertising.[25]

General practitioners, as already noted, formed a large portion of the British Gynaecological Society's membership. During the 1860s and 1870s general practitioners had looked at specialists as a source of competition they would gladly do without; by the late 1880s, a different mood was noticeable among the rank and file of the profession. Specialists were beginning to be seen as the experts from whom the general practitioner might profitably learn, signalling the emergence of a hierarchy of functions between specialist and general practitioner. The trend was foreseen in 1890 by Dr Thomas Dolan, a general practitioner associated with the Halifax Union and North-East representative of the BGS: 'By linking themselves closer with such a Society as the British Gynaecological, and by digesting the experience which the leaders in gynaecological practice so readily place at their disposal,' he argued,

general practitioners can thereby better qualify themselves for that position which, if I read rightly the signs of the times, they are likely to hold in the future. It is nothing new when I say that the prospect of the future appears to hold out almost a certainty, that the differentiation in the ranks of the profession will be of such a nature that we shall have two orders: first, a family physician or medical attendant, who shall have the general care of the public; and, secondly, that we shall have behind them an order who devote themselves exclusively to the study of a single part or parts of the body.[26]

For Dolan the division between gynaecological specialist and GP contained the seeds for a fruitful co-operation between mutually dependent parties. The GP needed the gynaecologist's advice and skills; gynaecologists on their part may have been skilled operators and diagnosticians, but they were ill acquainted with the early stages of gynaecological disease and the social circumstances of patients, which were better known to the GP. Dolan might also have added that, as specialists increasingly relied on GPs for referrals, their success as individual practitioners depended on the GP's confidence and goodwill.

Pelvic surgery, however, was one area of gynaecology which the leaders of the BGS were unwilling to share with the general practitioner. Speaking on the place of gynaecology in general practice, in 1901 Dr John Lycett, then surgeon to out-patients at the Wolverhampton Hospital for Women, pleaded not only for better and more comprehensive training in the diseases of women, but also for practical instruction in the details of abdominal surgery and the post-operative management of such cases. Lycett rightly argued that specialist skills were not always available to patients, but the specialists were not impressed. Dr Bantock claimed that few places in Britain were so remote from a skilled operator as to justify the performance of abdominal surgery by inexperienced men. Dr Fenton maintained that the necessity for a general practitioner to do major operations seldom arose, as abdominal sections were not to be done on the spur of the moment; there was thus no need to instruct general practitioners in the details of ovariotomy.[27]

In the right context, though, gynaecological surgery had to be encouraged, and the discussion of surgical topics played a dominant part in the Society's activities. At the fortnightly meetings of the Society, pathological specimens were presented and papers on surgical questions were read and discussed. In 1886 John Bland-Sutton was employed to take charge of all the specimens and make microscopical preparations (these had become very important in the diagnosis of surgical diseases since the introduction of cellular pathology into surgery).[28] In 1887 a museum of instruments and specimens illustrating the practical aspects of gynaecology was established.[29] The question of setting up a gynaecological school was raised at one of the meetings of the Council in 1886. Tait, Meadows, Aveling, Bantock and Travers were appointed to investigate the matter, but the proposal did not come to fruition.[30] Encouragement for the study of gynaecology at the student level was provided the following year by Lawson Tait, who offered a prize of ten guineas to medical students for proficiency in gynaecology.[31] The Society further sponsored an investigation into the pathology and physiology of menstruation, a question that was central to the scientific study of femininity.[32] In 1883 there was an attempt to assert the separate status of gynaecology within medicine, as a specialism distinguished from obstetrics. A letter was sent to the President of the Council of the British Medical Association, suggesting that a separate section of gynaecology be formed at the Association's forthcoming meeting at Cardiff. The letter was not received unfavourably, but it was argued that the Obstetrical Section would include gynaecological subjects and that unnecessary duplication was to be avoided.[33]

Little did the leaders of the BGS realise that, by their polemical insistence on severing the links with obstetrics, they were doing a disservice to the obstetricians in whose interest the Society had been founded. To some extent *because of* Robert Barnes' efforts, the Surgeons continued to monopolise gynaecological surgery in the capital. Their professional dominance in gynaecology was reflected by changes in the qualifications taken by the metropolitan obstetricians. In the second half of the nineteenth century the leading obstetricians in London had been Fellows of the Royal College of Physicians, but by the beginning of the twentieth century it had become common for the young gynaecologist to take both the MRCP and the FRCS.[34]

The emphasis on the surgical aspects of the specialism gradually undermined the unity of obstetrics and gynaecology: increasingly, surgeons argued that gynaecology was a special branch of general surgery rather than the twin sister of obstetrics. The very existence of a specialist gynaecological association which had grown up to foster abdominal surgery in antagonism to the Obstetrical Society played in the hands of the surgeons; so did the increasing import-ance of the women's hospitals in the training of gynaecologists. With their marked bias towards operative intervention, the gynae-cological hospitals inevitably encouraged young trainees to adopt a surgical approach to women's diseases.

At the same time, the application of operative and surgical pro-cedures was being extended to obstetrics, bringing to an end the conservative phase which had characterised English midwifery since the days of William Hunter. Episiotomy became more common in the 1930s, and the usual delivery position on the left side was replaced by the lithotomy position which made obstetric surgery easier.[35] The increasing influence of the surgeons on obstet-ric departments was notable, for example, at the Middlesex Hospi-tal in the early 1900s. When in 1908 Comyns Berkeley and Victor Bonney, two of the leading lights of Edwardian gynaecology, were appointed to the midwifery department, they acknowledged its growing emphasis on surgery by taking up the titles of surgeon and assistant surgeon respectively instead of those of physician and assistant physician, which had been customary until then. Signifi-cantly, Bonney was one of the propounders of the idea that obstet-rics was a 'pure surgical art': pregnancy was a 'state induced by the growth of a neoplasm', labour a 'process accompanied by self-inflicted wounds' and the puerperium 'the period of healing'.[36]

Critics of obstetric interventionism at the time attributed this trend to the growth of abdominal surgery. 'Since the development of pelvic surgery few obstetricians limit their practice to obstetrics', wrote in 1934 William Oxley, Medical Officer to the East End Maternity Hospital in London; 'they have all become operating gynaecologists, and I suggest that the surgical bias which this has given to their minds has swept them away from the sound foundations of midwifery laid down by Smellie and his successors.'[37] The extent to which Oxley's claim was justified calls for further investigation. It is beyond the scope of this book to explore the influence of gynaecological surgery on obstetrics; however, it seems in order to analyse the attempt to extend the 'active management of labour' in childbirth in the light of the social relations of dominance and conflict between surgeons and obstetric physicians from the late nineteenth century onwards.

By the beginning of the twentieth century the BGS was in decline and none of the rising stars of gynaecology can be found on its rolls. When the Royal Society of Medicine was founded in 1907, it was amalgamated with the Obstetrical Society of London to form the Section of Obstetrics and Gynaecology. It was hoped at the time that the 'friendly rivalry' between the members of the two societies would be harnessed into the production of a large amount of scientific work.[38] Such optimism was ill-founded, for the antagonism between obstetric physicians and gynaecological surgeons was about to enter its most virulent phase.

A College of Obstetricians and Gynaecologists

The period between the two World Wars was marked by the rise of specialties that wanted to advance their own status *vis-à-vis* general medicine and surgery. Increasingly from the 1920s onwards, specialists demanded greater representation within the organisation of the Royal Colleges and sought to assert their right to control standards of training and education in their specialty. If the Colleges failed to serve the needs of these groups, there was a danger that specialists would be encouraged to set up professional organisations outside their jurisdiction, a step which the radiologists, for example, considered in 1936. The technical and professional advance of radiology had proceeded in concert in the early part of the century, resulting in the establishment of specialist diplomas and associations. In spite of this progress, the radiologists were not satisfied, and in 1936 they attempted to found a College; they eventually had to settle for an independent Faculty, in the face of strong opposition from the Royal Colleges.

Of the two Colleges, it was that of Surgeons which felt these pressures more keenly: specialist groups within the Royal College of Surgeons, from the ophthalmologists to the ear–nose–throat surgeons, were more vociferous, more concerned about their status and more demanding of specialist examinations than the specialties of general medicine. By 1948, the Royal College of Surgeons had been forced to accommodate the demands of its four major sub-specialties, establishing separate fellowship examinations for ophthalmology and otolaryngology, and creating semi-autonomous faculties for dentistry and anaesthetics. It was only a matter of time before the Royal College of Physicians would be faced with similar problems in relation to paediatrics, psychiatry and pathology.[39]

Obstetrics and gynaecology registered these trends with particular force. After the First World War a movement began within the gynaecological profession, the principal object of which was the creation of a Faculty of Gynaecology within the Royal College of Surgeons. The initiator of the campaign was Victor Bonney, a loyal supporter of the Royal College of Surgeons and the only gynaecologist ever to be elected on to its Council. His views deserve special attention, as they provide the key to understanding the effort to bring gynaecology and obstetrics together under the aegis of a third College. Born in 1872, Bonney had been trained in gynaecological surgery at the Chelsea Hospital for Women under Sir John Bland-Sutton. At the Middlesex and other hospitals, Bonney established his reputation as the leading gynaecological surgeon of his time: he developed a special technique for the removal of uterine fibroids and became the chief exponent of radical pelvic surgery for cervical cancer, known as the Wertheim operation.

Bonney traced the genealogy of gynaecology through Spencer Wells, Lawson Tait and Bland-Sutton – the general surgeons who had developed abdominal surgery – overlooking the contribution made by late nineteenth-century obstetricians to the fields of vaginal and pelvic surgery; indeed he spoke with contempt of the 'inert, inept "men-midwives"' who had previously 'treated' women's ailments. Although he shared the obstetricians' dissatisfaction with the lowly status accorded to their profession, he did not believe that the key to raising it was to make obstetrics and gynaecology the third branch of medicine, as William Tyler Smith and James Aveling had suggested in the previous century. He feared that any movement aimed at asserting the separate status of the subject would widen the 'deplorable gap' which existed between general medicine and surgery on the one hand, and obstetrics and gynaecology on the other. The only way to advance the obstetrical and gynaecological profession, he argued, was to train all gynaecologists as abdominal surgeons; gynaecological surgery and operative obstetrics should become a concern of the Royal College of Surgeons, while medical obstetrics could remain under the care of the College of Physicians. Two universities accepted this suggestion and went so far as to separate obstetrics and gynaecology, although in each, at succeeding elections, the decision was reversed.[40]

Bonney's proposals touched a raw nerve in the obstetrical profession. Among obstetric physicians, commented the Liverpool Professor of Obstetrics and Gynaecology William Blair Bell (1871–1936), co-founder and first President of the British College of Obstetricians and Gynaecologists,

there had long been a strong feeling against the performance of gynaecological operations by general surgeons, and against the regulations in certain hospitals which required gynaecologists to seek the help of their colleagues in General Surgery for abdominal operations.[41]

As the other founder of the College, the Manchester Professor of Obstetrics and Gynaecology William Fletcher Shaw (1878–1962), wrote in 1954, obstetricians realised that, 'carried to its logical conclusion, the movement afoot would separate obstetrics from gynaecology and that, in all probability, the ablest men would be attracted to gynaecology, while obstetrics would be left to the second-rate'.[42]

Opposition to Bonney's ideas was strongest in the provinces. Outside London the dominance of the English Colleges was weak. Gynaecology in the provinces had been able to grow free from restrictions by physicians and surgeons, developing closer ties with obstetrics than was the case in London. Unlike their London colleagues, who took both the MRCP and the FRCS examinations, provincial obstetricians served a long period of clinical apprenticeship; the majority held university degrees, with or without a Fellowship of either the Scottish or Irish Colleges. Metropolitan and provincial practitioners were also divided by a long history of professional rivalries which, from Charles Clay to Lawson Tait, had coloured controversy in gynaecology. London obstetricians were apt to distrust and ridicule the achievements of their extra-metropolitan colleagues; provincial obstetricians on their part vehemently resented the socio-economic power of the capital and of the London Colleges. The prospect of delivering their specialty into the hands of the Royal College of Surgeons was anathema to them.

Obstetricians advanced various arguments in support of the unification of obstetrics and gynaecology. As Kerr *et al.* maintained in their *Combined Text-Book of Obstetrics and Gynaecology* (1923), anyone practising gynaecology should be an obstetrician, first because a large proportion of gynaecological conditions were ultimately due to the complications of labour, secondly because it was often very difficult to distinguish the symptoms of pelvic disease from those of pregnancy.[43] At a time of widespread anxiety about the continuing decline in the birth rate, obstetricians also emphasised the dangers of entrusting women to men trained as abdominal surgeons, with a bias towards operative measures and scanty knowledge of medical gynaecology. There was no doubt in the mind of Fletcher Shaw that, if this were allowed to happen, 'many women in the plenitude of their powers would be debarred from the motherhood that more knowledge and patience might have procured'.[44]

The foundation of a College of Obstetricians *and* Gynaecologists in 1929 was the provincial obstetricians' answer to the London gynaecological surgeons. As Fletcher Shaw explained in 1929 to Wentworth Alexander Taylor (1900–68), Assistant Master at the Rotunda Hospital, Dublin, 'the primary object of the College is to bind obstetrics and gynaecology and to prevent gynaecology from becoming a mere subdivision of surgery while obstetrics is left to those who have nothing better to do'.[45] The College was to form a single portal through which all those who desired to practise as consultants in obstetrics and gynaecology must pass: this would eventually enable the obstetricians to control entry into the profession and undermine the surgeons' dominance of gynaecology. An independent College could determine standards of training, speak as the representative body of all obstetricians and enhance their status and public visibility.

The realisation of the project was facilitated by a climate in which the question of maternal mortality had taken on political significance. At a time when the value of motherhood was emphasised, the government's own reports began to draw attention to the maternal mortality rate, which had not changed since the middle of the nineteenth century. The number of maternal deaths in England and Wales was between four and five per 1,000 live births; in

Scotland, the rate actually increased between 1900 and 1930 from just under five to well over six. A number of investigations were undertaken to discover the causes, but the results proved inconclusive. One of the problems was that women passed through many hands during the ante-natal period, labour and the puerperium: hospital specialists, general practitioners, independent and institutional midwives and local authority clinics all provided maternity services. Death could be caused by complications arising in any one or more stages of pregnancy and labour, and different attendants could be involved each time.

Some of the evidence seemed to indict the general practitioner. General practice had come into focus as the black spot of the maternity services as early as 1898, when Cullingworth's investigation of maternal deaths in London had revealed the existence of a reverse relationship between social class and maternal mortality.[46] These findings suggested that the standards of maternity care provided by the general practitioner were inadequate, since high rates of maternal mortality in the professional and managerial classes appeared to be associated with a high percentage of deliveries by medical practitioners, while low rates were found in poor areas with deliveries by midwives. However, studies which examined regional differences showed a correlation between regions of high mortality and regions traditionally associated with poverty and deprivation: in 1926, for example, the maternal mortality in Wales was 4.92 per 1,000 deliveries, 4.75 in the north of England, 3.78 in the midlands and 3.43 in the south. In spite of this evidence, comparatively little attention was paid to the influence of poor nutrition, female employment and the environment on mortality; instead, health officials concentrated on the immediate clinical causes of death and attempted to isolate the 'primary avoidable factor' involved in each case – the point at which it was believed that the maternity services had fallen down.[47] The resulting focus on the clinical aspects of pregnancy and labour led to a redefinition of the problem as a question for the medical profession: thus an initiative which, like the College, could be seen to be working for the solution of the maternal mortality problem, was bound to find supporters in the government and the public.

Concern about the obstetrical training of medical students and general practitioners underlay the subsidiary aims of the College, namely, to institute special qualifications in obstetrics for general practitioners and to bind the teachers of obstetrics and gynaecology together, so as to demand adequate facilities for the teaching and examining of students. Anxiety about maternal mortality, however, was not the only reason why specialists were interested in the skills of general practitioners. The demand for improved teaching facilities in obstetrics was also a 'battle of the beds' which, if successful, would enhance the professional status of obstetricians in relation to their colleagues in general medicine and surgery. The specialists' recommendation that all medical students undertake a period of resident training in a maternity hospital could only be implemented by increasing the small number of beds allotted to lying-in cases in the medical schools. Beds in the voluntary hospitals, the London ones especially, were rigidly allocated, and neither the physicians nor the surgeons were willing to give them up to the obstetricians until required to do so by the examining bodies.[48]

The crucial question with regard to the training of medical students was the direction in which teaching had to be improved – and this depended on the way in which obstetricians envisaged the role of the generalist in obstetric practice. Relations between specialists and general practitioners were not harmonious, since both considered themselves experts in the same field. General practitioners firmly denied any suggestion that they were responsible for the high maternal mortality. Indeed for Dr William Oxley, a generalist attached to the East End Maternity Hospital, general practitioners were the 'real obstetric specialists of the country'. It was a general practitioner, said Oxley at a symposium on the 'Future of the maternity services' in 1929,

who had taught in the middle of the last century that diagnosis should be made abdominally and that vaginal examinations were undesirable. It was a general practitioner – the late Dr Cursham Corner – who had inaugurated antenatal work on a large scale 15 years before Ballantyne. It was a general practitioner who had first drawn attention to the grave dangers of puerperal fever. Nothing whatever had been done by the obstetric specialists until the report of the Ministry of Health had alarmed the country.[49]

The British Medical Association stressed that the general practitioner was the bedrock on which the midwifery services should be built; its scheme for a national maternity service, published in 1929, minimised both the need for specialist hospital care and the role of the midwife in domiciliary practice. These proposals were strongly resisted by consultant obstetricians: they pressed for an extension of institutional midwifery, under the control of specialists, and argued for a more clearly defined division of labour between general practitioners and consultant obstetricians. Specialists needed the general practitioner as the 'first line of defence' in domiciliary practice, but the scope of his intervention in childbirth had to be limited to the attendance of minor complications.

The specialists' views on this score were spelled out in the *Memorandum on the Training of Medical Students in Midwifery and Gynaecology*, published by the British College of Obstetricians and Gynaecologists in 1932. In this report it was stated that the medical student should be thoroughly trained in antenatal care, the management of normal labour, the after-care of the mother and new-born infant, the recognition of the early signs of abnormality and the performance of the minor obstetrical procedures:

In the more serious obstetrical complications, he should be taught that the proper course is the immediate transference of the patient, whenever possible, to hospital unless the services of someone with special obstetrical experience are available.[50]

After instituting its own diploma for general practitioners, the College would begin to insist that every general practitioner wishing to practise midwifery should spend a period of postgraduate clinical training in obstetrics, as laid down by the diploma regulations. This would have created a grade of obstetric practitioner half way between the fully fledged specialist and the GP; it would also have automatically reduced the number of general practitioner-obstetricians, since resident posts in obstetrics were few and far between, and the general practitioner would be faced with stiff competition from trainee obstetricians. F. J. Browne (1879–1968), the first Director of the Obstetric Unit opened at University College Hospital in 1926, claimed that midwifery was incompatible with general practice, both because of the postgraduate training that he believed was necessary and because of the irregular hours it demanded. No wonder general practitioners were left with the impression that specialists were intent on banishing midwifery from general practice, thus creating a monopoly shared between themselves and the midwives.[51]

The provinces take the lead

According to Blair Bell, the idea of a college of obstetrics and gynaecology was suggested to William Fletcher Shaw by Sir William Sinclair, founder of the *Journal of Obstetrics and Gynaecology of the British Empire*. Shaw was very much taken with this idea, but he recognised that it was fraught with difficulties: it was not easy to see how a profession divided by so many jealousies and rivalries could be brought together. There was one association, though, which had done much to establish ties of friendship and mutual appreciation amongst the various schools of gynaecology: this was the Gynaecological Visiting Society founded by William Blair Bell in 1911. Unlike the medical societies that had sprung up since the beginning of the eighteenth century, the GVS was organised as a club to which members were elected by strict ballot, on the combined basis of professional ability and likeable personality. Its purpose was to promote research into the methods of clinical gynaecology at centres in Britain and overseas and into scientific topics of relevance to the specialism. In 1911 the original members of the Society were all comparatively young practitioners from the medical schools of Britain; by the early 1920s these same men filled the chairs in obstetrics and gynaecology in all but two of the universities in the British Isles. The GVS was thus an influential association and the only one capable of galvanising the profession into action on a national scale.[52]

Shaw, who was himself a member of the GVS, eventually realised the potential of this Society as the seeding ground for the College plan. In order to enlist its help, it was essential that he should gain the support of William Blair Bell, the autocratic leader of the Society. Shaw and Blair Bell did not know each other well, but a series of circumstances brought them together in 1923–24 and led to a friendship which, despite many ups and downs, was to last until Blair Bell's death in 1936. Thus encouraged in his resolve to involve the Liverpool professor, Shaw finally outlined his plans to him in October 1924.[53]

Blair Bell's initial reaction was one of cautious interest, but once he had been persuaded, he threw himself into the cause with characteristic fervour. In December 1924 he discussed the matter with two members of the GVS who acted as external examiners in obstetrics to Liverpool University. One was Sir Ewen Maclean, the first

Professor of Obstetrics and Gynaecology in the University of Wales; the other was Comyns Berkeley, Bonney's senior at the Middlesex, who was to play a very important part in the early history of the College. Fletcher Shaw's idea was accepted, and it was agreed that he should bring up the matter at the next meeting of the GVS in Cardiff on 2 February 1925. At this meeting there was great interest in the plan, and Blair Bell, Berkeley, Maclean and Shaw were elected to form a committee with the brief of drawing up a detailed scheme.[54]

It soon became apparent that the project stood little chance of success. At a meeting of the founding committee in April 1925, Berkeley informed his colleagues that a Royal Charter was never given to any organisation to which there was opposition – and the Royal Colleges were certain to oppose the proposed College. Up until then, specialities had not constituted a big problem for the Colleges. Specialisation followed on from the MRCP and FRCS, or through the new diplomas instituted by the universities or by the Conjoint Board. University diplomas did not challenge the authority of the Colleges, but the creation of a new College, with its own qualifications, did.

Berkeley had done some research, and he had discovered an alternative. He suggested that the College might be founded as a Limited Liability Company, registered by the Board of Trade, but with the permission to omit the word Limited from its title. This privilege was usually granted to companies from which no profits were derived, and which were brought into existence for the public weal. Berkeley was confident that the College would be able to obtain a Royal Charter at a later date, once it was established on a sound foundation.[55] After some hesitation, this advice was accepted and the first proposals for the College were submitted to the GVS.

In June 1926 the name of Russell Andrews was added to the founding committee, which then became the Executive Committee of the proposed College. Later that year, the first officers of the College were appointed. Berkeley and Shaw became Treasurer and Secretary respectively, Blair Bell insisted upon being elected Chairman; in this capacity he was to claim sole authority to conduct the negotiations with the Royal Colleges.[56] Before setting to work on the Memorandum and Articles of Association, the Executive Committee deemed it politically expedient to approach a number of leading London gynaecologists who were not members of the

GVS. It was anticipated that London practitioners would resist the idea of the new College, both because the proposal came from the provinces and because all the metropolitan obstetricians already had an allegiance to either of the two Colleges. Thus in July 1926 Sir Francis Champneys, Sir George Blacker (1865–1948), Dr Thomas Watts Eden (1863–1946), Dr John Fairbairn (1865–1944), Dr Herbert Spencer (1860–1941) and Dr Archibald Donald (1860–1937) were invited to meet the Executive Committee at Comyns Berkeley's house in London.[57]

As expected, the London obstetricians had many reservations about the plan. Herbert Spencer, the first president of the Section of Obstetrics and Gynaecology in the Royal Society of Medicine, was the most uncompromising. He saw no need for a new College, as he thought that the Section of Obstetrics and Gynaecology was already contributing to the improvement of the specialty through the work of its individual members. He did concede that the Colleges were guilty of neglecting obstetrics and gynaecology, but argued that the solution was to amalgamate the Colleges into a Royal Academy of Medicine and foster interest in the specialism under the aegis of this new body.[58] George Blacker, obstetrician at University College Hospital, London, strongly criticised the venture on the grounds that it threatened the vested interests of the Colleges. In fact, Blacker was opposed to all Colleges and argued that in an ideal world universities alone would grant medical qualifications. Under the circumstances, he thought it would have been wiser to ask the older Colleges to grant special diplomas in obstetrics and gynaecology.[59]

The greatest controversy arose over whether the new institution should be an association or a College with the powers to be an examining body. Blair Bell was adamant that it should be a College enjoying the same powers and privileges of the older corporations. He wanted the College to have the right to grant certificates of proficiency in obstetrics and gynaecology to candidates for the MRCS, LRCP, jointly with the other two Colleges and with an equal share in the fees, and to institute a post-graduate diploma. His London colleagues Champneys, Eden and Fairbairn took the opposite view. The difference of opinion was in part one of tactics. Some thought the first object of the College should be the improvement of midwifery training and practice, and that the College should seek further powers later if necessary. Others felt that the Royal Colleges would oppose the project if its full powers were stated.[60] The Ministry of Health was of the opinion that the issue of the diploma should be dropped. As the Principal Medical Officer of Health George Newman said to Comyns Berkeley in February 1927, no certificate for public purposes was worth anything unless it was recognised by Parliament or by a Royal Charter – and this might take the obstetricians several years to obtain.[61]

For the older Colleges the question was one of financial interests as well as of prestige. The Royal Colleges made a large income from the MRCS and LRCP examinations and they were naturally loath to share it with a third party. The gynaecologists and obstetricians who were Fellows of either or both the London medical corporations were the examiners in obstetrics and gynaecology for the Conjoint Diploma and were thus anxious not to be seen to be furthering the interests of a rival organisation. The argument was finally settled when all the Professors of Obstetrics and Gynaecology in the United Kingdom, with the exception of the two in London, declared themselves in favour of a College. Blair Bell welcomed the decision with a comment which sums up both his character and his feelings about his metropolitan colleagues: 'It is useless to have anything to do with "Associations", and the provinces must apparently keep the matter in their own hands or at least leave out those in London who are so stupid.'[62]

The Executive Committee very much hoped that Victor Bonney might be persuaded to give his support to the College. Bonney has been portrayed as the most uncompromising adversary of the obstetricians, but this is undoubtedly a gross oversimplification of his position: as a founding member of the GVS, Bonney was on good terms with the nucleus of obstetricians who were promoting the idea of the College and he sympathised with some of their aims. In 1927 he signified his intention to join the College as soon as it was founded. A year later, as the Royal Colleges opposed the new venture, he promised Blair Bell that he would endeavour to appease his colleagues on the Council of the College of Surgeons:

I will do my best to help the College of Obstetrics and Gynaecology. I am not antagonistic to the project by any means, and see quite well the good it might do, but on the other hand, I have not been enthusiastic about it, because I feel that unless it is very judiciously managed it will widen the deplorable gap which still exists between General Medicine and Surgery on the one hand, and Obstetrics and Gynaecology on the other . . . I look upon myself as representing all you fellows on the Council of the College of Surgeons, and as such I intend to do the best I can for you.[63]

By 1929, though, Bonney's attitude had changed. Shortly after the foundation of the College, the names of those elected to the first Council were announced to the papers. By an oversight, Bonney had been included in the list without his knowledge or consent; to add insult to injury, he had been described as 'Dr', a title which suggested humble links with general practice. Outraged, Bonney immediately penned a stiff note of protest:

I have for years been hoping for the time when Obstetrics and Gynaecology would be accounted as special branches of Surgery and obstetricians and gynaecologists would be considered as surgeons and not as physicians, and reading my name among a list which must give to the public the idea of a gathering of respectable apothecaries has fairly made me wince![64]

He was later to turn down the Fellowship of the College, in spite of Blair Bell's entreaties. Regrettably for Bonney's old associates, the establishment of the College of Obstetricians and Gynaecologists coincided with Bonney's ascent to the highest offices of the College of Surgeons. The ambitious gynaecologist aspired to the Presidency and he would not spoil his chances by siding with Blair Bell and Shaw. He was duly elected Vice-President in 1936, but his hopes to become the Surgeons' leader were never to be fulfilled. The obstetricians could not easily bring themselves to forgive Bonney, and it was not until 1946 that amicable relations were officially restored with the acceptance by Bonney of the Honorary Fellowship of the College.[65]

At the beginning of 1927 the Memorandum and Articles of Association of the proposed College were circulated to the members of the GVS. The Board of Trade required applications for incorporation to carry nine signatures, thus at a meeting of the GVS in February 1927 Dr H. Russell Andrews, Professor Blair Bell, Mr Comyns Berkeley, Sir Francis Champneys, Dr T. Watts Eden, Sir Ewen Maclean, Professor Fletcher Shaw, Professor J. Munro Kerr (representing Scotland) and Professor C. G. Lowry (for Ireland) were chosen to sign the Articles. At this point it was thought advisable to sever the connection between the GVS and the College. The GVS aroused many jealousies among those who were not invited to join, and it was feared that the College would not receive general support if it was closely identified with the Society.[66]

In April 1927, the Articles of Association were submitted to a general meeting of consultant obstetricians and gynaecologists in Manchester. Champneys and Eden finally agreed that the College should hold examinations for students and for general practitioners, provided it was 'duly authorised by competent authority' (that is to say the Royal Colleges). This amendment was accepted by the Executive Committee in order to avoid a split, and it seemed then that the chief bone of contention between London and the provinces had been removed; but more trouble was in store. The lawyers did not like the proviso: they pointed out that the Royal Colleges might use it as an excuse for not asking the obstetricians to co-operate, and insisted on deleting it. Unfortunately they circulated the text of their amendment rather than the document accepted in Manchester, thus precipitating a violent row between Shaw and Blair Bell on the one hand, and the London-men on the other. Berkeley and his metropolitan colleagues were convinced that they had been double-crossed, and it was not until they had been given an opportunity to reconsider the original clause that they finally agreed to accept the lawyers' suggestion.[67]

In June 1928 the nine signatories announced their intention to apply to the Board of Trade for incorporation as a Company. On the eve of the last day on which objections could be lodged, the Royal Colleges signified their opposition to the proposed College of Obstetricians and Gynaecologists. The Colleges objected to the articles concerning the examination of finalists and the postgraduate diploma. They viewed them as detrimental to the interests of medical education, as encroaching on their privileges, and as impairing public confidence in their own diplomas. The Scottish and the Irish Colleges for their part remained silent.[68] The signatories were advised that they could go ahead and apply for registration in spite of the objections, but there was general agreement that an open confrontation should be avoided; it was thus resolved that Blair Bell, as Chairman of the Executive Committee, should open negotiations with Rose Bradford, President of the Royal College of Physicians, and Lord Moynihan, President of the Royal College of Surgeons. Of the two, Moynihan would prove the more obdurate, and with good reason. Moynihan was an abdominal surgeon of international repute, and one can appreciate his hostility to a project which directly threatened his professional interests.

Several months of intense discussion ensued, during which the birth of the new College was obstructed not only by the medical corporations, but also by differences of opinion between the signatories. To Fletcher Shaw it seemed at times that Blair Bell's impetuous and domineering temperament would alienate the medical corporations to the point of killing off any support the project might ever have enjoyed; Blair Bell for his part disliked Fletcher Shaw's conciliatory attitude and deeply resented other people having a hand in the negotiations. Berkeley and Eden especially were 'interfering' and taking 'individual action'; they would soon begin to complain that the College had become a 'one-horse show', and they turned into Blair Bell's most implacable critics within the College.

As there was opposition to the new College, the Board of Trade decided to hold an inquiry into the case. After the hearing in March 1929, further attempts were made at composing the differences with the Royal Colleges, but no agreement could be reached. Finally in May 1929 the Board of Trade refused to grant registration.[69] Just when the battle seemed to be lost, the Baldwin government suddenly resigned, and the question of maternal mortality became one of the chief issues of the Conservative electoral platform. This political denouement provided the obstetricians with an unexpected trump card. In a letter to Sir Boyd Merriman, a contact in the government who had worked with the Minister of Health Neville Chamberlain, Fletcher Shaw was able to put the case for a College of obstetrics and gynaecology in the light of the Conservative electoral campaign. 'I do not wish it to sound as though I had a pistol to his head', Shaw later wrote to Blair Bell, 'but at the same time parliamentarians, being what they are, will only grant this if they are afraid of their own seats'.[70] Boyd Merriman's reply was not long in coming: Mr Chamberlain felt strongly that nothing should be left undone 'in the interest of the Public Health' to secure agreement on the point of controversy.[71]

Chamberlain put pressure on the Presidents of the two Royal Colleges, and he was instrumental in bringing about a meeting of the three parties involved in the controversy. On 16 May a formula was finally agreed, according to which the College of Obstetricians and Gynaecologists was empowered firstly

to take part (if invited) in the examination of candidates for admission to the British Register of Medical Practitioners in co-operation with teaching and/or examining bodies

and secondly

to grant to Registered Medical Practitioners certificates or other equivalent recognition of special knowledge in Obstetrics and Gynaecology either alone or in co-operation with teaching and/or examining bodies . . . But should the Royal College of Physicians, London, and the Royal College of Surgeons, England, jointly agree to invite the co-operation of the College of Obstetricians and Gynaecologists . . . and for so long as this arrangement shall remain in force the College alone shall not grant a diploma . . . but shall not be debarred from entering into a similar arrangement with other bodies authorised to grant such certificates.[72]

The first clause was a victory for the Physicians and Surgeons, as it enabled them to exclude the College from the final examination (it was not until 1943, during the negotiations for a National Health Service, that the Royal College of Surgeons invited the Royal College of Obstetricians and Gynaecologists to take part in the Conjoint Board examinations). The second clause gave an edge to the obstetricians, in that it provided them with an opportunity to set up their own diploma for general practitioners, should the Royal Colleges prove unco-operative.

The crucial issue of course was how the word 'co-operation' should be interpreted. Blair Bell believed that the new College should appoint examiners and share the exam fee equally.[73] The Royal Colleges had other plans: their idea was that the diploma should be granted by the Physicians and Surgeons alone, and that the College of Obstetricians and Gynaecologists should co-operate by nominating a panel of examiners. To this end, in June 1929 Moynihan summoned the examiners in obstetrics for the Conjoint Diploma, together with the obstetric Fellows of the College of Physicians. The outcome of this meeting was that a committee of Bradford, Moynihan, Berkeley, Eden, Blair Bell and Shaw was formed to draw up regulations for a new Diploma in Obstetrics and Gynaecology of the two Colleges.[74]

In June 1929 the agreement between Blair Bell and the Presidents of the two Colleges was ratified by the Council of the Royal

College of Surgeons; the Comitia of the Royal College of Physicians unanimously followed suit at the beginning of July. The matter was practically concluded when the Colleges made a further attempt at amending the disputed clause. The suggested formula implied that the diploma would be granted by the two Colleges alone: this was unacceptable to Blair Bell, and the Surgeons then retaliated by refusing to withdraw their objections.[75] The Board of Trade, however, was not prepared to re-open the case, and on 26 August 1929 the signatories were informed that registration had been finally granted: the British College of Obstetricians and Gynaecologists was born.

Restructuring the profession

One of the first tasks to which the founders of the College turned their attention was the construction of rules for the election of Foundation Fellows and Members, thus spelling out the meaning they attached to the title 'specialist in obstetrics and gynaecology'. Membership was restricted to those who held honorary appointments as obstetricians and gynaecologists on the staffs of teaching hospitals and other carefully selected institutions: practitioners on the senior staff were invited to become Foundation Fellows, while those at the assistant level were offered the Foundation Membership. Both surgeons and general practitioners were debarred from the Foundation Membership and Fellowship.[76] Various attempts were made to devise a formula which would not exclude Victor Bonney, but no satisfactory alternative could be found; it was thus resolved to approach Bonney informally and invite him to join the first Council. As noted already, Bonney refused. The decision to exclude GPs from the Membership was sharply criticised by Comyns Berkeley as a 'retrograde step'. As Berkeley justly pointed out to Shaw in 1932, most provincial obstetricians were also general practitioners; the rule would have forced the Council to strike such practitioners off its Rolls, thus weakening the influence of the College outside London.[77] The College's policy on this score was not to change, but exception had to be made for GPs like William Oxley, who was doing valuable work for the maternity services in the East End of London. Oxley was invited to be a Foundation Member in 1929, and two years later he was elevated to the Fellowship.

After the initial nucleus of Founding Fellows and Members had been recruited, much thought had to be given to the question of standardising education and training requirements for aspirants to the Membership (MCOG until 1938, when the granting of the title 'Royal' changed it to MRCOG). The founders originally envisaged a College of definitely established specialists in obstetrics and gynaecology, all of whom were attached to the honorary staffs of hospitals. Shaw suggested that candidates should be selected by means of three tests: the completion of a period of postgraduate clinical training, the submission of a prescribed number of case-records and an examination. Of the three tests, the first and the second were an innovation; the third was the usual method by which higher medical diplomas were granted at the time. Shaw feared that these suggestions might prove too radical for the veteran teachers and examiners who formed the first Council; he was thus surprised when his colleagues accepted the idea of a prescribed period of training, but turned down the examination part of his proposals. Most believed that the MCOG was unlikely to replace the MRCP or the FRCS as a route to specialisation in obstetrics and gynaecology and they did not want to frighten off candidates by making the Membership requirements too burdensome: senior practitioners were unlikely to have the time and inclination to prepare for a further examination, nor could they run the risk of failing it.[78]

Shaw's insistence upon postgraduate training was motivated by the desire to exclude general practitioners from the Membership. As most doctors settled in general practice immediately upon quali-fication, they would have found it very difficult to comply with the clinical requirements laid down by the College. Shaw objected to examinations as a means of selection because exams were open to 'all and sundry' and especially to the 'young general practitioners, who merely wish to show the general public that they are a little above their neighbour simply because they have the ability to pass examinations'. This, Shaw thought, was where the Fellowship of the Royal College of Surgeons of Edinburgh, which was awarded on the results of an examination only, 'had done so much harm'.[79] The Membership had to be restricted to the handful of committed specialists who were willing to forgo the financial security of gen-eral practice and chance the hospital system.

Shaw did not spare his criticisms for the recently reformed

MRCP. 'In the old days the MRCP had an extraordinarily high standard', he wrote to Thomas Watts Eden in 1930, 'and this I think is due to its regulations which made it difficult for men in general practice to conform to it and now that it has been reduced to a mere examination I think its standard will decrease.'[80] As it now stood, Shaw would argue two years later in a letter to Berkeley, the MRCP simply meant

that a man is a good examinee, whereas before it was a guarantee that a man was in the firect [sic] line for a physician's post and a gentleman. Now it is the clever Jew in the neighbourhood who does the MRCP easily while the really good man with clinical training and good general education is sometimes overlooked.[81]

These words reflected the growing anti-semitism of British practitioners as refugee doctors from Nazi Germany began to arrive in England in ever-increasing numbers. In the middle of the Great Depression, the medical profession could not afford to be generous: even socialist practitioners argued that they would reject their own relatives if they tried to compete.[82]

To the danger of competition from GPs and immigrant Jewish doctors there was added the threat posed by the Royal Colleges. In December 1929 the RCP and the RCS instituted a Conjoint Diploma in Obstetrics and Gynaecology (DGO) for general practitioner-obstetricians, thus raising fears that younger practitioners intending to specialise might take this qualification rather than wait until they could apply for the MCOG. Louis Carnac Rivett (1887–1947), Consultant Obstetrician at the Middlesex Hospital and Members' Representative on the Council of the BCOG, thought that this danger might be averted by opening the Membership to practitioners of registrar rank, those who were hoping to apply for staff appointments. This, however, re-opened the tricky question of selection. How could the College make sure that only committed specialists would gain admission? Two alternatives were considered: one was to establish a diploma by examination only which specialists would have to take before the Membership – the latter being given only to people who were on the staffs of hospitals. The other was to give the Membership by examination as well as by a record of appointments.[83] Shaw for one was not over-enthusiastic about the latter option because he thought that the College would then have to admit 'all sorts of coloured people' (who would compete with white men) and those in Great Britain who had no intention of practising solely obstetrics and gynaecology.[84] Never-theless, the second method was finally accepted, and in June 1930 the rules for admission were revised: candidates of senior rank were allowed to join without further formality, while younger prac-titioners were required to take an oral examination and to submit the records of twenty-five obstetrical and ten gynaecological cases. A year later, a clinical examination was added, and in March 1932 it was decided to introduce commentaries on one obstetrical and one gynaecological case to test a candidate's ability to use a library and digest the literature relevant to a particular case. But initially the examination was not as stringent as the MRCP or the FRCS: it merely consisted of an interview upon the candidate's case-records and the discussion of a few pathological specimens.[85] In a few cases the regulations were stretched, and candidates were admitted with-out examination: the College simply had to do all it could to attract promising young obstetricians.

Recruitment problems dictated compromises also with regard to the length of training required of candidates. It was widely felt that resident posts in both general medicine and surgery should be required in addition to a period of clinical experience in special hospitals and ante-natal clinics, but the scarcity of junior appoint-ments in general medicine and surgery would have drastically reduced the number of applicants for the Membership. If the Col-lege insisted upon both a house physicianship and a house sur-geonship, many candidates would be induced to take the DGO, which did not require any general training in either medicine or surgery. Similar problems were experienced in respect of obstetrics and gynaecology. As the London teaching hospitals had inadequate facilities for the training of students in obstetrics and gynaecology, only a short period of training in resident appointments could be required if all of these hospitals were to be included in the scheme. A standard of training below that which was desired thus had to be accepted – namely, six months in either medicine or surgery, and six months each of obstetrics and gynaecology.

This policy undoubtedly helped the young College build up its membership, but it also generated two major problems. First, as Shaw had forecast, it widened the professional base from which members were drawn, so that in the event some GPs were included. Secondly, it pitched the standard for the MCOG at too low a level in relation to the FRCS. Six years after the foundation of the

College, the MCOG had not diminished the value of the FRCS for staff appointments at London hospitals, and Shaw was forced to acknowledge that the 'intellectual value' of the Membership needed raising.[86] In the meantime, the College had instituted its own diploma in obstetrics for general practitioners, thus bringing the obstetric training of general practitioners under its aegis; once the danger of competition from the Royal Colleges had been elim- inated, it became possible to raise the standards of the MCOG and draw a clearer distinction between general practitioner–obstetrician and obstetric specialist.[87]

Everybody agreed that the MCOG should contain a written paper, so as to bring it to a standard equivalent to the FRCS and MRCP. Shaw believed that a paper common to all candidates would be most useful in shaping their training and standardising the exam: as he pointed out to Blair Bell in 1935, it was possible to get the Membership without any knowledge of the advanced physi- ology of the female reproductive organs or of endocrinology – a most undesirable state of affairs.[88] However, he hoped that the exam would never become of a type 'which lets in the good exam- inee and keeps out the better practical man'.[89] He thus supported an examination which would emphasise the clinical, rather than the theoretical aspects of the subject – a handicap for GPs, who had limited access to hospitals. The first full Membership examination, held in 1937, fulfilled these aims by introducing two written papers (in anatomy, pathology, physiology, obstetrics and gynaecology), and a clinical examination which included two viva voce exam- inations, one in pathology and the other in obstetrics and gynaecology.[90]

The question of the diploma for general practitioners was bound up with the College Membership, not only because the diploma was potentially a rival to the Membership, but also because the two qualifications had to define more tightly the professional relations between generalists and specialists. When the Royal Colleges re- solved to establish a diploma in obstetrics and gynaecology for general practitioners, they sought the advice of a small committee consisting of William Blair Bell, Thomas Watts Eden, Comyns Berkeley and William Fletcher Shaw – all of them being Signatories of the new College. The committee believed that the BCOG would subsequently be asked to take part in the examination, but it soon became apparent that this was not to be. At the beginning of 1930, there was widespread agreement within the Council of the College that the obstetricians should institute their own diploma in the event of co-operation not being offered. That it should have taken the College four years to put the plan into action was due to two factors: first, a growing desire on the part of the London men not to alienate the Royal Colleges by setting up a rival qualification; secondly, differences of opinion as to the relation between the Membership (for specialists) and the diploma (for general practitioner-obstetricians).

In February 1930 Fletcher Shaw formally asked the Royal Colleges if they intended to invite the BCOG to co-operate in the examination. The Surgeons, still smarting with disappointment after their failure to amend the diploma clause, answered in the negative. The Physicians were more accommodating: they hoped the College would co-operate by appointing a panel of examiners. There was no suggestion of full partnership, and the College was free, therefore, to institute its own diploma. The Examination Committee immediately set about drafting the regulations, but pressure from the London men, especially Thomas Watts Eden, soon persuaded the Council to accept the offer of the College of Physicians. Thus in May 1930, three examiners (one from London and two from the provinces) were appointed to form the panel: these were Eardly Holland (1879–1967), Obstetric Physician at the London Hospital, Munro Kerr and Bethel Solomons (1885–1965), Master of the Rotunda Hospital.[91] The medical corporations hoped to cut the ground from under the feet of their rivals by setting up the DGO, but the obstetricians managed to sabotage the diploma by making its standards only a little less stringent than those of the College Membership.[92] The result of this clever manoeuvre was that only seven candidates were granted this qualification between 1930 and 1935, the year in which the diploma was withdrawn.

The question of the diploma was laid to rest while Blair Bell devoted his energy to an abortive Maternity Scheme; it was not until January 1931 that the issue was raised again. After some discussion, the Council of the College agreed to set up a diploma sub-committee, on condition that the draft scheme be 'pigeon-holed until needed'.[93] The diploma was at first conceived of as a qualification in both obstetrics and gynaecology, aimed primarily at general practitioners acting as local consultants at municipal and county hospitals. The proposals for the diploma were discussed at a meeting of Council in July 1931, marking the beginning of a long and complex debate over the standards and scope of obstetrical training for general practitioners. Thomas Watts Eden strongly criticised the recommendations of the sub-committee, the standards proposed being much lower than those of the DGO. The College could not accept less stringent requirements and say that its diplomates were qualified to act as local obstetric consultants; furthermore, there was a 'gentlemanly agreement' not to enter into competition with the Royal Colleges. Fletcher Shaw did not like the scheme much either, as it played into the hands of untrained general practitioners who were encroaching upon gynaecological surgery. Serious reservations about the idea of a diploma were once again voiced by all the London obstetricians, who were anxious to heal the breach with the Royal Colleges.[94] In spite of widespread doubt and criticism, Blair Bell stuck to his guns: one day the diploma would be registrable, he argued, and if the College were invited to take part in the Conjoint examination, as he was convinced that it should be, then the diploma would rank on a par with the MRCS and LRCP.

In the event the Council resolved to make one last attempt at co-operation with the Royal Colleges: it was thought that the Colleges might be more amenable now, since their diploma was proving to be a failure. Thus in May 1932, a deputation of obstetricians led by Blair Bell met representatives of the two Royal Colleges to discuss the problem. Blair Bell reiterated the terms on which the BCOG was prepared to co-operate; he intimated that the College would go ahead with its own diploma if these were not complied with. As a result, a special committee of the two Colleges was appointed to reconsider the question.

For a brief moment it seemed that co-operation was much closer than anyone could have expected, but Sir Henry Simson's (1872–1932) endeavours to gain Royal support for the College before an agreement had been reached, led to a breakdown in the negotiations. In October 1932, the committee issued a statement in which the possibility of co-operation was ruled out; at the same time, they recommended that the DGO be withdrawn. This decision was strongly criticised by Victor Bonney: he thought that it put the final seal on the divorce of obstetrics and gynaecology from medicine and surgery and he regretted that the Surgeons should abandon their interest in advancing the specialty.[95] When the recommendation of the committee was brought before the Council of the RCS they would not confirm it, so the examination was continued for three more years.

During this interval, the College was busy finalising its own scheme. Following representations from the Dominions, in 1931 the regulations for the diploma had been stiffened, but in the meantime the question of gynaecological surgery in general practice had emerged as a central problem for the College. Since 1920 general practitioners had made inroads into surgery, and it had not taken the gynaecologists long to join the surgeons and the orthopaedists in a battle against the general practitioners who strayed into surgery.[96] It was essential that the College's diploma should not appear to endorse the generalists' pretensions to operative gynaecology.

In 1929 Shaw and Blair Bell had considered the possibility of instituting a diploma in obstetrics only for general practitioners, 'the idea being', explained Blair Bell to Thomas Watts Eden, 'that it is Obstetrics in General Practice that really requires encouragement and not Gynaecology; for we do not want to make the general practitioner imagine that he is a specialist in Gynaecology because he has a Diploma.'[97] Beckwith Whitehouse (1882–1943), Professor of Obstetrics and Gynaecology at Birmingham University, heartily agreed:

The general practitioner of to-day is anxious at all costs to obtain some authority which will give him the opportunity to practice [sic] Surgery and unless we are *very* careful this Diploma will be accepted by him in that spirit and will be used as a lever for ulterior motives whatever we may say, think or wish.[98]

Thus in April 1933 an alternative scheme was submitted which made no provision for gynaecology – except insofar as it may be related to childbearing.

But how could the College *both* exclude general practitioners from gynaecological surgery *and* preserve the unity of obstetrics and gynaecology, the principle upon which the whole idea of a College of Obstetricians and Gynaecologists turned? John Fairbairn, the second President of the College, suggested that this might be done by splitting the Membership into two parts: part one (the diploma) would be a preliminary for the Membership; it would be aimed at non-specialists and comprise obstetrics only. Part two would consist of gynaecology and would be open to those who wished to specialise. But other members of Council, notably Eardly Holland, Fletcher Shaw and Miles Phillips (1875–1965) wanted to widen the gap between specialist and general practitioner and argued that the Membership examination should be differentiated from the diploma as much as possible.[99]

Finally, at the end of 1933 it was decided that the diploma should be quite separate from the Membership and that it should be in obstetrics only. Emergencies were far more frequent in obstetrical than gynaecological practice, argued Carnac Rivett in support of these provisions, thus it was more important to create competent obstetric consultants than gynaecological surgeons; gynaecological surgery could remain in the hands of 'trained people'.[100] Not everyone agreed, though. Thomas Watts Eden pointed out that under the scheme practitioners would not be trained in abdominal surgery and would thus be unable to perform emergency caesareans. This meant that in rural districts where there were no Members or Fellows of the College, gynaecological surgery would be abandoned in the hands of the local surgeons: 'Such an attitude would leave an unfortunate impression that the College desired to make gynaecological surgery the special preserve of its Fellows and Members', observed Eden in July 1933.[101] He forgot to mention that the interests of patients were not well served by these provisions: women living in the outlying areas of the country had no immediate access to specialist help and often it was not possible to get a consultant to a patient until the need for his services had passed.

In order to retain the unity of obstetrics and gynaecology in the title of the diploma, it was resolved to call the new qualification the Diploma in Obstetrics of the College of Obstetricians and Gynaecologists (DCOG). This strategy badly misfired: in a few instances practitioners with the DCOG posed as consultants, and in some Commonwealth countries they even got hospital appointments on the strength of the diploma. Thus in 1945, in the wake of criticism from the younger Members, the title was changed to D. Obst. RCOG.[102] In 1976, however, the original letters were re-instated as the GP's involvement in obstetrics declined and the emphasis on non-surgical gynaecology and family planning in general practice increased.

With the establishment of a formal organisation, the definition of specialist status and the restriction of entry into the profession to those who met prescribed criteria, obstetricians and gynaecologists were fashioned into a recognisably modern profession. But there was still a long way to go before the internecine conflicts which had stimulated the establishment of the College could be resolved. Cracks in the friendship between Blair Bell and Berkeley were already in evidence before the foundation of the College; by 1930 this quarrel had degenerated into an acrimonious dispute which had the effect of splitting the Council into a provincial camp led by Blair Bell and a metropolitan group supporting Berkeley. The row between the two gynaecologists was caused chiefly by differences of opinion over the manner of dealing with Lord Riddell (1865–1934), a newspaper tycoon who gave munificent donations to the young College. Lord Riddell viewed the College as a commercial enterprise and he thought that it should raise funds by playing upon the public's anxiety about maternal mortality: he suggested that a manifesto should be drawn up emphasising the good a College of Obstetricians and Gynaecologists might do for maternal health and a copy sent to every rich patient. Berkeley thought the College would do well to heed this advice, but Blair Bell and Shaw were 'very averse to collecting money for a College on a charitable basis and with a plea that it is to save the women and children. If the College is a success', wrote Shaw to Blair Bell in 1927, 'it will certainly improve the teaching and practice of obstetrics, but it will be a slow business and I do not see any justification for asking for money for this particular purpose.'[103] When Lord Riddell gave the College a seven-years covenant for £600 annually, Berkeley wrote to him an extravagant thank-you letter in which he equated Riddell to the benefactors of Caius College in Cambridge, where Berkeley had been a student. Blair Bell condemned Berkeley's expressions of gratitude as 'undignified grovellings' and Berkeley promptly resigned his post as Honorary Treasurer in a storm of protest.

The founders of the College were determined that the provinces should always retain control of the Council; to this end they had arranged that the Council be elected on a territorial basis, with so many members from London, the provinces, Scotland and Ireland. During the presidency of Blair Bell's successor, the London obstetrician John Fairbairn, the metropolitan practitioners who sat on the Council attempted to alter the Articles governing the election of the Council, so as to gain increased representation for London. The matter was referred to a sub-committee which in the end did recommend some increase in London representation, but when the proposed changes were submitted to the Council they were emphatically turned down.

In *The Medical Profession in Mid-Victorian London*, Peterson has argued that 'the modern professions – whose archetype is medicine – fostered group solidarity, loyalty, and exclusiveness, regardless of differences in general education, ascribed social rank, or economic standing'.[104] The foundation of the BCOG suggests that, on the contrary, medicine is a divided profession, in which groups and individuals vie with each other for the protection of sectional and personal interests. The ev·lution of gynaecology in England cannot be fully understood without reference to the intra-professional rivalries that have shaped its theory and practice.

Despite these divisions, one central assumption has underpinned gynaecology throughout its long history: this is the belief that woman is dominated by her sexual functions. During the early twentieth century the development of gynaecological endocrinology, of which Blair Bell was a pioneer, was to give a new twist to the 'science of woman'. In the *Sex Complex*, published in 1916, Blair Bell maintained that femininity depended on all the glands of internal secretion interacting together. He argued that the secretions of the ovaries bent the metabolism of the female body to serve the needs of the reproductive function, at the same time as the other glands regulated the development and activity of the sexual system. Echoing Van Helmont and Chéreau, he enunciated this concept: 'Propter secretiones internas totas mulier est quod est' (it is because of all the internal secretions that woman is what she is).[105] For the scientist, the march of progress had pushed the boundaries of gynaecology forward. The historian will be more inclined to view this development as the expression of an enduring ideology.

Appendix

Table 1. *Hospital for Women, Soho Square. Protheroe Smith's case-book, 1869–1870*

	Paying patients: occupation and marital status	
Occupation	Married	Single
National school mistress		1
Governess		1
Draper's daughter		1
Clergyman's daughter		1
Laceworker		1
Hospital Clerk	1	
Total	1	5

All paying patients	22
Married	8
Single	11
Widowed	2
Unstated	1

Table 2. *Hospital for Women, Soho Square. Protheroe Smith's case-book, 1869–70*

Occupation	Charity Patients: occupation and marital status		
	Married	Single	Widowed
Cook		1	
Traveller in drapery		1	
Plate-layer	1		
Laundress	1		
General servant		3	
Bootmaker	1		
Confectioner	1		
Upholsterer	1		
Mantle-maker		1	
'No occupation'		1	
Sewing-machine maker	na		
Cabinet-maker's wife	1		
Washer	1		
?-maker	1		
Missionary		1	1
Ladies' maid		1	
Waistcoat-maker	1		
Ironer			1
House messenger	1		
Lithographer	1		
Nurse		1	
Dressmaker	1		1
Housewife	3		
Total	15	10	3

All charity patients	50
Married	29
Single	12
Widowed	3
Not stated	4

Table 3. *Middlesex Hospital – Prudhoe Ward. June 1863–October 1866*

Occupation	Patients' occupation and marital status		
	Married	Single	Widowed
Housewife	58		
Servant	1	20	
Dressmaker	3	3	
Nurse	2	3	
Cook		3	1
Nursery Governess		2	
Housemaid		2	
Shop girl		1	1
Needlewoman		1	2
Laundress			1
Housekeeper		1	
Cloth-cap maker		1	
Stewardess			1
Companion		1	
Charwoman	1		
Workwoman	1		
Total	66	38	6

All patients	175
Married	101
Single	45
Widowed	19
Not stated	10

210

Table 4. *Rate of mortality after surgical operations, 1844*

Operation	Total number of cases	Deaths	Rate of mortality (%)
Amputations	3586	1146	31.9
Tying large arteries	199	66	33.1
Lithotomy	5900	765	12.9
Hernia	545	260	47.7
Ovariotomy	42	14	33.3
Caesarean section	321	172	53.5

Source: T. Inman, 'Tables of the mortality after operations', *Lancet*, 2 (1844), 39–40. The figures refer to all known cases.

Table 5. *Chelsea Hospital for Women: ovariotomy 1873–89*

Year	No. of admissions	Cases of ovarian disease	No of ovariotomies
1873	21	2	1
1874	37	0	0
1875	16	0	0
1876	10	0	0
1877	43	0	0
1878	13	0	0
1879	73	4	2
1884	296	13	6
1889	403	32	25[a]

[a] In three cases ovariotomy was recommended, but the patient refused the operation.
All figures refer to the extant case-records and are compiled for the calendar year.

Notes

Introduction

1 T. S. Wells, *Modern Abdominal Surgery: The Bradshaw Lecture Delivered at the Royal College of Surgeons of England. With an Appendix on the Castration of Women* (London, 1891), p. 51.
2 M. Bloch and J. H. Bloch, 'Women and the dialectics of nature in eighteenth-century French thought', in C. MacCormack and M. Strathern (eds.), *Nature, Culture, and Gender* (Cambridge, 1980), 25–41; J. B. Elshtain, *Public Man, Private Woman: Women in Social and Political Thought* (Oxford, 1981), pp. 100–46.
3 T. Laqueur and L. Schiebinger have examined the development of a discourse of sex differences in respect of reproductive biology and anatomy. T. Laqueur, 'Orgasm, generation, and the politics of reproductive biology', *Representations*, 14 (1986), 1–41; L. Schiebinger, 'Skeletons in the closet: the first illustrations of the female skeleton in eighteenth-century anatomy', *ibid.*, 42–82.
4 See Bloch and Bloch, 'Women and the dialectics of nature'.
5 L. Jordanova, 'Naturalizing the family: literature and the bio-medical sciences in the late eighteenth century', in L. Jordanova, *Languages of Nature: Critical Essays on Science and Literature* (London, 1986), pp. 86–116. For an account of the way in which the private/public boundaries could become blurred, see L. Davidoff, 'The separation of home and work? Landladies and lodgers in nineteenth- and twentieth-century England', in S. Burman (ed.), *Fit Work for Women* (London, 1979), pp. 64–93. In an article on the turn-of-the-century debate on health visiting as an appropriate occupation for women, C. Davies had argued that ideas about gender and class shaped the way in which women's role in the public sphere was perceived; 'The health visitor as mother's friend: a woman's place in public health, 1900–14', *Social History of Medicine*, 1 (1988), 39–59. A Marxist critique of the private/public distinction is provided by E. Fox-Genovese, 'Placing women's history in history', *New Left Review*, 133 (1982), 5–29. Fox-Genovese's analysis of women's economic role as producers of use-values (i.e. non-commodities) echoes Jordanova's discussion of women and the family in the late eighteenth century.

6 G. Weber, 'Science and society in nineteenth-century anthropology', *History of Science*, 12 (1974), 260–83; Schiebinger, 'Skeletons in the closet'. As J. de Groot has shown in her analysis of nineteenth-century 'orientalist' paintings, sexual metaphors were used to characterise the orient and justify the need for the 'inferior' colonial races to be controlled by the 'civilised' European countries; J. de Groot, '"Sex" and "race": the construction of language and image in the nineteenth century', in S. Mendus and J. Rendall (eds.), *Sexuality and Subordination: Interdisciplinary Studies of Gender in the Nineteenth Century* (London and New York, 1989), pp. 89–128.

7 Jordanova, *Languages of Nature*, pp. 34–6.

8 Quoted in J. L. Newton, M. P. Ryan, J. R. Walkowitz, *Sex and Class in Women's History* (London, Boston, Melbourne and Henley, 1983), p. 5. This volume provides an excellent introduction to the questions involved. See also Fox-Genovese, 'Placing women's history'. For an example of a study which puts class back into gender, see K. Figlio, 'Chlorosis and chronic disease in nineteenth-century Britain: the social constitution of somatic illness in a capitalist society', *Social History*, 3 (1978), 167–97.

9 G. Rosen, *The Specialization of Medicine, with Particular Reference to Ophthalmology* (New York, 1944).

10 T. Gelfand, 'The origins of a modern concept of medical specialization: John Morgan's *Discourse* of 1765', *Bulletin of the History of Medicine*, 50 (1976), 511–35.

11 D. Armstrong, *Political Anatomy of the Body: Medical Knowledge in Britain in the Twentieth Century* (Cambridge, 1983).

12 L. Jordanova, 'Medicalisation and modernisation: some problems in the historical sociology of medicine', unpublished paper, April 1980.

13 M. Pelling, 'Medical practice in the early modern period: trade or profession?' *Society for the Social History of Medicine Bulletin*, 32 (1983), 27–30. See also R. Dingwall and P. Lewis (eds.), *The Sociology of the Professions* (London and Basingstoke, 1983). R. Porter has suggested that late eighteenth-century 'professionals' (e.g. William Hunter) should be seen as entrepreneurs. R. Porter, 'William Hunter: a surgeon and a gentleman', in W. Bynum and R. Porter (eds.), *William Hunter and the Eighteenth-Century Medical World* (Cambridge, 1985), pp. 7–34.

1 The problem of femininity

1 J. Craig, *A New Universal Etymological, Technological, and Pronouncing Dictionary of the English Language: Embracing All the Terms Used in Art, Science and Literature*, 2 vols. (London, 1849).

2 C. Wall, *A History of the Worshipful Society of Apothecaries of London*, vol. I, 1617–1815 (no further vols. published). Abstracted and arr. by H. C. Cameron; rev., annotated, and ed. by E. A. Underwood (London, 1963), pp. 109–10. On gynaecological theory in the early

modern period, see A. Eccles, *Obstetrics and Gynaecology in Tudor and Stuart England* (London and Canberra, 1982).

3 L. Bourgeois, *Observations diverses sur la stérilité, perte de fruit, foecondité, accouchements, et maladies des femmes et enfants nouveaux naiz* (Paris, 1642).

4 J. Sharp, *The Midwives Book* (London, 1671).

5 J. H. Aveling, *English Midwives: Their History and Prospects*, ed. J. L. Thornton (1872; London, 1967), pp. 41–2.

6 S. Stone, *A Complete Practice of Midwifery* (London, 1737), p. xix.

7 A. L. Wyman, 'The surgeoness: the female practitioner of surgery 1400–1800', *Medical History*, 28 (1984), 22–41, p. 37.

8 *Ibid.*, p. 31; see also A. Clark, *Working Life of Women in the Seventeenth Century* (London and New York, 1919), pp. 253–65.

9 J. V. Ricci, *The Genealogy of Gynaecology: History of the Development of Gynaecology Throughout the Ages* (Philadelphia, 1943), p. 423. On quack doctresses, R. Porter, 'Female quacks', unpublished paper, November 1988.

10 Ricci, *Genealogy*, p. 521.

11 I. S. L. Loudon, *Medical Care and the General Practitioner 1750–1850* (Oxford, 1986), pp. 11–28. On the development of man-midwifery, see J. Donnison, *Midwives and Medical Men: A History of Inter-Professional Rivalries and Women's Rights* (London, 1977); A. Wilson, *A Safe Deliverance: Conflict and Ritual in English Childbirth, 1600–1750* (Cambridge, forthcoming); A. Wilson, 'William Hunter and the varieties of man-midwifery', in W. F. Bynum and R. Porter (eds.), *William Hunter and the Eighteenth-Century Medical World* (Cambridge, 1985), 343–69, pp. 344–53.

12 G. Rosen, *From Medical Police to Social Medicine: Essays on the History of Health Care* (New York, 1974), esp. pp. 120–41; 159–75.

13 P. Buck, 'People who counted: political arithmetic in the eighteenth century', *Isis*, 73 (1982), 28–45. See also L. Jordanova; 'Policing public health in France', in T. Ogawa (ed.), *Public Health* (Tokyo, 1981), pp. 12–32, and C. Hannaway, 'From private hygiene to public health: a transformation in Western medicine in the eighteenth and nineteenth centuries', *ibid.*, pp. 108–28.

14 K. Figlio, 'The metaphor of organisation: an historiographical perspective on the bio-medical sciences of the early nineteenth century', *History of Science*, 14 (1976), 17–53, pp. 25ff.; F. Delaporte, *Le second règne de la nature: essai sur les questions de la végétalité au XVIIIᵉ siècle* (Paris, 1979); J. Roger, *Les sciences de la vie dans la pensée Français du XVIIIᵉ siècle* (Paris, 1963).

15 W. Cadogan, *An Essay on the Management of Children, from Their Birth to Three Years of Age*, 6th edn. (London, 1753; 1st publ. 1748), p. 3.

16 J. Leake, *Introduction to the Theory and Practice of Midwifery* (London, 1787), pp. 6–7. For an account of how the debate on *naissances tardives* in eighteenth-century France established the role of medical men in cases where the legitimacy of a child was being disputed, see L. B.

Wilson, 'Les maladies des femmes: women, charlatanry, and professional medicine in eighteenth-century France' (Ph.D. thesis, University of Stanford, 1982). Wilson however does not discuss the significance of the debate to the development of man-midwifery.

17 M. Schurig, *Gynaecologia historico-medica hoc est congressus muliebris consideratio physico-medico-forensis. Qua utriusque sexus salacitas et castitas deinde coitus ipse eiusque voluptas et varia circa hunc actum occurrentia nec non coitus ob atresiam seu vaginae uterinae imperforationem et alias causas impeditus et denegatus, item nefandus et sodomiticus raris observationibus et aliquot casibus medico-forensibus exhibentur* (Leipzig and Dresden, 1730). On Lotichius, see Ricci, *Genealogy*, pp. 362–3. Interestingly, Schurig also wrote a medico-legal text entitled *Embryologia*, but I know of no historical work which analyses the relations between embryology and legal medicine.

18 For an example, see W. Alexander, *The History of Women, from the Earliest Antiquity, to the Present Time; Giving Some Account of Almost Every Interesting Particular Concerning That Sex, among All Nations, Ancient and Modern* (London, 1779). The emergence of this discourse in France is examined by Y. Knibiehler, 'Les médecins et la "nature féminine" au temps du code civil', *Annales: E.S.C.*, 31 (1976), 824–45.

19 On the science of Man, see e.g. S. Moravia, *La scienza dell'uomo nel Settecento* (Bari, 1970); S. Moravia, *Filosofia e scienze umane nell'età dei lumi* (Florence, 1982); E. A. Williams, 'The science of Man: anthropological thought and institutions in nineteenth-century France' (Ph.D. thesis, Indiana University, 1983); G. Weber, 'Science and society in nineteenth century anthropology', *History of Science*, 12 (1974), 260–83; G. Stocking, Jr., 'French anthropology in 1800', *Isis*, 5 (1964), 134–50; C. Blanckaert, 'Médecine et histoire naturelle de l'homme: l'anthropologie française dans la seconde moitié du XIX siècle', in J. Poirier and J. L. Poirier (eds.), *Médecine et philosophie à la fin du XIXe siècle* (Paris, 1981), pp. 101–16.

20 D. K. van Keuren, 'Human science in Victorian Britain: anthropology in institutional and disciplinary formation, 1863–1908' (Ph.D. thesis, University of Pennsylvania, 1982).

21 J. Jamieson, 'Sex, in health and disease', *Australian Medical Journal*, n.s., 9 (1887), 145–58, p. 145.

22 *Ibid.*, p. 146.

23 See E. Fee, 'Science and the "Woman Question", 1860–1920: a study of English scientific periodicals' (Ph.D. thesis, University of Princeton, 1978); R. Rosenberg, *Beyond Separate Spheres* (New Haven and London, 1982) looks at the feminist contribution to the debate. For a comprehensive overview of the themes encompassed by the 'Woman Question', see E. K. Helsinger, R. L. Sheets, W. Veeder (eds.), *The Woman Question: Social Issues, 1837–1883*, 3 vols. (Manchester, 1983).

24 E. Clarke, *Sex in Education; Or, a Fair Chance for the Girls* (Boston, 1873), p. 12.

25 van Keuren, 'Human science in Victorian Britain', pp. 116–42.

26 1757–1808. One of the French *idéologues* who proposed the new 'science of Man'; P. J. G. Cabanis, *Oeuvres philosophiques*, 2 vols. (Paris, 1956).

27 J. Oliver, 'Woman physically and ethically considered', *Liverpool Medico-Chirurgical Journal*, 9 (1889), 219–26, p. 219.

28 C. Pears, 'The case of a full grown woman in whom the ovaria were deficient', *Philosophical Transactions of the Royal Society of London*, 115 (1805), 225–7. See also E. Goujon, 'A study of incomplete hermaphroditism in a man', in M. Foucault (ed.), *Hérculine Barbin* (Brighton, 1980), 128–144, pp. 138–9; A. Tardieu, *Question médico-légale de l'identité* (Paris, 1874).

29 G. J. Romanes, 'Mental differences between men and women', in Romanes, *Essays*, ed. C. Lloyd Morgan (London, 1897), 113–151, p. 113.

30 Blanckaert, 'Medécine et histoire naturelle de l'homme'. On the question of interbreeding in relation to the monogenism versus polygenism debate, see G. W. Stocking Jr., 'Polygenist thought in post-Darwinian anthropology', in Stocking, *Race, Culture, and Evolution: Essays in the History of Anthropology* (1968; Chicago and London, 1982), pp. 42–68. The political dimensions of the debate are discussed by van Keuren, 'Human science in Victorian Britain'; W. Bynum, 'The great chain of being after forty years: an appraisal', *History of Science*, 13 (1975), 1–28.

31 Laqueur has argued that the homologies drawn by ancient medical writers were rejected in the nineteenth century, signalling a radical reinterpretation of the female body in relation to the male from a 'metaphysics of hierarchy' to 'an anatomy and physiology of difference'. While agreeing that the concept of sexual difference became fundamental to the analysis of femininity and masculinity during the nineteenth century, I want to argue that the notion of kinship was no less important. T. Laqueur, 'Orgasm, generation, and the politics of reproductive biology', *Representations*, 14 (1986), 1–41.

32 For a comprehensive table of homologies, see J. Y. Simpson, 'Hermaphroditism', in W. G. Simpson (ed.), *The Works of Sir J. Y. Simpson*, 3 vols. (Edinburgh, 1871), II, 407–542, pp. 509–10.

33 A. Farre, 'Uterus and its appendages', in R. B. Todd (ed.), *The Cyclopaedia of Anatomy and Physiology*, 5 vols. (London, 1835–59), V, 545–725, p. 623.

34 See R. Barnes, 'On vicarious menstruation', *British Gynaecological Journal*, 2 (1886–7), 151–83; A. Wiltshire, 'Clinical lecture on vicarious or ectopic menstruation, or menses devii', *Lancet*, 2 (1885), 513–17.

35 Wiltshire, 'Vicarious or ectopic menstruation', p. 514.

36 *Ibid.*, pp. 513; 517.

37 V. O. King, 'Case of menstruation in the male', *Canada Medical Journal*, 2 (1867), 472–3, p. 472.

38 Laycock elaborated his doctrine in a series of articles published in the *Lancet* in the early 1840s. T. Laycock, 'Evidence and arguments in proof of the existence of a general law of periodicity in the phenomena of life', *Lancet*, 1 (1842–3), 124–9; 160–4; 'Further development of a general law of vital periodicity; being a second contribution to proleptics', *ibid.*, 423–7; 'On some of the causes which determine the minor periods of vital movements', *ibid.*, 929–33; 'On the influence of the moon on the atmosphere of the earth, and on the pathological influence of the seasons', *Lancet*, 2 (1842–3), 826–30; 'On lunar influence; being a fourth contribution to proleptics', *ibid.*, 438–44; 'On annual vital periods, being a fifth contribution to vital proleptics', *Lancet*, 1 (1843–4), 85–9; 'On the major periods of development in man, being a sixth contribution to proleptics', *ibid.*, 253–8.

39 T. Laycock, *A Treatise on the Nervous Diseases of Women* (London, 1840), p. 218.

40 Wiltshire, 'Vicarious or ectopic menstruation', p. 516.

41 Quoted in F. J. Sulloway, *Freud, Biologist of the Mind* (New York, 1979), p. 140.

42 Quoted *ibid.*, p. 144. On Freud and bisexuality, see *ibid.*, esp. pp. 222–23.

43 Simpson, 'Hermaphroditism', pp. 491–2.

44 *Ibid.*, p. 490.

45 *Ibid.*, pp. 481–2.

46 *Ibid.*, p. 490. Simpson argued that when the female approximated the male it was by excess, whereas the male approximated the female by defect. Even this however was not unambiguous, as he also remarked that while in certain respects the female was developed less than it was proper in the species, in other respects she was developed in greater degree. However, later in the treatise Simpson maintained that the enlargement of the breasts was a character peculiar to the species in general.

47 C. Darwin, *The Descent of Man and Selection in Relation to Sex*, 2nd edn. (1871; London, 1909).

48 C. Gegenbaur, *Elements of Comparative Anatomy* (London, 1878), p. 54.

49 Darwin, *Descent of Man*, p. 322.

50 *Ibid.*, p. 858.

51 Tait's relationship with Darwin is narrated by J. A. Shepherd, *Lawson Tait: The Rebellious Surgeon (1845–1899)* (Lawrence, Kansas, 1980), pp. 109–37.

52 *Ibid.*, p. 109.

53 The paper was republished in R. L. Tait, *Two Essays on the Law of Evolution* (Birmingham, 1885). Tait made the point that the law of natural selection may operate adversely in civilised societies.

54 Shepherd, *Lawson Tait*, pp. 132–3.

55 Jamieson, 'Sex, in health and disease', p. 151.

56 See L. Jordanova, 'Earth science and environmental medicine: the

synthesis of the late Enlightenment', in L. Jordanova and R. Porter (eds.), *Images of the Earth* (Chalfont St Giles, 1979), pp. 119–46.

57 For a particularly good example of this perspective, see C. Waller, 'Lectures on the functions and diseases of the womb', *Lancet*, 1 (1839–40), 393. See also A. Raciborski, *De la puberté et de l'âge critique chez la femme* (Paris, 1844), pp. 4–27; 34–52; 'Woman in her psychological relations', *Journal of Psychological Medicine and Mental Pathology*, 4 (1851), 36; R. Barnes and F. Barnes, *A System of Obstetric Medicine and Surgery*, 2 vols. (London, 1884), I, p. 42; D. B. Hart and A. H. F. Barbour, *Manual of Gynaecology* (Edinburgh and London, 1886), p. 82.

58 J. Roberton, 'On the period of puberty in Esquimaux women', *Edinburgh Medical and Surgical Journal*, 63 (1845), 57–65.

59 Weber, 'Science and society', pp. 276–9. J. Calder, *Women and Marriage in Victorian Fiction* (London, 1976), pp. 72–3.

60 H. Mayhew, *London Labour and the London Poor: A Cyclopaedia of the Conditions and Earnings of Those That Will Work, Those That Cannot Work, and Those That Will Not Work*, 4 vols. (London, 1861).

61 H. H. Ploss, M. Bartels and P. Bartels, *Woman: An Historical, Gynaecological and Anthropological Compendium*, ed. E. J. Dingwall, 3 vols. (London, 1935). P. Weideger, *History's Mistress: A New Interpretation of a Nineteenth-Century Ethnographic Classic* (Harmondsworth, 1985) contains a selection from *Das Weib* and a conceptually disappointing introduction to this work.

62 J. Power, *Essays on the Female Economy* (London, 1821), esp. pp. ii; 9; 14–27; 35.

63 F.-A. Pouchet, *Théorie positive de l'ovulation spontanée et de la fécondation des mammifères et de l'espèce humaine* (Paris, 1847), pp. 233; 244. His ideas echoed the Malthusian argument that civilisation had increased the power of human beings to reproduce.

64 C. Darwin, *The Variation of Animals and Plants under Domestication*, 2 vols. (London, 1868).

65 A. Wiltshire, 'Lectures on the comparative physiology of menstruation', *British Medical Journal*, 1 (1883), 395–8.

66 J. B. Hicks, 'On the differences between the sexes in regard to the aspect and treatment of disease', *British Medical Journal*, 1 (1877), 318–20; 347–9; 377–9; 413–15; 447–9; 475–6, p. 319. Hicks seems to have subscribed to a notion of infantile sexuality: cf. *ibid.*, 348, where he argues that sexual differences and feelings exist 'almost from the cradle', becoming more marked at the time of puberty.

67 *Ibid.*, p. 414. He was referring to the characters developed through sexual selection.

68 *Ibid.*, p. 414.

69 W. R. Williams, *The Influence of Sex in Disease* (London, 1885), p. 3.

70 Jamieson, 'Sex, in health and disease', p. 152. On sex and life-expectancy, see also J. Stockton-Hough, 'Longevity, or the relative vitality of the sexes', *Medical Recorder*, 8 (1873), 297–301; 353–5.

71 Oliver, 'Woman physically and ethically considered', p. 223.

72 H. Ellis, *Man and Woman: A Study of Human Secondary Sexual Characters*, 4th edn. (1894; London, 1904), pp. 440–1.

73 E. Fee, 'Nineteenth-century craniology; the study of the female skull', *Bulletin of the History of Medicine*, 53 (1979), 415–33, and J. Haller and R. Haller, *The Physician and Sexuality in Victorian America* (Urbana, 1974), pp. 48–61. On the use of cranial capacity, brain weight and language as indices of the development and complexity of the intellectual faculties, see for example C. Bolt, *Victorian Attitudes to Race* (London, 1971), 11–16; Figlio, 'The metaphor of organisation'; Weber, 'Science and society'. By the turn of the century, the problem had been reformulated in terms of what brains could do rather than how much they weighed. P. Jorion, 'The downfall of the skull', *Royal Anthropological Institute Newsletter*, 48 (1982), 8–11; R. Rosenberg, *Beyond Separate Spheres* (New Haven, 1982) examines the feminist contribution to the field.

74 W. Balls-Headley, *The Evolution of the Diseases of Women* (London, 1894), p. 1.

75 T. B. Curling, 'Testicles', in Todd, *The Cyclopaedia of Anatomy and Physiology*, IV, part II, 976–1016, p. 992.

76 *Ibid.*, pp. 985; 994.

77 Jordanova, 'Natural facts', pp. 42–5; R. Williams, *The Country and the City* (St Albans, 1975).

78 V. C. Medvei, *A History of Endocrinology* (Lancaster, 1982), p. 406.

79 M. Bloch and J. H. Bloch, 'Women and the dialectics of nature in eighteenth-century French thought', in MacCormack and Strathern (eds.), *Nature, Culture and Gender*, pp. 25–41.

80 Jamieson, 'Sex, in health and disease', p. 146.

81 R. L. Tait, *Diseases of Women and Abdominal Surgery* (Leicester, 1889), I, 3.

82 R. Barnes, 'Women, diseases of', in R. Quain (ed.), *A Dictionary of Medicine: Including General Pathology, General Therapeutics, Hygiene, and the Diseases Peculiar to Women and Children*, 2 vols. (London, 1882), II, 1789.

83 On Michelet, see e.g. L. Orr, *Jules Michelet: Nature, History and Language* (Ithaca, New York, 1976).

84 R. Smith, *Trial by Medicine: Insanity and Responsibility in Victorian Trials* (Edinburgh, 1981), pp. 143–60.

85 van Keuren, 'Human science in Victorian Britain'; Stocking, *Race, Culture, and Evolution*, pp. 110–32; Figlio, 'The metaphor of organisation'; W. Bynum, 'The great chain of being after forty years: an appraisal', *History of Science*, 13 (1975), 1–28. On the maleness of reason in Western philosophical thought, G. Lloyd, *The Man of Reason: 'Male' and 'Female' in Western Philosophy* (London, 1984).

86 'Andrology as a specialty', *Journal of the American Medical Association*, 17 (1891), 631. For an alternative view about men's diseases, see E. Shorter, *A History of Women's Bodies* (London, 1983).

87 K. Walker, *Diseases of the Male Organs of Generation* (London, 1923). I

know of no study of andrology, alias urology, between the Wars. The question of male sterility has been woefully neglected by historians. One notable exception is N. Pfeffer, 'Pronatalism and sterility' (Ph.D. thesis, University of Essex, 1988).

88 M. Warner, *Alone of All Her Sex: The Myth and the Cult of the Virgin Mary* (London, 1976), pp. 255–69; A. Rich, *Of Woman Born* (London, 1977), pp. 84–109.

89 Wiltshire, 'Lectures on the comparative physiology of menstruation', p. 396. On the imagery of man disrobing woman as nature, see Jordanova, 'Natural facts', pp. 54–8.

90 The first proponents of the 'ovular theory' of menstruation were J. Power, R. Lee, T. L. W. Bischoff, A. Raciborski and F.-A. Pouchet. R. Lee, 'Lectures on the structure and physiology of the ovaria', *Medical Times and Gazette*, 14 (1857), 305–7; 329–30; 637–8 contains a brief historical note on the development of the theory. For a discussion, see H. H. Simmer, 'Pflüger's nerve reflex theory of menstruation: the product of analogy, teleology and neurophysiology', *Clio Medica*, 12 (1977), 57–90, esp. pp. 60–7; Laqueur, 'Orgasm, generation, and the politics of reproductive biology'.

91 C. West, *Lectures on the Diseases of Women*, 3rd edn. (London, 1864), p. 5.

92 A. Chéreau, *Memoires pour servir à l'étude des maladies des ovaires* (Paris, 1844), p. 91.

93 Barnes and Barnes, *System of Obstetric Medicine*, I, pp. 202–3.

94 M. Weber, quoted in L. Davidoff, 'Class and gender in Victorian England', in J. L. Newton, M. P. Ryan, J. R. Walkowitz (eds.), *Sex and Class in Women's History* (London, 1983), 17–71, p. 20.

95 However, not all pleasures were permissible within marriage – an emphatic line was drawn between the wife and the prostitute. On sex and the conjugal tie in western culture, see M. Foucault, *Histoire de la sexualité*, 3 vols. (Paris, 1977–84), III, pp. 173–216.

96 Jordanova, 'Natural facts', p. 50.

97 'Woman in her psychological relations', *Journal of Psychological Medicine and Mental Pathology*, 4 (1851), 18–50, pp. 18–19 *passim*. It is probable that the author of this essay was A. Walker, see below, note 100.

98 *Ibid.*, p. 20.

99 *Ibid.*, pp. 19–20 *passim*.

100 A. Walker, *Beauty Illustrated by an Analysis and Classification of Beauty in Woman* (London, 1852), pp. 72–84. His aim was to improve the population by teaching men to choose a beautiful and fit wife. On Walker's ideas about femininity and his gendering of aesthetics, see R. Cooper, 'Alexander Walker's woman', unpublished paper, 1988. I am grateful to Robyn Cooper for letting me read a copy of this paper.

101 'Woman in her psychological relations', p. 35. Eunuchs and effeminate men were also unattractive because wanting in the masculine attributes.

102 See e.g. A. Douglas, "The fashionable diseases": women's complaints and their treatment in nineteenth-century America', *Journal of Interdisciplinary History*, 4 (1973), 25–52. For a critique R. Morantz, 'The lady and her physician', in M. S. Hartmann and L. Banner (eds.), *Clio's Consciousness Raised* (New York, 1974), pp. 38–51.

103 'Sex in occupation', *Obstetrical Journal of Great Britain and Ireland*, 2 (1874–5), 157–8.

104 J. Roberton, *Essays and Notes on the Physiology and Diseases of Women, and on Practical Midwifery* (London, 1851), pp. 1–2.

105 'Woman in her social relations, past and present', *Journal of Psychological Medicine and Mental Pathology*, 9 (1856), pp. 536–40; Romanes, 'Mental differences between men and women', pp. 121–3.

106 'Woman in her psychological relations', p. 18.

107 M. Girouard, *The Return to Camelot: Chivalry and the English Gentleman* (New Haven and London, 1981), pp. 197–218.

108 Darwin, *Descent of Man*, p. 858.

109 Jamieson, 'Sex, in health and disease', pp. 147; 149.

110 R. Barnes, 'An address on obstetric medicine, and its position in medical education', *Obstetrical Journal of Great Britain and Ireland*, 3 (1875–6), p. 294.

111 *Ibid.*

112 On pelvimetry, see G. Vrolik, *Considerations sur la diversité des bassins de differentes races humaines* (Amsterdam, 1826); W. A. Lane, 'Which are the chief factors which determine the differences which exist in the form of the male and female pelves?', *British Medical Journal*, 2 (1887), 832; W. Turner, 'The index of the pelvic brim as a basis of classification', *Journal of Anatomy and Physiology*, 20 (1885–6), 125–43; J. G. Garson, 'Pelvimetry', *Journal of Anatomy and Physiology*, 16 (1881–2), 106–134; 'Sexe', in A. Bertillon *et al.*, *Dictionnaire des sciences anthropologiques* (Paris, 1884). The gendering of anatomy is discussed by L. Schiebinger, 'Skeletons in the closet: the first illustrations of the female skeleton in eighteenth-century anatomy', *Representations*, 14 (1986), 42–82.

113 Barnes and Barnes, *System of Obstetric Medicine*, I, pp. 170–1.

114 *Ibid.*, p. 173.

115 H. Maudsley, 'Sex in mind and in education', *Fortnightly Review*, 21 (1874), 446–83; E. G. Anderson, 'Sex in mind and education, a reply', *ibid.*, 582–94.

116 Clarke, *Sex in Education*, p. 13.

117 *Ibid.*, p. 14.

118 *Ibid.*, pp. 114–15. The quotation is from H. Maudsley, *Body and Mind: An Inquiry into Their Connection and Mutual Influence, Specially in Reference to Mental Disorders* (London, 1870), pp. 32–3.

2 Men-midwives and medicine

1 J. Donnison, *Midwives and Medical Men: A History of Inter-Professional Rivalries and Women's Rights* (London, 1977), p. 3; A. Wilson, 'Participant or patient? Seventeenth century childbirth from the mother's point of view', in R. Porter (ed.), *Patients and Practitioners: Lay Perceptions of Medicine in Pre-Industrial Society* (Cambridge, 1985), pp. 129–44; A. Wilson, *A Safe Deliverance: Conflict and Ritual in English Childbirth, 1600–1750* (Cambridge, forthcoming).

2 Donnison, *Midwives and Medical Men*, p. 8.

3 *Ibid.*, pp. 5–7. According to the seventeenth-century midwife Elizabeth Cellier, a break in the system occurred in London between 1642 and 1662, during which period midwives were licensed by the Surgeons; J. H. Aveling, *English Midwives: Their History and Prospects* (1872; London, 1967), p. 89.

4 Wilson, *A Safe Deliverance*.

5 Donnison, *Midwives and Medical Men*, p. 6.

6 For an example of the midwife's oath, see Aveling, *English Midwives*, pp. 153–5.

7 Even J. Donnison's ideologically sensitive study hints that men-midwives may have brought improvements to the crude craft of women.

8 A. Bourne, *A Doctor's Creed: The Memoirs of a Gynaecologist* (London, 1962), p. 22.

9 Wilson, 'Participant or patient?', p. 136.

10 See P. Willughby, *Observations in Midwifery*, ed. H. Blenkinsop (Warwick, 1863), pp. 40; 49; 66; 82.

11 *Ibid.*, p. 184.

12 A. Wilson, 'William Hunter and the varieties of man-midwifery', in W. F. Bynum and R. Porter (eds.), *William Hunter and the Eighteenth-Century Medical World* (Cambridge, 1985), pp. 342–69, esp. p. 353.

13 D. Harley, 'Ignorant midwives – a persistent stereotype', *Society for the Social History of Medicine Bulletin*, 28 (1981), 6–9; B. Boss and J. Boss, 'Ignorant midwives – a further rejoinder', *Society for the Social History of Medicine Bulletin*, 32 (1983), 71.

14 Wilson, 'William Hunter', esp. pp. 349–57.

15 I. S. L. Loudon, 'Nature vs. intervention in obstetrics: a historical survey', unpublished paper, May 1986.

16 O. H. Wangensteen and S. D. Wangensteen, *The Rise of Surgery: From Empiric Craft to Scientific Discipline* (Folkestone, 1978), p. 206.

17 For a history of the forceps, see K. Das, *Obstetric Forceps* (Calcutta, 1929).

18 W. Radcliffe, *Milestones in Midwifery* (Bristol, 1967), p. 30.

19 Willughby, *Observations*, pp. 151–3.

20 S. Stone, *A Complete Practice of Midwifery* (London, 1737).

21 Aveling, *English Midwives*, p. 127.

22 A. L. Wyman, 'The surgeoness: the female practitioner of surgery,

1400–1800', *Medical History*, 28 (1984), 22–41; S. Young, *The Annals of the Barber Surgeons* (London, 1890), p. 260. It would appear that women continued to be members of the Barbers' Company after the separation from the Surgeons.

23 Quoted in H. R. Spencer, *The History of British Midwifery from 1650 to 1800* (London, 1927), pp. 72–3.

24 Wilson, *A Safe Deliverance*.

25 H. van Deventer, *The Art of Midwifery Improv'd. Fully and Plainly Laying down Whatever Instructions are Requisite to Make a Compleat Midwife . . . Also a New Method, demonstrating, how Infants Ill Situated in the Womb . . . May, by the Hand Only . . . be Turned into Their Right Position . . . To Which is Added a Preface Giving Some Account of This Work, by an Eminent Physician* (London, 1716).

26 J. Douglas, *Short Account of the State of Midwifery in London, Westminster, &c.* (London, 1736).

27 J. Maubray, *Midwifery Brought to Perfection by Manual Operation* (London, 1725). See Donnison, *Midwives and Medical Men*, p. 31.

28 Spencer, *The History of British Midwifery*, pp. 52–3. In late twentieth-century Britain, a forceps rate of 20 to 50 per 1000 is usual amongst a healthy population of low-risk mothers. For a detailed account of Smellie's use of the forceps, see J. Glaister, *Dr. William Smellie and His Contemporaries: A Contribution to the History of Midwifery in the Eighteenth Century* (Glasgow, 1894), pp. 226–57. Outside London, man-midwifery developed long before the use of the forceps became general: when Dr. J. Toogood arrived in Bridgwater in 1800, he was surprised to find that the forceps was unknown; I. S. L. Loudon, *Medical Care and the General Practitioner 1750–1850* (Oxford, 1986), n. 44, p. 90.

29 Wilson, 'William Hunter'.

30 This is how Thomas Young, the first Professor of Midwifery at Edinburgh University, described the evolution of the man-midwife; C. Hoolihan, 'Thomas Young, M.D. (1726?–1783) and obstetrical education at Edinburgh', *Journal of the History of Medicine and Allied Sciences*, 40 (1985), 327–45, p. 339.

31 L. Jordanova, 'Medicalisation and modernisation: some problems in the historical sociology of medicine', unpublished paper, April 1980.

32 P. Lomas, 'An interpretation of modern obstetric practice', in S. Kitzinger and J. A. Davis (eds.), *The Place of Birth: A Study of the Environment in Which Birth Takes Place with Special Reference to Home Confinements* (Oxford, 1978), pp. 174–84.

33 Hoolihan, 'Thomas Young, M.D.'.

34 The first lying-in ward was established by Sir Richard Manningham in 1739. See M. C. Versluysen, 'Midwives, medical men and "poor women labouring of child": lying-in hospitals in eighteenth century London', in H. Roberts (ed.), *Women, Health, and Reproduction* (London, 1981), pp. 18–49.

35 Wilson, *A Safe Deliverance*.

36 See G. Clark, *A History of the Royal College of Physicians of London*, 2 vols. (London, 1966).

37 C. Wall, *The History of the Surgeons' Company* (London, 1937); Z. Cope, *The Royal College of Surgeons of England: A History* (London, 1959).

38 C. Wall, *A History of the Worshipful Society of Apothecaries of London*, vol. I, 1617–1815 (no further vols. published). Abstracted and arr. by H. C. Cameron; rev., annotated, and ed. by E. A. Underwood (London, 1963).

39 D. Hamilton, *The Healers: A History of Medicine in Scotland* (Edinburgh, 1981).

40 R. S. Roberts, 'The personnel and practice of medicine in Tudor and Stuart England. Part I: the provinces', *Medical History*, 6 (1962), 363–82; Roberts, 'The personnel and practice of medicine in Tudor and Stuart England. Part II: London', *Medical History*, 8 (1964), 217–34.

41 Roberts, 'The personnel and practice of medicine. Part II: London', esp. pp. 221; 224. Most medical practitioners also combined the practice of surgery or physic with other occupations. M. Pelling, 'Surgeons, Barbers, and Barber-Surgeons: an occupational group in an English provincial town, 1550–1640', *Society for the Social History of Medicine Bulletin*, 28 (1981), 14–16.

42 In the winter of 1699–1700 John Seale, a butcher of Hungerford Market, was given medicine by William Rose, apothecary, without the intermediary of a physician. The case was reported to the College of Physicians, and legal proceedings were brought against Rose. The apothecary was found guilty and was fined; he later appealed to the House of Lords, which reversed the judgment given in the Queen's Bench. The Lords argued it was not only contrary to custom, but also against the interest of the public to prevent apothecaries from giving medical advice. See Clark, *A History of the Royal College of Physicians of London*, II, pp. 437–47.

43 R. Porter, 'William Hunter: a surgeon and a gentleman', in W. F. Bynum and R. Porter (eds.), *William Hunter and the Eighteenth-Century Medical World* (Cambridge, 1985), p. 18.

44 Wall, *The History of the Surgeons' Company*, p. 54.

45 On the licentiates, see Clark, *A History of the Royal College of Physicians of London*, II, pp. 552–73.

46 L. G. Stevenson, 'The siege of Warwick Lane, together with a brief history of the Society of Collegiate Physicians, 1767–98', *Journal of the History of Medicine*, 7 (1952), 105–21; I. Waddington, 'The struggle to reform the Royal College of Physicians, 1767–1771: a sociological analysis', *Medical History*, 17 (1973), 107–26.

47 On the new statutes, see Clark, *A History of the Royal College of Physicians of London*, II, pp. 565–6.

48 *Ibid.*, pp. 502–3.

49 I am grateful to Adrian Wilson for supplying information about the political sympathies of Walker and Birch.

50 For a critique of the concept of marginality, see P. Weindling, 'The British Mineralogical Society: a case study in science and social improvement', in I. Inkster and J. Morrell (eds.), *Metropolis and Province: Science in British Culture 1780–1850* (London, 1983), pp. 120–50.

51 This view was emphasised by the famous cartoon which portrayed the man-midwife as half-man, half-woman. See Donnison, *Midwives and Medical Men*, pl. 3.

52 Porter, 'William Hunter'.

53 Clark, *A History of the Royal College of Physicians*, II, pp. 588–9.

54 The other midwifery licentiates were: Louis Poignard (1746–1809); Robert Batty (1763–1849); John Cooper; Thomas Savage (1724–1804); Charles Combe (1743–1817); John Clarke and John Squire (1732–1816).

55 Clark, *A History of the Royal College of Physicians of London*, II, p. 637. This is thought to be the earliest occurrence of the phrase 'general practice'.

56 Donnison, *Midwives and Medical Men*, pp. 43–4.

57 Clark, *A History of the Royal College of Physicians of London*, II, p. 637; Donnison, *Midwives and Medical Men*, p. 44.

58 On obstetrics and general practice, see Loudon, *Medical Care*, pp. 85–99.

59 For an alternative interpretation, see I. S. L. Loudon, 'The concept of the family doctor', *Bulletin of the History of Medicine*, 58 (1984), 347–62.

60 M. J. Peterson, *The Medical Profession in Mid-Victorian London* (Berkeley, 1978), pp. 5–20; D. L. Cowen, 'Liberty, laissez-faire and licensure in nineteenth-century Britain', *Bulletin of the History of Medicine*, 43 (1969), 30–40. The first case concerned Dr Paris T. Dick, who was a Scottish graduate and was thus not legally qualified to practise in England. In 1809 the College reminded the Fellows that they would be fined if they consulted with him, only to find that Dr Pemberton, a fellow, had consulted with Dick no less than nine times. Dick was prosecuted and fined £50, but he did not become a licentiate till 1823. The second case involved the medical reformer Dr Harrison, also a Scottish graduate, who had set up practice as a physician in London without the College's licence. The legal action brought against him in 1828 failed. Clark, *A History of the Royal College of Physicians of London*, II, pp. 507–16; 641–2.

61 On the rise of the druggist and medical reform, see Loudon, *Medical Care*, pp. 129–37. For an account of the debates on medical reform, see I. Waddington, *The Medical Profession in the Industrial Revolution* (Dublin, 1984); C. Newman, *The Evolution of Medical Education in the Nineteenth Century* (London, 1957), esp. pp. 56–193.

62 Cowen, 'Liberty, laissez-faire and licensure'; M. Ramsey, 'The politics of professional monopoly in nineteenth-century medicine: the

French model and its rivals', in G. L. Geison (ed.), *Professions and the French State, 1700–1900* (Philadelphia, 1984), 225–305, pp. 245–50.

63 However, certain disabilities were imposed on practitioners who were not on the Register, i.e. they could not be exempted from military, community and jury duties; they could not hold government appointments, nor could they sue for fees.

64 See Loudon, *Medical Care*, pp. 138–46; Clark, *A History of the Royal College of Physicians of London*, II, pp. 627–32; Newman, *The Evolution of Medical Education*, pp. 59–65.

65 Loudon, *Medical Care*, pp. 152–88. On the apothecaries' proposals for the control of midwifery, see Aveling, *English Midwives*, pp. 153–5.

66 Cope, *The History of the Royal College of Surgeons of England*, pp. 38–9.

67 Donnison, *Midwives and Medical Men*, p. 46.

68 Clark, *A History of the Royal College of Physicians of London*, II, p. 664.

69 *Ibid.*

70 *Ibid.*

71 Donnison, *Midwives and Medical Men*, p. 47.

72 *Report from the Select Committee on Medical Education*, PP. 1834, vol. XIII, evidence of Sir H. Halford, Q.232.

73 *Ibid.*, evidence of Charles Clarke, Q.4220.

74 Cope, *The History of The Royal College of Surgeons of England*, p. 129.

75 *Ibid.*, pp. 42–56.

76 *Ibid.*, pp. 129–30.

77 *Ibid.*, p. 131.

78 *Ibid.*, pp. 131–2.

79 Clark, *A History of the Royal College of Physicians of London*, II, p. 721.

80 Waddington, *The Medical Profession*, p. 91.

81 Donnison, *Midwives and Medical Men*, p. 57.

82 J. M. Kerr, R. W. Johnstone and M. H. Phillips (eds.), *Historical Review of British Obstetrics and Gynaecology* (Edinburgh, 1954), pp. 296–8.

83 Newman, *The Evolution of Medical Education*, pp. 229–30.

84 *Lancet*, 1 (1842), 664.

85 'A former pupil' (pseud.), 'St Marylebone Infirmary', *Lancet*, 1 (1841), 64.

86 See e.g. 'Medical practitioner unjustly indicted for manslaughter', *Lancet*, 1 (1846), 393.

87 See the *Lancet*, *Medical Times* and *London Medical Gazette* for 1844–5. Midwives and irregular practitioners were seen by qualified medical men to form a single group.

88 'Restrictions on the practice of midwifery', *London Medical Gazette*, n.s., 1 (1845), 779–82.

89 See chapter 6.

90 W. Tyler Smith, 'Introductory lecture to a course of lectures on obstetricy (delivered at the Hunterian School of Medicine)', *Lancet*, 2 (1847), 371–4, p. 371.

91 W. T. Smith's obituary, *Lancet*, 1 (1873), 825–7.

92 Cope, *The Royal College of Surgeons of England*, pp. 146–9.
93 'The teaching of midwifery and Mr Syme's Committee on Medical Education', *Lancet*, 2 (1868), 708–9.
94 M. Poovey makes a similar point with regard to the mid-nineteenth-century debate on anaesthesia in childbirth; ' "Scenes of an indelicate character": the medical "treatment" of Victorian women', *Representations*, 14 (1986), 137–68, p. 149.
95 R. Barnes, 'An address on obstetric medicine and its position in medical education', *Obstetrical Journal of Great Britain and Ireland*, 3 (1875–6), 289–99.
96 Memorial from the Obstetrical Society of London, *Special Report from the Select Committee on the Medical Act (1858) Amendment Bill*, PP. 1879, vol. XII, pp. 402–9.
97 *Select Committee on the Medical Act (1858) Amendment Bill*, evidence of Dr Acland, Q.265, 437–9; recommendations of the GMC on education and examinations, p. 392. See also S. Butler, 'Science and medicine in the nineteenth century: changing conceptions of medical practice', *Society for the Social History of Medicine Bulletin*, 37 (1985), 35–7.
98 *Select Committee on the Medical Act (1858) Amendment Bill*, evidence of Dr Acland, Q.187.
99 See pp. 79–81.
100 *Select Committee on the Medical Act (1858) Amendment Bill*, evidence of Mr Waters, Q. 1913–15.
101 *Ibid.*, evidence of Dr Acland, Q.190–2.
102 'Report of the Infantile Mortality Committee of the Obstetrical Society of London', *Transactions of the Obstetrical Society of London*, 12 (1870), 132–49; 13 (1871), 388–403.
103 J. H. Aveling, 'Instruction of midwives' (letter), *British Medical Journal*, 1 (1874), 433.
104 Peterson, *The Medical Profession*, pp. 99–100.
105 F. B. Smith, *The People's Health 1830–1910* (London, 1979), p. 44.
106 J. H. Aveling, 'Instruction of midwives' (letter), *British Medical Journal*, 1 (1874), 252–3, p. 253.
107 Donnison, *Midwives and Medical Men*, p. 83.
108 *Ibid.*, pp. 80–2.
109 Aveling, 'Instruction of midwives', pp. 252, 433.
110 For an account of women's entry into medicine, see e.g. E. M. Bell, *Storming the Citadel: The Rise of the Woman Doctor* (London, 1953).
111 Cope, *The Royal College of Surgeons of England*, pp. 121–8.
112 J. H. Aveling, 'The College of Surgeons of England, and obstetric medicine', *Obstetrical Journal of Great Britain and Ireland*, 3 (1875–6), 732–6, p. 732.
113 *Ibid.*, p. 734.
114 J. Manton, *Elizabeth Garrett Anderson* (London, 1965), p. 236.
115 Aveling, 'The College of Surgeons of England', p. 736.
116 See chapter 6.

117 Donnison, *Midwives and Medical Men*, pp. 159–74.
118 Cope, *The Royal College of Surgeons of England*, pp. 150–4.
119 R. R. Rentoul, 'The training of the medical student in midwifery', *Lancet*, 1 (1891), 875–6, p. 876.

3 The rise of the women's hospitals

1 These figures are drawn from M. J. Peterson, *The Medical Profession in Mid-Victorian London* (Berkeley, 1978), pp. 262–3.
2 Other specialisms followed the same pattern. See Peterson, *The Medical Profession*, pp. 259–80; L. Granshaw, '"Fame and fortune by brick and mortar": the medical profession and specialist hospitals in Britain, 1800–1948', unpublished paper, 1986.
3 B. Abel-Smith, *The Hospitals 1800–1948: A Study in Social Administration in England and Wales* (London, 1964), p. 6; Peterson, *The Medical Profession*, pp. 154–5.
4 On the growth of medical schools, see C. Newman, *The Evolution of Medical Education in the Nineteenth Century* (London, 1957), pp. 112–22; W. R. Merrington, *University College Hospital Medical School: A History* (London, 1976); Z. Cope, *The History of St. Mary's Hospital Medical School, or a Century of Medical Education* (Toronto, 1954).
5 Abel-Smith, *The Hospitals*, p. 152.
6 *Ibid.*, pp. 152–3.
7 This could be an expensive business: for example, at the Aldersgate Street Dispensary in 1824 two competing applicants paid six hundred guineas between them in the hope of being elected as surgeon; Granshaw, '"Fame and fortune by brick and mortar"'.
8 E. T. Collins, *The History and Tradition of Moorfields Eye Hospital* (London, 1929), pp. 1–16.
9 Granshaw, '"Fame and fortune by brick and mortar"'.
10 Hospital for Women, Committee Minutes, 1/4/1880.
11 *Ibid.*, 16/12/1880.
12 Abel-Smith, *The Hospitals*, pp. 5–6.
13 C. Morson, *St. Peter's Hospital for Stone, 1860–1960* (Edinburgh and London, 1960).
14 W. Martin, 'Special hospitals', *British Medical Journal*, 2 (1861), 301–4, p. 304.
15 D. Armstrong, *Political Anatomy of the Body: Medical Knowledge in Britain in the Twentieth Century* (Cambridge, 1983), pp. 54–63.
16 The letter was published in the *British Medical Journal*, 1860, 583.
17 'Hospital distress', *British Medical Journal*, 1860, pp. 458–9, 459.
18 *Ibid.*, p. 458.
19 'Special hospitals', *British Medical Journal*, 1860, 625–9, p. 628.
20 Peterson, *The Medical Profession*, p. 276.
21 W. R. Bett, *Sir John Bland-Sutton 1855–1936* (Edinburgh and London, 1956), p. 28.
22 Morson, *St. Peter's Hospital*, p. 21.

23 C. West to the Medical Committee, Nov. 5, 1846 (letter), Middlesex Hospital Fair Minute Book, February 1845–April 1847.

24 S. Ashwell, 'Testimonial', Hospital for Women Reports, 1842, p. 11.

25 Peterson, *The Medical Profession*, pp. 145–7. Peterson describes Harrison as the 'archetypal figure of lay authority in the early nineteenth-century medical world'.

26 Smith's biographical data are drawn from his obituary, *British Medical Journal*, 2 (1889), 849, and from W. R. Winterton, 'The story of the London gynaecological hospitals', *Proceedings of the Royal Society of Medicine*, 54 (1961), 191–8, p. 193.

27 P. Smith, *Scriptural Authority for the Mitigation of the Pains of Labour by Chloroform and Other Anaesthetic Agents* (London, 1848).

28 P. Smith, 'Medical Testimony on the expediency of establishing a hospital for the diseases of women', HW Reports, 1842, 1–6, p. 3.

29 See chapter 4.

30 Dispensary practice involved a substantial amount of home visiting; this may have made Smith more sensitive to the environment of his patients. See I. S. L. Loudon, 'The origins and growth of the dispensary movement in England', *Bulletin of the History of Medicine*, 55 (1981), 322–42.

31 E. Rigby, *On Dysmenorrhoea and Other Uterine Affections in Connection with Derangements of the Assimilating Functions* (London, 1844); E. Rigby, *On the Constitutional Treatment of Female Disorders* (London, 1856). The doctrine competed with the local theory of uterine disease, according to which uterine affections were idiopathic and could engender constitutional derangements.

32 E. Rigby, 'Reports on uterine disease', *Medical Times*, 10 (1844), 505–6, p. 505.

33 *Ibid.*, p. 505.

34 E. Rigby, 'Reports on uterine disease', *Medical Times*, 12 (1845), 263–4, p. 264.

35 Smith, 'Medical Testimony', p. 3.

36 *Ibid.*, p. 3.

37 J. H. Davis, 'Testimonial', HW Reports, 1842, p. 14.

38 This attitude is exemplified by H. Mayhew, *London Labour and the London Poor: A Cyclopaedia of the Condition and Earnings of Those That Will Work, Those That Cannot Work, and Those That Will Not Work*, 4 vols. (London, 1861). At bottom, the problem of urban health mediated middle-class anxieties about the close proximity of the poor; see A. S. Wohl, *Endangered Lives: Public Health in Victorian Britain* (London, 1983); G. S. Jones, *Outcast London: A Study of the Relationship between Classes in Victorian Society* (Oxford, 1971); H. Himmelfarb, 'The culture of poverty', in H. J. Dyos and M. Wolff (eds.), *The Victorian City: Images and Reality*, 2 vols. (London, 1973), II, pp. 707–36.

39 F. Engels, *The Condition of the Working Class in England* (1845; Oxford, 1958). Engels discusses the disruption of family life caused by women's factory work on pp. 160–2.

40 Quoted in J. M. Eyler, 'Mortality statistics and Victorian health policy: programme and criticism', *Bulletin of the History of Medicine*, 50 (1976), 335–55, p. 336. See also W. Coleman, *Death is a Social Disease: Public Health and Political Economy in Early Industrial France* (Madison WI, 1982). Florence Nightingale's programme for hospital reform was founded on the assumption that disease stemmed from moral disorder; C. E. Rosenberg, 'Florence Nightingale on contagion: the hospital as a moral universe', in C. E. Rosenberg (ed.), *Healing and History: Essays for George Rosen* (New York and Folkestone, 1979), pp. 117–36.

41 For a case-study, see K. Figlio, 'Chlorosis and chronic disease in nineteenth-century Britain: the social constitution of somatic illness in a capitalist society' *Social History*, 3 (1978), 167–97. On the diseases of poverty, see G. Rosen, 'Disease, debility and death', in Dyos and Wolff (eds.), *The Victorian City*, II, pp. 625–68.

42 S. Alexander, 'Women's work in nineteenth-century London: a study of the years 1820–1850', in J. Mitchell and A. Oakley (eds.), *The Rights and Wrongs of Women* (Harmondsworth, 1976), pp. 59–111. On women's work, see also J. W. Scott and L. A. Tilly, *Women, Work and Family* (New York, 1978); M. Hewitt, *Wives and Mothers in Victorian Industry* (Westport CT, 1958).

43 'The sanitary condition of the milliners and dressmakers of London', *Lancet*, 1 (1853), 519–20, p. 520.

44 For general works on the Evangelical movement, see I. Bradley, *The Call to Seriousness: the Evangelical Impact on the Victorians* (London, 1976). The role played by the Evangelical movement in the creation of the ideology of domesticity is discussed by C. Hall, 'The early formation of Victorian domestic ideology', in S. Burman (ed.), *Fit Work for Women* (London, 1979), pp. 15–32. Chadwick devoted a great deal of attention to bad domestic management as a source of disease among the poor: E. Chadwick, *Report on the Sanitary Condition of the Labouring Population in Great Britain* (London, 1842). For a discussion of how this ideology functioned in relation to occupational diseases in France, see A. Farge, 'Work-related diseases of artisans in eighteenth-century France', in R. Forster and O. Ranum (eds.), *Medicine and Society in France: Selections from the 'Annales'* (Baltimore and London, 1980), pp. 89–103.

45 See R. L. Schoenwald, 'Training urban man: a hypothesis about the sanitary movement', in Dyos and Wolff (eds.), *The Victorian City*, II, pp. 669–92. On the emergence of a disciplined society, see E. P. Thompson, 'Time, work-discipline, and industrial capitalism', *Past and Present*, 35 (1967), 56–97. M. Foucault has analysed the extension of discipline to the details of human action: M. Foucault, *Discipline and Punish: the Birth of the Prison* (Harmondsworth, 1979).

46 L. Davidoff, 'Class and gender in Victorian England', in J. L. Newton, M. P. Ryan and J. R. Walkowitz (eds.), *Sex and Class in Women's History* (London, 1983), pp. 17–71, p. 21.

47 The hospital was opposed at first, but I have not been able to find out who objected to it and why.
48 HW Reports, no. 7, 1850, p. 6.
49 HW Reports, no. 1, 1844.
50 HW Reports, no. 2, 1845, p. 5.
51 'Unprofessional advertisements', *Lancet*, 2 (1853), opp. p. 68.
52 HW Reports, no. 13, 1856, pp. 6–7.
53 HW Reports, no. 15, 1858, p. 12.
54 HW Reports, no. 3, 1846, p. 6.
55 *Ibid.*, p. 7.
56 HW Reports, no. 7, 1850, pp. 11–12.
57 On the training of Magdalens, see S. B. P. Pearce, *An Ideal in the Working: The Story of the Magdalen Hospital 1758 to 1958* (London, 1958), pp. 52–8 *passim*; H. F. B. Compston, *The Magdalen Hospital: The Story of a Great Charity* (London, 1917), esp. pp. 170–86.
58 HW Reports, no. 30, 1873, p. 10.
59 *Ibid.*, 18; p. 29.
60 *Ibid.*, p. 24.
61 C. Cappe, *Thoughts on the Desirableness and Utility of Ladies Visiting the Female Wards of Hospitals and Lunatic Asylums* (London, 1816). On the role played by upper-class women in philanthropic activities, see F. K. Prochaska, *Women and Philanthropy in Nineteenth-Century England* (Oxford, 1980); A. Summers, 'A home from home: women's philanthropic work in the nineteenth century', in Burman (ed.), *Fit Work for Women*, pp. 33–63.
62 Cappe, *Thoughts on the Desirableness and Utility of Ladies Visiting the Female Wards of Hospitals and Lunatic Asylums*, p. 376. The lady nurses who went out to the Crimea adopted exactly the same system in their relations with their working-class sisters; A. Summers, 'Pride and prejudice: ladies and nurses in the Crimean war', *History Workshop Journal*, 16 (1983), pp. 33–56, esp. pp. 46–7.
63 HW Reports, no. 7, 1850, p. 10. The implications for the family must have been dramatic.
64 HW Reports, no. 4, 1847, p. 5.
65 These data are compiled on the basis of Protheroe Smith's case-notes, Oct. 1869–Nov. 1870.
66 Data based on the records of gynaecological cases, Prudhoe Ward, Middlesex Hospital, June 1863–Oct. 1866.
67 R. Pinker, *English Hospital Statistics 1861–1938* (London, 1966), p. 121.
68 HW, Committee Minutes, 8 Jan. 1873.
69 'The authorities of the Hospital for Women and their honorary medical officers', *Medical Times and Gazette*, 1 (1874), 374–5, p. 375.
70 Abel-Smith, *The Hospitals*, p. 27.
71 'The authorities of the Hospital for Women', p. 374.
72 *Ibid.*

73 HW, Committee Minutes, 17 March 1881.
74 HW, Committee Minutes, 7 April 1881.
75 HW, Committee Minutes, 2 March 1882; 8 Jan. 1885.
76 HW, Committee Minutes, 1 Oct. 1885.
77 'The authorities of the Hospital for Women', p. 374.
78 H. Burdett, 'Home hospitals: their scope, object and management',
    British Medical Journal, 2 (1877), 243–5.
79 *Lancet*, 1 (1877), 913–15.
80 HW Reports, no. 24, 1864, p. 8.
81 *Lancet*, 2 (1877), 914.
82 Abel-Smith, *The Hospitals*, p. 148.
83 HW Reports, no. 27, 1870, p. 11.
84 *Ibid.*, pp. 4–5.
85 HW Reports, no. 28, 1871, p. 5.
86 Aveling's biographical data are drawn from his obituary, *British
    Medical Journal*, 2 (1892), 1349–50, and from the preface to J. H.
    Aveling, *English Midwives: Their History and Prospects*, ed. J. L.
    Thornton (1872; London, 1967), pp. xi–xxxi.
87 Chelsea Hospital for Women Reports, 1871–3, p. 21.
88 A. J. Hammerton, 'Feminism and female emigration, 1861–1886', in
    M. Vicinus (ed.), *A Widening Sphere: Changing Roles of Victorian
    Women* (London, 1977), pp. 52–71, discusses the problem of 'surplus'
    women in relation to female emigration.
89 M. J. Peterson, 'The Victorian governess: status incongruence in
    family and society', in M. Vicinus (ed.), *Suffer and Be Still* (Bloo-
    mington and London, 1972), pp. 3–19.
90 'The hospital for ladies', *The Times*, 22 May 1865, p. 9.
91 H. C. Burdett, 'Home hospitals: their scope, object, and manage-
    ment', *British Medical Journal*, 2 (1877), 243–5.
92 CHW Reports, 1871–3, p. 21.
93 *Ibid.*, pp. 5–6.
94 CHW Reports, 1882–3, p. 25.
95 CHW Reports, 1884–5, pp. 11, 17; 1885–6, p. 13.
96 'The Chelsea Hospital for Women', *Lancet*, 1 (1894), p. 365.
97 H. C. Burdett, *Hospitals and Asylums of the World: Their Origin,
    Construction, Administration, Management, and Legislation*, 4 vols.
    (London, 1891–3), IV, p. 317.
98 'The Chelsea Hospital for Women', *Lancet*, 2 (1894), 200–1.
99 *Ibid.*, p. 201.
100 H. E. Wright, 'The Chelsea Hospital for Women' (letter), *Lancet*, 1
    (1894), 631–2.
101 'The Chelsea Hospital for Women', *Lancet*, 2 (1894), 1299.
102 See chapter 6. On the exclusion of GPs from hospital work, see F.
    Honigsbaum, *The Division in British Medicine: A History of the Separ-
    ation of General Practice from Hospital Care 1911–1968* (London, 1979),
    esp. chapter 13.

103 R. D. French, *Antivivisection and Medical Science in Victorian Society* (Princeton, 1975), p. 325; M. A. Elston, 'Women and anti-vivisection in Victorian England, 1870–1900', in N. A. Rupke (ed.), *Vivisection in Historical Perspective* (London, 1987), 259–94, p. 279. The feminist and antivivisectionist opposition to surgical gynaecology is explored in chapters 4 and 5.
104 Bett, *Sir John Bland-Sutton.*
105 Abel-Smith, *The Hospitals*, p. 159.
106 *British Medical Journal*, 1 (1889), 1412.
107 Abel-Smith, *The Hospitals*, p. 157.
108 *Ibid.*, p. 159.
109 'Special hospitals', *British Medical Journal*, 1860, 627.

4 Woman and her diseases

1 R. Barnes, 'Women, diseases of', in R. Quain (ed.), *A Dictionary of Medicine: Including General Pathology, General Therapeutics, Hygiene, and the Diseases Peculiar to Women and Children*, 2 vols. (London, 1882), II, p. 1790.
2 W. T. Smith, 'Lectures on parturition, and the principles and practice of obstetricy', *Lancet*, 2 (1848), 119.
3 There is a vast literature on this issue. See e.g. T. Laycock, *A Treatise on the Nervous Diseases of Women* (London, 1840); S. W. D. Williams, 'Cases illustrating the action of amenorrhoea as a cause of insanity', *Journal of Mental Science*, 9 (1863–4), 344–53; R. Barnes, 'On the correlations of the sexual functions and mental disorders of women', *British Gynaecological Journal*, 6 (1890–1), 390–413; 416–30.
4 Laycock, *A Treatise on the Nervous Diseases of Women*, p. 83.
5 J. B. Hicks, 'On the difference between the sexes in regard to the aspect and treatment of disease', *British Medical Journal*, 1 (1877), 413.
6 *Ibid.*, p. 476.
7 See J. Schiller, *La notion d'organisation dans l'histoire de la biologie* (Paris, 1978); G. Canguilhem, 'Le tout et la partie dans la pensée biologique', *Etudes d'histoire et de philosophie des sciences* (Paris, 1968), pp. 319–33.
8 Barnes, 'Women, diseases of', p. 1788.
9 This question is discussed in chapter 6.
10 R. Barnes, 'Observations introductory to clinical lectures on the diseases of women', *Lancet*, 1 (1880), 4–6, p. 5. See also A. Edis, 'On the relations of gynaecology to general therapeutics', *British Gynaecological Journal*, 4 (1888–9), 7–23 and C. D. Palmer, 'Gynaecology and general medicine: their reciprocal relations', *American Journal of Obstetrics and the Diseases of Women and Children*, 34 (1896), 83; 375–9.
11 L. Jordanova, 'Naturalizing the family: literature and the bio-medical sciences in the late eighteenth century', in L. Jordanova (ed.), *Languages of Nature: Critical Essays on Science and Literature* (London, 1986), 86–116, esp. pp. 108–9.

12 E. Clarke, *Sex in Education: Or, a Fair Chance for the Girls* (Boston, 1873), p. 41.

13 H. Maudsley, 'Sex in mind and in education', *Fortnightly Review*, 21 (1874), 466–83. This theory applied to men as well as to women: thus the loss of semen in masturbation was regarded as a powerful cause of male insanity.

14 R. Smith, 'Scientific thought and the boundary of insanity and criminal responsibility', *Psychological Medicine*, 10 (1980), 22–3.

15 On the mental disorders of women's life-cycle, see H. Maudsley, *Body and Mind* (London, 1873), pp. 90–2. See also R. Barnes, 'Lumleian lectures on the convulsive diseases of women', *British Medical Journal*, 1 (1873), 391–4; 421–5; 453–5; 483–5. For a historical critique of psychiatric theories about female insanity, see E. Showalter, *The Female Malady: Women, Madness and English Culture, 1830–1980* (London, 1987). The importance of ideological notions of femininity in medico-legal discourse is discussed by R. Smith, *Trial by Medicine: Insanity and Responsibility in Victorian Trials* (Edinburgh, 1981), pp. 143–60.

16 'The Obstetrical Society's charges and Mr Baker Brown's reply', *Lancet*, 1 (1867), 427–41.

17 See chapter 5.

18 A. T. Hobbs, 'Surgical gynaecology in insanity', *British Medical Journal*, 2 (1897), 769–70; E. Hall, 'Gynaecology among the insane in private practice', *British Gynaecological Journal*, 14 (1898), 571–6.

19 J. C. Bucknill and D. H. Tuke, *A Manual of Psychological Medicine: Containing the History, Nosology, Description, Statistics, Diagnosis, Pathology, and Treatment of Insanity* (London, 1858), pp. 275–6.

20 T. Claye Shaw, 'The sexes in lunacy', St Bartholomew's Hospital Reports, 24 (1888), 1–15, pp. 4–15 *passim*.

21 Smith, *Trial by Medicine*, p. 151.

22 R. Barnes, 'Lectures on the diseases of women', *Lancet*, 1 (1880), 155–7, p. 156.

23 W. R. Williams, *The Influence of Sex in Disease* (London, 1885).

24 *Ibid.*, p. 10; C. Locock, 'Amenorrhoea', in J. Forbes, A. Tweedie and J. Conolly (eds.), *The Cyclopaedia of Practical Medicine*, 4 vols. (London, 1833–5), I, p. 68.

25 For a historical study of medico-legal issues in gynaecology, see S. Edwards, *Female Sexuality and the Law: A Study of Constructs of Female Sexuality as They Inform Statute and Legal Procedure* (Oxford, 1981); on the development of 'medical police' in late eighteenth-century France, see L. Jordanova, 'Policing public health in France, 1780–1815', in T. Ogawa (ed.), *Public Health* (Tokyo, 1981), pp. 12–32.

26 H. Macnaughton-Jones 'A gynaecological question of importance in forensic medicine relating to the hymen', *British Gynaecological Journal*, 10 (1894–5), 38–48, pp. 38–9 *passim*; J. W. Underhill, 'The female

generative organs in their medico-legal relations', *American Journal of Obstetrics*, 12 (1879), 91–111.

27 E. G. Anderson, 'Sex in mind and education, a reply', *Fortnightly Review*, 21 (1874), 582–94.

28 F. P. Cobbe, 'The little health of ladies', *Contemporary Review*, 31 (1877), 276–96.

29 For overviews of the development of gynaecological theory and therapy, see R. A. Leonardo, *History of Gynaecology* (New York, 1944); J. V. Ricci, *The Genealogy of Gynaecology* (Philadelphia, 1943); J. V. Ricci, *The Development of Gynaecological Surgery and Instruments* (Philadelphia and Toronto, 1949); H. Speert, *Obstetric and Gynaecologic Milestones* (New York, 1958); J. M. M. Kerr, R. W. Johnstone, M. H. Phillips (eds.), *Historical Review of British Obstetrics and Gynaecology 1800–1950* (Edinburgh and London, 1954).

30 O. Temkin, 'The role of surgery in the rise of modern medical thought', *Bulletin of the History of Medicine*, 25 (1951), 248–59; T. Gelfand, *Professionalising Modern Medicine: Paris Surgeons and Medical Science and Institutions* (Westport CT, 1980). On the development of medical technology see S. Reiser, *Medicine and the Reign of Technology* (Cambridge, 1978).

31 On Magendie's physiology, see W. R. Albury, 'Experiment and explanation in the physiology of Bichat and Magendie', *Studies in the History of Biology*, 1 (1977), 47–131. On the rise of vivisectionist experimentation, P. Elliott, 'Vivisection and the emergence of experimental physiology in nineteenth-century France', in N. A. Rupke (ed.), *Vivisection in Historical Perspective* (London, New York, Sydney, 1987), pp. 48–77. K. Figlio has discussed the increasingly analytical approach in physiology in relation to the rise of therapeutic interventionism during the nineteenth century. K. Figlio, 'The historiography of scientific medicine: an invitation to the human sciences', *Comparative Studies in Society and History*, 19 (1977), 262–86. On Claude Bernard see R. Virtanen, *Claude Bernard and His Place in the History of Ideas* (Lincoln, Nebraska, 1960); J. Schiller, *Claude Bernard et les problèmes scientifiques de son temps* (Paris, 1967).

32 J. Murphy, 'The influence of surgery on gynaecology', *Provincial Medical Journal*, 10 (1891), 403–4, p. 403.

33 *Ibid.*, p. 404.

34 J. Berger, *Ways of Seeing* (Harmondsworth, 1972), pp. 45–64.

35 H. P. Newman, 'Woman and her diseases vs. gynaecology', *American Gynaecological and Obstetrical Journal*, 2 (1896), 417–22, pp. 421–2. See also W. O. Priestley, 'On over-operating in gynaecology', *British Medical Journal*, 2 (1895), 284–7.

36 Newman, 'Woman and her diseases', p. 421.

37 V. Deneffe, *Le spéculum de la matrice à travers les âges* (Anvers, 1902).

38 J. V. Ricci, 'The vaginal speculum and its modifications throughout the ages', *Contributions from the Department of Gynaecology of the City Hospital, New York, 1848–1949* (n.p., n.d.), pp. 1–55.

39 J. Hirsin, *Policing Prostitution in Nineteenth-Century Paris* (Princeton, 1985).

40 W. Jones, *Practical Observations on Diseases of Women* (London, 1839), pp. 79–80.

41 R. Lee, 'On the use of the speculum in the diagnosis and treatment of uterine diseases', *Medico-Chirurgical Transactions*, 33 (1850), 261–78.

42 *Ibid.*, p. 269.

43 'Royal Medico-Chirurgical Society: the speculum in uterine diseases' *Lancet*, 1 (1850), 704. It was well known that the integrity of the hymen did not prove a woman's virginity. J. B. Hicks urged obstetricians not to issue certificates of virginity on the basis of a gynaecological examination, as there were women with naturally open hymens in whom coitus produced no sign. J. B. Hicks, 'Notes of cases in obstetric jurisprudence', *Lancet*, 2 (1885), 243. Macnaughton-Jones, 'A gynaecological question of importance', pp. 38–48.

44 M. Hall, 'On a new and lamentable form of hysteria', *Lancet*, 1 (1850), 660–1, p. 661.

45 R. B. Carter, *On the Pathology and Treatment of Hysteria* (London, 1853), p. 69.

46 Hall, 'On a new and lamentable form of hysteria', p. 661.

47 'The speculum in uterine diseases', p. 702.

48 *Ibid.*, p. 704.

49 *Ibid.*, pp. 703–4.

50 *Ibid.*, p. 705.

51 'Pudor' (pseud.), 'The speculum committee' (letter), *Medical Times*, 22 (1850), 45.

52 'Censor' (pseud.), 'Use of the speculum vaginae' (letter), *Lancet*, 1 (1845), 105.

53 'Censor' (pseud.), 'Use of the speculum vaginae' (letter), *Lancet*, 1 (1845), 223.

54 R. Porter, 'A touch of danger: the man–midwife as sexual predator', unpublished paper, June 1987.

55 F. Nicholls, *The Petition of the Unborn Babes to the Censors of the Royal College of Physicians* (London, 1751), p. 6. See also P. Thicknesse, *Man-Midwifery Analysed* (London, 1764).

56 G. Morant, *Hints to Husbands: A Revelation of the Man-Midwife's Mysteries* (London, 1857), p. 24. It was no coincidence that Morant was a member of the Female Medical Society (founded 1862), which hoped to secure the admission of women to the medical profession.

57 *Ibid.*, p. 65.

58 *Ibid.*, pp. 10–14. See also J. Stevens, *Man-Midwifery Exposed, or the Danger and Immorality of Employing Men in Midwifery Proved: and the Remedy for the Evil Found* (London, 1850), p. 5.

59 For general works on prostitution, see J. Walkowitz, *Prostitution and Victorian Society: Women, Class, and the State* (Cambridge, 1980); P. McHugh, *Prostitution and Victorian Social Reform* (London, 1980). On child prostitution, see M. Pearson, *The Age of Consent: Victorian*

Prostitution and Its Enemies (Newton Abbot, 1972); A. Robson, 'The Significance of the "Maiden Tribute of Modern Babylon"', *Victorian Periodicals Newsletter*, 11 (1978), 50–7; D. Gorham, 'The "Maiden Tribute of Modern Babylon" re-examined: child prostitution and the idea of childhood in late-Victorian England', *Victorian Studies*, 21 (1977–8), 353–79.

60 Cf. Freud's idea of infant sexuality. L. Jordanova has examined the ambiguous status of children in terms of the ideology of separate spheres and ideas about the 'natural' status of the family; 'Naturalizing the family', esp. pp. 112–16. It must be noted that gynaecologists did not refer to an 'age' of consent, they just drew a broad distinction between the married and the unmarried. There was in fact considerable debate as to the age that should be selected.

61 Gorham, 'The "Maiden Tribute" re-examined', pp. 363–4; Edwards, *Female Sexuality and the Law*, pp. 31–4. Consortium actions also embraced a husband's rights over the services of a wife. Thus a husband could bring an action for the loss of his wife's consortium (i.e. sexual congress and household duties) against her seductor.

62 Quoted in Gorham, 'The "Maiden Tribute" re-examined', p. 368.

63 Hall, 'On a new and lamentable form of hysteria', p. 661.

64 'The Obstetrical Society's charges', p. 430.

65 *Ibid.*

66 On the crime and tort of battery in medical practice, see P. D. G. Skegg, *Law, Ethics and Medicine: Studies in Medical Law* (Oxford, 1984), pp. 29–40. Cf. the Eliza Armstrong case (1885), in which the obstetrician Heywood Smith was accused of carrying out a vaginal examination on a child of thirteen without the consent of her father; the scandal wrecked Smith's career. See Royal Society of Medicine MSS I, 41, British Gynaecological Society, Minutes of Council, pp. 24–7; Heywood Smith to the Council of the B.G.S., 11/11/1885, *ibid.*; A. Plowden, *The Case of Eliza Armstrong: 'A Child of 13 Bought for £5'* (London, 1974). The question of a minor's consent to bodily touchings is a complex one. In a number of legal cases during the early Victorian period, the consent of a minor to bodily touchings of a sexual nature was effective in preventing a conviction for assault, thus implying that minors were sometimes capable of consenting to bodily touchings, including those that occurred in medical practice; Skegg, *Law, Ethics, and Medicine*, p. 53, n. 25. The Family Law Act (1969) removed some of the ambiguity by reducing the age of majority from eighteen to sixteen years for the purpose of medical treatment, and allowing anyone over that age to consent to his or her medical treatment. Under the age of sixteen the situation is less clear and conflicts of interest have arisen between medical responsibility and parental rights.

The problem was highlighted by the Gillick case in relation to contraception and abortion. In 1980 the Department of Health and Social Security (DHSS) advised that if a girl under the stated age does not wish her parents to know that she has requested contraception, her wishes should be respected. Mrs Gillick disagreed and in 1982 she went to court. Her case was rejected, but the Court of Appeal reversed the judgment. The DHSS then appealed to the House of Lords, and the Department's original guidance was upheld as lawful by a very narrow margin; C. James, 'Contraceptive practice: some medico-legal questions answered', *Journal of the Medical Defence Union*, 11 (1988), 30–1. For a discussion of medical procedures on minors, see Skegg, *Law, Ethics and Medicine*, pp. 49–71.

67 Cf. the definition of child abuse as an abuse of authority. It was not until 1877 that fraudulently obtained consent to sexual intercourse was recognised as grounds for rape; Edwards, *Female Sexuality and the Law*, p. 39.

68 'The Plymouth speculum case', *Medical Times and Gazette*, 26 (1852), 294.

69 T. Litchfield, 'On the use and abuse of the speculum' (letter), *Lancet*, 1 (1850), 705. See also R. Hull, 'On the speculum vaginae', *London Medical Gazette*, 13 (1851), 493–5.

70 Edwards, *Female Sexuality and the Law*, pp. 56–7.

71 M. A. Elston, 'Women and anti-vivisection in Victorian England', in N. A. Rupke (ed.), *Vivisection in Historical Perspective* (London, 1987), 259–93, p. 280.

72 Elston, 'Women and anti-vivisection', esp. pp. 274–6. Morantz-Sanchez has analysed the opposition of Elizabeth Blackwell to bacteriology; R. M. Morantz-Sanchez, *Sympathy and Science: Women Physicians in American Medicine* (New York and Oxford, 1985), p. 190.

73 C. B. Taylor, *The Contagious Diseases Acts (Women), from a Sanitary Point of View* (London, 1870), pp. 37–8. See also C. B. Taylor, *Observations on the Contagious Diseases Acts (Women, not Animals)* (Nottingham, 1870); J. J. G. Wilkinson, *The Forcible Introspection of the Women for the Army and Navy by the Oligarchy Considered Physically* (London, 1870). For works on anti-vivisection, see R. D. French, *Antivivisection and Medical Science in Victorian Society* (Princeton, 1975); Rupke (ed.), *Vivisection*.

74 E. Blackwell, 'Scientific method in biology', *Essays in Medical Sociology* (1902; New York, 1972), pp. 119–20. On science, morality and women doctors, see the excellent discussion by Morantz-Sanchez, *Sympathy and Science*, esp. pp. 184–202. On anti-vivisection and the opposition to gynaecological surgery, see C. Lansbury, *The Old Brown Dog: Women, Workers and Vivisection in Edwardian England* (Madison WI, 1985), pp. 83–111; Elston, 'Women and anti-vivisection', p. 275.

75 Elston, 'Women and anti-vivisection', p. 279.

76 Lansbury, *The Old Brown Dog*, p. 59.

77 Elston, 'Women and anti-vivisection', p. 280.

78 Lansbury, *The Old Brown Dog*, pp. 83–111.

79 *Ibid.*, pp. 63–82.

80 P. Elliott, 'Vivisection and the emergence of experimental physiology in nineteenth-century France', in Rupke (ed.), *Vivisection*, 48–77, p. 52; Schiller, *Claude Bernard*, p. 35.

81 M. S. Pernick, *A Calculus of Suffering: Pain, Professionalism, and Anesthesia in Nineteenth-Century America* (New York, 1985), p. 174.

82 *Ibid.*, p. 86.

83 C. H. F. Routh, 'On the etiology and diagnosis, considered especially from the medico-legal point of view, of those cases of nymphomania which lead women to make false charges against their medical attendants', *British Gynaecological Journal*, 2 (1886–7), 485–511. Medical fears about false allegations of rape led to the creation of the police surgeon; Edwards, *Female Sexuality and the Law*, pp. 126–9. A fine analysis of the debate over the use of anaesthesia in obstetrics is provided by M. Poovey, '"Scenes of an indelicate character": the medical "treatment" of Victorian women', *Representations*, 14 (1986), 137–68.

84 See C. Rosenberg and C. Smith-Rosenberg, 'The female animal: medical and biological views of woman and her role in nineteenth-century America', *Journal of American History*, 60 (1973), 332–56; C. Smith-Rosenberg, 'The hysterical woman: sex roles conflict in nineteenth-century America', *Social Research*, 39 (1972), 652–78; C. Smith-Rosenberg, 'Puberty to menopause: the cycle of femininity in nineteenth-century America', in M. S. Hartman and L. Banner (eds.), *Clio's Consciousness Raised: New Perspectives on the History of Women* (New York, 1974), pp. 23–37; G. J. Barker-Benfield, *The Horrors of the Half-Known Life: Male Attitudes Toward Women and Sexuality in Nineteenth-Century America* (New York, 1976).

85 A. Douglas, '"The fashionable diseases": women's complaints and their treatment in nineteenth-century America', *Journal of Interdisciplinary History*, 4 (1973), 25–52, p. 13.

86 Morantz-Sanchez, *Sympathy and Science*, p. 209.

87 J. Manton, *Elizabeth Garrett Anderson* (London, 1965), pp. 228–30.

88 Morantz-Sanchez, *Sympathy and Science*, pp. 225–31.

89 HW Reports, 7, 1850, p. 6.

90 See Showalter, *The Female Malady*, pp. 129–34.

91 Morantz-Sanchez has noticed a similar discrepancy in her comparison of male and female obstetric practice in Boston. Male physicians were not as meticulous in recording patients' social background as their female colleagues. Morantz-Sanchez argues that men in overcrowded teaching hospitals tended to lump the poor together; *Sympathy and Science*, pp. 227–8.

92 P. Smith, Case-book, cases no. 21; 30; 59; 60; 65; 73.

93 Gynaecological cases, Prudhoe Ward, Middlesex Hospital, June 1863–Oct. 1866, cases no. 9; 13; 25; 30; 37; 38; 40; 45; 59; 60; 68; 93; 111; 115; 145; 195. Case 111 was a re-admission. Ovariotomy was attempted in cases 93 and 111; in case 68 it was attempted to remove the tumour by an incision through the uterus. The patient died.

94 Case 115.
95 J. Bland-Sutton, *The Story of a Surgeon* (London, 1930), p.65.
96 Chelsea Hospital for Women Reports, 1871–3, p. 6.
97 T. Chambers, Medical Register B, 1879, case no. 347.
98 *Ibid.*, 1877, case no. 210.
99 CHW Reports, 1887–8, p. 19; 1894, p. 21.
100 CHW Reports, 1887–8, p. 19; 1893, p. 19.
101 J. Aveling, Medical Register A–1, 1884, case no. 918.
102 F. Barnes, Medical Register A–13, 1889, case no. 2781.
103 W. Travers, Medical Register A–15, 1889, case no. 2693.
104 G. Apostoli, *Sur un nouveau traitement de la métrite chronique et en particulier de l'endométrite par la galvano-caustique chimique intra-utérine* (Paris, 1887).
105 W. Travers, Medical Register A–15, 1889, case no. 2821.
106 HW Committee Minutes, 30 July 1885.
107 HW Reports, 35, 1878, p. 13.
108 HW Committee Minutes, 1 November 1883; 15 May 1884; 2 July 1885.
109 *Ibid.*, 7 May 1885; 4 February 1886.

5 The 'unsexing' of women

1 The phrase 'extirpation of the ovaria' was at first used to describe ovariotomy. The term 'ovariotomy' was apparently coined by J. Y. Simpson, who suggested it to Charles Clay. The nomenclature is misleading, as the operation did not consist in 'incising' an ovary as suggested by the etymology of the term, but in excising one or both ovaries. The etymologically more accurate term 'oöphorectomy', introduced in 1872, defined a different kind of surgical procedure, in which non-cystic ovaries were removed for the cure of insanity, epilepsy and dysmenorrhoea. See pp. 157–8.
2 J. Murphy, 'The influence of surgery on gynaecology', *Provincial Medical Journal*, 10 (1891), 404.
3 J. Hunter, 'Lectures on the principles of surgery', in *The Works of John Hunter*, ed. J. F. Palmer, 4 vols. (London, 1835–7), I, p. 573.
4 J. V. Ricci, *One Hundred Years of Gynaecology 1800–1900* (Philadelphia, 1945), pp. 48–56.
5 P. Pott, *The Chirurgical Works* (London, 1775), pp. 791–2.
6 M. R. Ridenbaugh, *The Biography of Ephraim McDowell, M.D.* (New York, 1890), pp. 70–84.
7 J. Johnson, 'Extirpation of the ovaria', *Medico-Chirurgical Review*, 2 (1825), 215–17.
8 J. Lizars, 'Observations on extirpation of the ovaria, with cases', *Edinburgh Medical and Surgical Journal*, 22 (1824), 247–56.
9 A. B. Granville, 'Removal of the ovarium', *London Medical Gazette*, 31 (1843), 539–40.
10 W. Jeaffreson, 'A case of ovarian tumour successfully removed',

Transactions of the Provincial Medical and Surgical Association, 5 (1837), 239–45.

11 R. Lee, 'An analysis of one hundred and eight cases of ovariotomy which have occurred in Great Britain', *Medico-Chirurgical Transactions*, 16 (1851), 10–35, p. 12.

12 C. West, *Lectures on the Diseases of Women*, 3rd edn. (London, 1864), p. 587.

13 J. Y. Simpson, 'Is ovariotomy justifiable?' *Monthly Journal of Medical Science*, 61 (1846), 53–67, p. 56.

14 T. S. Wells, *Diseases of the Ovaries: Their Diagnosis and Treatment* (London, 1872), p. 86.

15 Simpson, 'Is ovariotomy justifiable?', p. 59; J. Y. Simpson, 'Discussion on a case of ovariotomy', *Edinburgh Medical Journal*, 2 (1856–7), 755. On the use of the 'numeric method' in medicine, see U. Tröhler, 'Quantification in British medicine and surgery 1750–1830' (Ph.D. thesis, University of London, 1978).

16 J. Finlaison (1783–1860) was actuary and statistician to the government. His life-expectancy tables in 1829 were the first to show the difference between male and female lives.

17 'On the diagnosis and treatment of ovarian disease, with the history of one hundred and fifty-six cases, by Robert Lee', *Lancet*, 2 (1851), 536–40, p. 537.

18 These arguments are summarised in 'Discussion sur les kystes ovariques', *Bulletin de l'Académie Impériale de Médecine*, 22 (1856–7), esp. pp. 20–113. See also 'Supplement to a paper entitled "An analysis of one hundred and sixty-two cases of ovariotomy which have occurred in Great Britain"', Dr Lee's intervention, *Lancet*, 2 (1862), 568–9.

19 'Discussion on a case of ovariotomy', J. M. Duncan's intervention, pp. 753–4.

20 'Is ovariotomy justifiable?', J. R. Cormack's intervention, p. 54; 'Discussion on a case of ovariotomy', J. M. Duncan's intervention, pp. 752–3; 'Discussion on Robert Lee's "Analysis of one hundred and eight cases of ovariotomy which have occurred in Great Britain"', C. Hawkins' intervention, *Lancet*, 2 (1850), 585.

21 'Clay on *Extirpation of Diseased Ovaria*' (review article), *British and Foreign Medical Review*, 16 (1843), 402.

22 'Supplement to a paper', Dr Lee's intervention, p. 569.

23 'Discussion on Robert Lee's "Analysis of one hundred and eight cases of ovariotomy which have occurred in Great Britain"', Lancet, 2 (1850), 584–7.

24 *Ibid.*, B. Phillips' intervention, p. 585.

25 See e.g. 'Discussion sur les kystes ovariques', P.-C. Huguier's intervention, p. 113; 'Supplement to a paper', R. Lee's intervention, p. 568. For a history of the caesarean section, see J. H. Young, *Caesarean Section: The History and Development of the Operation from the Earliest Times* (London, 1944). The French practice of the operation is

reviewed by J. P. Pundel, *Histoire de l'opération césarienne* (Brussels, 1969).

26 Pundel, *Histoire de l'opération césarienne*, pp. 200–2.

27 W. T. Smith, 'Introductory lecture to a course of lectures in obstetricy (delivered at the Hunterian School of Medicine), 1847–8', *Lancet*, 2 (1847), 371–4, p. 373. Tyler Smith was one of the early opponents of craniotomy.

28 See J. Y. Simpson, *Obstetric Memoirs and Contributions* ed. W. O. Priestley and H. R. Storer. 2 vols. (Edinburgh, 1871), I, pp. 661–2; Young, *Caesarean Section*, pp. 73–8.

29 W. T. Smith, 'On the abolition of craniotomy from obstetric practice, in all cases where the foetus is living and viable', *Transactions of the Obstetrical Society of London*, 1 (1859), 21–50, p. 21.

30 The question of the legitimacy of performing a caesarean section was submitted by the Physicians to the Doctors of Theology of the Paris Faculty in 1733. They replied that, as a general rule, the operation was justifiable; however, if it was certain to cause the mother's death, it should not be performed. In practice, the deliberation left the matter to the discretion of the physician. Pundel, *Histoire de l'opération césarienne*, pp. 92–4. See also Young, *Caesarean Section*, p. 75.

31 Smith, 'On the abolition of craniotomy'. See also R. Dyce, 'Case of caesarean section', *Edinburgh Medical Journal*, 7 (1861–2), 895–900.

32 Cf. the argument put forward by T. Radford, one of the advocates of the caesarean section in Britain: if the mother was diseased, and thus unfit to perform her domestic duties (which he claimed was always the case in mothers who could not be delivered *per vias naturales*), then it was legitimate to sacrifice her life. T. Radford, *Observations on the Caesarean Section and on Other Obstetric Operations* (Manchester, 1855), p. 57; T. Radford, *On the Value of Embryonic and Foetal Life, Legally, Morally, and Socially Considered* (n.p. 1848), p. 19.

33 See L. Rose, *The Massacre of the Innocents: Infanticide in Britain 1800–1939* (London, 1986), pp. 86–7.

34 'Clinical Midwifery, with the Histories of Four Hundred Cases of Difficult Labour, by R. Lee' (review article), *Medico-Chirurgical Review and Journal of Practical Medicine*, n.s., 38 (1843), 242–3.

35 W. Campbell, *Introduction to the Study and Practice of Midwifery, and the Diseases of Women and Children* (Edinburgh, 1833), p. 266.

36 See 'Discussion sur les kystes ovariques'.

37 J. Rochard, *Histoire de la chirurgie française au XIXᵉ siècle* (Paris, 1875), p. 394.

38 *Ibid.*, p. 394.

39 C. Bernard, *Introduction à l'étude de la médecine expérimentale* (Paris, 1865), p. 182.

40 *Ibid.*, pp. 176–7.

41 R. Barnes, 'On the correlations of the sexual functions and mental disorders of women', *British Gynaecological Journal*, 6 (1890–1), 392.

42 R. D. French, *Antivivisection and Medical Science in Victorian Society* (Princeton, 1975), pp. 37–40.

43 On the Bell-Magendie controversy, see G. Gordon-Taylor and E. W. Walls, *Sir Charles Bell, His Life and Time* (Edinburgh and London, 1958); L. Deloyers, *François Magendie: précurseur de la médecine expérimentale* (Brussels, 1970); W. R. Albury, 'Experiment and explanation in the physiology of Bichat and Magendie', *Studies in the History of Biology*, 1 (1977), 47–131. In his analysis of the vitalism versus materialism debate of the 1820s, Figlio has argued that although English physiologists accused their French counterparts of materialism, their conceptualisation of the living organism was highly compatible with the views of Magendie. K. Figlio, 'The metaphor of organisation: an historiographical perspective on the bio-medical sciences of the early nineteenth century', *History of Science*, 14 (1976), 17–53. It must be pointed out that ovariotomists were divided over vivisection. Tait and Clay were antivivisectionists, whereas Spencer Wells used living animals in a series of experiments aimed at improving the technique of ovariotomy. R. L. Tait, *The Uselessness of Vivisection as a Method of Scientific Research* (London, 1882); T. S. Wells, 'Vivisection and ovariotomy' (letter) *British Medical Journal*, 2 (1879), 794. For a defence of vivisection, see also S. Gamgee, *The Influence of Vivisection on Human Surgery* (London, 1882). Wells' methods were fiercely condemned by the Society for the Total Abolition of Vivisection. Society for the Total Abolition of Vivisection, *Correspondence with T. Spencer Wells, F.R.C.S., on Ovariotomy* (London, 1882).

44 See note 32 of this chapter.

45 R. Lee, 'Ovaria, diseases of', in J. Forbes, A. Tweedie and J. Conolly (eds.), *The Cyclopaedia of Practical Medicine*, 4 vols. (London 1833–5), III, 225–31, pp. 228–9; A. Farre, 'Uterus and its appendages', in R. B. Todd (ed.), *The Cyclopaedia of Anatomy and Physiology*, 5 vols. (London, 1835–59), V, 545–725, pp. 590–1.

46 T. S. Wells, 'Ovaries, diseases of', in R. Quain (ed.), *A Dictionary of Medicine: Including General Pathology, General Therapeutics, Hygiene, and the Diseases Peculiar to Women and Children*, 2 vols. (London, 1882), II, 1073–8, p. 1073.

47 Middlesex Hospital, Prudhoe Ward, Jan. 1864, case no. 42.

48 Middlesex Hospital, Prudhoe Ward, October 1864, case no. 93.

49 R. Saundby, *Medical Ethics*, 2nd edn. (London, 1907), p. 104.

50 A. McLaren, *Birth Control in Nineteenth-Century England* (London, 1978), esp. pp. 116–40. See also R. Soloway, *Birth Control and the Population Question in England, 1877–1930* (Chapel Hill, 1982); L. Gordon, *Woman's Body, Woman's Right: A Social History of Birth Control in America* (Harmondsworth, 1977).

51 M. Julien, 'Recherches sur les suites éloignées de l'opération de la castration chez la femme, et sur la valeur de l'opothérapie ovarienne' (M.D. thesis, Lille University 1899), pp. 6–8.

52 On the social and political background of the novel, see J. M. Winter,

'Demography and international politics', in M. S. Teitelbaum and J. M. Winter, *The Fear of Population Decline* (Orlando, 1985), pp. 13–43.

53 E. Zola, *Fécondité*, 2 vols. (1899; Paris, 1925), II, pp. 41–52.

54 *Ibid.*, I, pp. 197–214.

55 *Ibid.*, II, pp. 1–22.

56 *Ibid.*, pp. 155–60.

57 A. Meadows, 'On certain obstetric and gynaecological operations', *British Medical Journal*, 2 (1886), 357.

58 R. L. Tait, 'The antiseptic theory tested by the statistics of one hundred cases of successful ovariotomy', *Medico-Chirurgical Transactions*, 63 (1880), 161–80, p. 168.

59 T. S. Wells, 'The revival of ovariotomy and its influence on modern surgery', *British Medical Journal*, 2 (1884), 893–6, p. 894.

60 J. A. Shepherd, *Spencer Wells: The Life and Work of a Victorian Surgeon* (Edinburgh, 1965), p. 96.

61 Wells, 'The revival of ovariotomy', p. 894.

62 'Supplement to a paper', Dr. Lee's intervention, p. 569.

63 *Ibid.*, pp. 566–8.

64 'Ovariotomy', *British Medical Journal*, 2 (1862), 494.

65 'Ovariotomy in the Royal Medical and Chirurgical Society', *ibid.*, 521–2, p. 522.

66 M. S. Pernick, *A Calculus of Suffering: Pain, Professionalism, and Anesthesia in Nineteenth-Century America* (New York, 1985), pp. 208–221.

67 J. M. D. Olmstead, *Claude Bernard, Physiologist* (London, 1939), p. 122.

68 The reception of the antiseptic method by the medical profession is discussed by A. J. Youngson, *The Scientific Revolution in Victorian Medicine* (London, 1979), pp. 157–211.

69 T. S. Wells, 'Abstract of six lectures on the diagnosis and surgical treatment of abdominal tumours', *Lancet*, 2 (1878), 134.

70 G. G. Bantock, 'Table of 238 cases of completed ovariotomy, (163 to 400 inclusive) with remarks', *British Gynaecological Journal*, 5 (1889–90), 344.

71 *Ibid.*, p. 344.

72 *Ibid.*, p. 345.

73 R. L. Tait, 'Cases treated antiseptically on Lister's method', *Lancet*, 1 (1871), 46.

74 R. L. Tait, 'Clinical lecture on the details necessary in the performance of abdominal section', *Lancet*, 2 (1891), 597.

75 'One hundred consecutive cases of ovariotomy, performed without any of the Listerian details', *British Medical Journal*, 2 (1882), 830–2.

76 Tait, 'The antiseptic theory tested', 164–6.

77 Tait, 'One hundred consecutive cases of ovariotomy', 830.

78 R. L. Tait, 'One hundred and thirty-nine consecutive ovariotomies performed between January 1st 1884 and December 31st 1885 without a death', *British Medical Journal*, 1 (1886), 923.

79 T. Keith, 'The history of ovariotomy', *British Medical Journal*, 2 (1880), 186.

80 Zola, *Fécondité*, II, pp. 17–18.

81 R. Battey, 'Is there a proper field for Battey's operation?', *Transactions of the American Gynaecological Society*, 2 (1877), 279–305; J. M. Sims, 'Normal ovariotomy: Battey's operation – oöphorectomy', *Medical Times and Gazette*, 2 (1877), 565–6. For a history of Battey's operation, see M. W. Butler, 'The British practice of Battey's operation 1872–1890' (M.Phil. thesis, University of Cambridge, 1982); L. D. Longo, 'The rise and fall of Battey's operation: a fashion in surgery', *Bulletin of the History of Medicine*, 53 (1979), 244–67.

82 A. Hegar, 'Castration in mental and nervous disease: a symposium', *American Journal of Medical Science*, 92 (1886), 455–90, pp. 472–3.

83 T. Savage, 'Oöphorectomy: being a series of twenty-five consecutive successful cases', *Birmingham Medical Review*, 10 (1881), 147–61, pp. 151–2.

84 French practitioners claimed that the population of Paris had decreased since the introduction of oöphorectomy. D. Pila, 'Etude critique de la castration chez la femme: ses résultats thérapeutiques, ses abus et ses conséquences sociales', (M.D. thesis, University of Paris, 1901). On population concerns in *fin de siècle* France and Britain, see Winter, 'Demography and international politics'; A. Davin, 'Imperialism and motherhood', *History Workshop Journal*, 5 (1978), 9–65.

85 'Normal ovariotomy: Battey's operation: Tait's operation', *British Medical Journal*, 1 (1887), 576–7, p. 577.

86 'Is there a "field" for Battey's operation?' *Lancet*, 2 (1881), 1115.

87 T. S. Wells, *Modern Abdominal Surgery: The Bradshaw Lecture Delivered at the Royal College of Surgeons of England. With an Appendix on the Castration of Women* (London, 1891), p. 43.

88 R. L. Tait, '"Spaying", or removal of the uterine appendages?' (letter), *Lancet*, 2 (1886), 557.

89 E. Blackwell, 'Scientific method in biology', *Essays in Medical Sociology* (1902; New York, 1972).

90 C. Lansbury, 'Gynaecology, pornography and the antivivisection movement', *Victorian Studies*, 28 (1985), 413–37, p. 431.

91 On maim, see W. Blackstone, *Commentaries on the Laws of England*, 4 vols. (Oxford, 1765–9), III (1768), p. 121; IV (1769), pp. 205–7. During the twentieth century the legality of sterilisation has come to the fore of public attention. Until the 1960s sterilisation for contraceptive reasons was held to be illegal and those who performed it were liable to charges of maim. In 1960, Mr Justice Stirling ruled that sterilisation for therapeutic or eugenic reasons was legal, provided there was a full and valid consent from the patient. Surgical operations rarely come within the scope of maim, since they are usually done for therapeutic reasons; the opponents of oöphorectomy as we have seen denied that the operation had any therapeutic value.

P. D. G. Skegg, *Law, Ethics, and Medicine* (Oxford, 1984), pp. 43–6; 'The legal aspects of sterilisation', *Lancet*, 1 (1929), 988; 'Legality of sterilisation', *British Medical Journal*, 1 (1970), 704–5.

92 Quoted in Lansbury, 'Gynaecology', p. 434. Lansbury does not comment on the symbolic meanings of 'unsexing'. Sarah Grand, *The Beth Book*, (1897; London, 1980).

93 Olmstead, *Claude Bernard*, pp. 123–5.

94 J. H. Shepherd, *Lawson Tait: The Rebellious Surgeon (1845–1899)* (Lawrence, Kansas, 1980), pp. 162–3.

95 'Special report of the committee submitted to the governors and subscribers of the Hospital for Women, 107 and 109 Shaw St.', *British Gynaecological Journal*, 1 (1885–6), 602–23; T. N. A. Jeffcoate, 'The precious ovary', *Transactions and Report of the Liverpool Medical Institution*, 1966, pp. 15–31.

96 Shepherd, *Lawson Tait*, p. 164.

97 'Special report', 602–3; Shepherd, *Lawson Tait*, p. 164.

98 'The action against Dr Imlach, of Liverpool', *British Medical Journal*, 2 (1886), 394–5.

99 See note 43 of this chapter.

100 'Special report', 604. The year in question was 1884–5 and the number of operations was 169, not 111.

101 Wellcome Library MSS., S. Wells A.7, T. S. Wells to E. Hart, 16/2/1886.

102 Shepherd, *Lawson Tait*, p. 165.

103 'Casey vs. Imlach', *Lancet*, 2 (1886), 304.

104 R. L. Tait, 'Casey vs. Imlach' (letter), *Lancet*, 2 (1886), 375–6.

105 'Special report', p. 614–15.

106 *Ibid.*, p. 618.

107 Shepherd, *Lawson Tait*, pp. 165–6.

6 From the BGS to the RCOG

1 'Ovariotomy at general hospitals', *Lancet*, 2 (1884), 282–3, p. 282.

2 *Ibid.*, p. 282.

3 *Ibid.*, p. 283.

4 *Ibid.*

5 See chapter 2.

6 R. Barnes, *On the Relations Between Medicine, Surgery, and Obstetrics in London* (New York, 1884), p. 14.

7 R. Barnes, 'The foundation of the British Gynaecological Society', *British Gynaecological Journal*, 1 (1885–6), 233–8, p. 234.

8 Barnes, *Relations Between Medicine, Surgery and Obstetrics*, p. 9.

9 *Ibid.*, pp. 13–14.

10 See chapter 5.

11 Barnes, *Relations Between Medicine, Surgery and Obstetrics*, p. 11.

12 'Ovariotomy at general hospitals', p. 282.

13 J. Gorham, 'Concerning the early days of ovariotomy', *Lancet*, 1 (1874), 440. On the income of medical practitioners in this period, see

M. J. Peterson, *The Medical Profession in Mid-Victorian London* (Berkeley, 1978), pp. 207–224.

14 F. B. Smith, *The People's Health 1830–1910* (London, 1979), pp. 27–8; Peterson, *The Medical Profession*, p. 212.

15 A. Bourne, *A Doctor's Creed: The Memoirs of a Gynaecologist* (London, 1962), p. 44.

16 Royal Society of Medicine [hereafter RSM], I 71, Obstetrical Society of London, Minutes of Council, 12 Dec. 1884, p. 489.

17 J. B. Potter's obituary, *Transactions of the Obstetrical Society of London*, 43 (1901), 64–7.

18 R. Barnes, 'The foundation of the British Gynaecological Society', *British Gynaecological Journal*, 1 (1885–6), 233–8, p. 237.

19 RSM, I 41, British Gynaecological Society, Minutes of Council, p. 2.

20 J. M. Duncan's obituary, *Lancet*, 2 (1890), 594–6.

21 W. R. Bett, *Sir John Bland-Sutton 1855–1936* (Edinburgh and London, 1956), p. 21.

22 A. W. Oxford, *History of the Samaritan Free Hospital* (Cambridge, 1931), p. 35.

23 Barnes, *Relations Between Medicine, Surgery, and Obstetrics*, p. 15.

24 See chapter 5.

25 RSM, I 51, British Gynaecological Society, Secretarial Correspondence, S. Mackenzie to Dr Shacht, 15/10/1895.

26 T. Dolan, 'Gynaecological specialism and general practice', *British Gynaecological Journal*, 5 (1889–90), 284–304; 327–31, pp. 284–5.

27 J. A. Lycett, 'Gynaecology in general practice', *British Gynaecological Journal*, 6 (1890–1), 208–31.

28 RSM, I 41, British Gynaecological Society, Minutes of Council, 1886, p. 36.

29 *Ibid.*, pp. 58–9.

30 *Ibid.*, p. 36.

31 *Ibid.*, p. 65.

32 *Ibid.*, pp. 18–19.

33 *Ibid.*, p. 14.

34 J. M. M. Kerr, R. W. Johnstone and M. H. Phillips (eds.), *Historical Review of British Obstetrics and Gynaecology* (Edinburgh, 1954), pp. 358–64. The first gynaecologist in London to take the FRCS was W.S.A. Griffiths. As a result, he was put on the full staff at St Bartholomew's in 1912 and permitted to do ovariotomy.

35 J. Lewis, *The Politics of Motherhood* (London, 1980), pp. 126–8.

36 V. Bonney's obituary, *Lancet*, 2 (1953), 93; V. Bonney, 'The continuing high maternal mortality of childbearing', *Proceedings of the Royal Society of Medicine*, 12 (1919), pt. III, 75–107, pp. 83–4.

37 W. H. F. Oxley, 'Prevention of puerperal sepsis in general practice', *British Medical Journal*, 1 (1934), 1017–19, p. 1017.

38 'The Obstetrical and Gynaecological Section of the Royal Society of Medicine', *Lancet*, 2 (1907), 1831.

39 R. Stevens, *Medical Practice in Modern England: The Impact of Specialization and State Medicine* (New Haven and London, 1966), esp. pp. 107–124.

40 See W. F. Shaw, *Twenty-Five Years: The Story of the Royal College of Obstetricians and Gynaecologists 1929–1954* (London, 1954), pp. 8–11; V. Bonney's obituaries, *British Medical Journal*, 2 (1953), 99–100; *Lancet*, 2 (1953), 93; *Journal of Obstetrics and Gynaecology of the British Empire*, 60 (1953), 566–69. A fuller account of the development of the RCOG from its foundation to the present day is provided in O. Moscucci, *The Royal College of Obstetricians and Gynaecologists, 1929–1989: A History*, (forthcoming).

41 W. Blair Bell, 'The history of the origin and rise of the Royal College of Obstetricians and Gynaecologists', 2 vols. (unpublished MSS, RCOG), p. 44.

42 W. F. Shaw, 'The College: its past, present and future. The William Meredith Fletcher Shaw Memorial Lecture', *Journal of Obstetrics and Gynaecology of the British Empire*, 61 (1954), 557–66, p. 559.

43 J. M. M. Kerr, J. H. Ferguson, J. Young, J. Hendry, *A Combined Text-Book of Obstetrics and Gynaecology* (Edinburgh, 1923), pp. 607–9.

44 Shaw, 'The College', p. 559.

45 RCOG A/31, W. F. Shaw to W. A. Taylor, 1/3/1929.

46 Lewis, *The Politics of Motherhood*, pp. 117–61; I. S. L. Loudon, 'Deaths in childbed from the eighteenth century to 1935', *Medical History*, 30 (1986), 1–41, esp. pp. 22–41. D. Palmer, 'The protracted foundation of a national maternity service: the failure to reduce maternal mortality in England and Wales, 1919–1939' (M.A. thesis, University of Warwick, 1978).

47 C. J. Cullingworth, 'On the undiminished mortality from puerperal fever in England and Wales', *Transactions of the Obstetrical Society of London*, 39 (1898), 91–114.

48 Stevens, *Medical Practice*, p. 43; Kerr *et al.*, *Historical Review*, pp. 301–2.

49 'Future of the maternity services', *Lancet*, 1 (1929), 609–11, p. 611.

50 British College of Obstetricians and Gynaecologists, *Memorandum on the Training of Medical Students in Midwifery and Gynaecology* (London, 1932).

51 A. Blair, 'The general practitioner and the maternity service' (letter), *British Medical Journal*, 2 (1924), 1177–8, p. 1177. See also Lewis, *The Politics of Motherhood*, pp. 145–9.

52 Kerr *et al.*, *Historical Review*, p. 319. Kerr *et al.* suggest that the structure of the GVS was inspired by that of the American Gynaecological Society.

53 Shaw, *Twenty-Five Years*, pp. 13–16.

54 RCOG, GVS Correspondence 1926–35.

55 Shaw, *Twenty-Five Years*, p. 17.

56 RCOG A1/1, Minute Book of the Executive Committee of the

Proposed College of Obstetricians and Gynaecologists of Great Britain [hereafter Executive Committee Minutes], 5/12/26; A4/4/3, W. F. Shaw to E. Holland, 25/2/1936.

57 RCOG A1/1, Executive Committee Minutes, 13/7/1926.

58 H. Spencer, 'A College of Obstetrics and Gynaecology' (letter), *British Medical Journal*, 1 (1929), 523.

59 RCOG A1/1, Executive Committee Minutes, 18/2/1927; A1/1, F. Champneys to R. Andrews, 7/2/1927; T. W. Eden to R. Andrews, 16/2/1927.

60 RCOG A1/1, Executive Committee Minutes, 6/4/1927.

61 Blair Bell, 'History', p. 103. The College obtained the Royal Charter in 1946, but for complicated reasons it was not until the early 1970s that the diplomas of the College were made registrable.

62 W. Blair Bell to F. Shaw, 4/8/26, quoted in Blair Bell, 'History', p. 63.

63 V. Bonney to Blair Bell, 25/8/28, quoted *ibid.*, p. 164.

64 RCOG A1/4, V. Bonney to Blair Bell, 28/9/1929.

65 In the same year the Council of the Royal College of Surgeons invited the RCOG to nominate a representative to attend the Council meetings, and the request was acceded to.

66 RCOG A1/1, Executive Committee Minutes, 18/2/1927.

67 *Ibid.*, 26/4/1927; W. F. Shaw, 'The birth of a College', *Journal of Obstetrics and Gynaecology of the British Empire*, 57 (1950), 876–90, pp. 886–7.

68 RCOG A1/27, Objections Lodged with the Board of Trade by the RCP and RCS. The reasons why the Scottish and Irish Colleges did not intervene are not clear.

69 RCOG A1/1, Executive Committee Minutes, 16/5/1929.

70 F. Shaw to Blair Bell, 30/4/1929, quoted in Blair Bell, 'History', p. 244.

71 Quoted in *ibid.*, p. 246.

72 RCOG A1/1, Executive Committee Minutes, 16/5/1929.

73 RCOG A1/15, 'Memorandum on Events and Policy of the College in Regard to the Granting of a Diploma', 19/3/1930.

74 RCOG A1/27, Moynihan–Blair Bell correspondence, June 1929.

75 Blair Bell, 'History', pp. 303–9.

76 RCOG A1/30, F. Shaw to Palmer, 25/11/1929.

77 RCOG A1/29, C. Berkeley to F. Shaw, 5/8/1932.

78 RCOG B1/7, F. Shaw to Cook, 17/2/1938; B1/8, F. Shaw to E. Holland, 19/10/1944.

79 RCOG B1/2, F. Shaw to T. W. Eden, 2/6/1930.

80 *Ibid.*

81 RCOG A1/29, F. Shaw to C. Berkeley, 9/8/1932.

82 F. Honigsbaum, *The Division in British Medicine: A History of the Separation of General Practice from Hospital Care 1911–1968* (London, 1979), pp. 275–7.

83 RCOG A2/1/5, F. Shaw to T. W. Eden, 22/5/1930.

84 *Ibid.*
85 RCOG B1/8, F. Shaw to E. Holland, 19/10/1944.
86 RCOG A4/4/5, F. Shaw to T. W. Eden, 23/10/1935.
87 RCOG B1/1, Examination Committee Minutes, 24/3/1933; 19/5/1933.
88 RCOG A4/2/2, F. Shaw to Blair Bell, 17/12/1935.
89 RCOG B1/5, F. Shaw to R. Andrews, 17/12/1935.
90 British College of Obstetricians and Gynaecologists, Annual Report, no. 8, 1936, pp. 92–4.
91 RCOG A2/1, Minutes of Council, 7/3/1930; 25/4/1930; 30/5/1930.
92 RCOG B1/1, Examination Committee Minutes, 24/9/1931.
93 *Ibid.*, 23/1/1931.
94 RCOG A2/1, Minutes of Council, 27/7/1931; B1/1, 24/9/1931.
95 RCOG A2/1, Minutes of Council, 6/12/1932.
96 Honigsbaum, *The Division in British Medicine*, p. 141.
97 RCOG A1/14, Blair Bell to T. W. Eden, 13/6/1929.
98 RCOG B1/1, B. Whitehouse to the Diploma Sub-Committee, n.d. [*c.* 1933].
99 See RCOG B1/1, Examination Committee Minutes, 29/9/1933; 20/10/1933; B1/1, W. Blair Bell, Notes on the Suggested Diploma, July 1933.
100 RCOG A2/2, Minutes of Council, 24/7/1933.
101 *Ibid.*
102 RCOG A2/4, Minutes of Council, 6/10/1945.
103 Quoted in Bell, 'History', I, p. 385.
104 Peterson, *The Medical Profession*, p. 287.
105 W. Blair Bell, *The Sex Complex* (London, 1916), p. 122.

Bibliography

MANUSCRIPT SOURCES

HOSPITALS
Chelsea Hospital for Women. Aveling, J. H., Medical Register, A–1, Jan.–Dec. 1884.
  Barnes, R. S. F., Medical Register, A–6, Jan.–Dec. 1884.
  Medical Register, A–13, Jan.–Dec. 1889.
  Chambers, T., Medical Register, A, Apr. 1873–June 1877.
  Medical Register, B, May 1877–Dec. 1879.
  Edis, A., Medical Register, A–5, Jan.–Dec. 1884.
  Medical Register, A–14, Jan.–Dec. 1889.
  Travers, W., Medical Register, A–15, Jan.–Dec. 1889.
  Hospital Reports, 1873–95.
  Minutes of Medical Staff Meetings, Oct. 1894–5.
Hospital for Women, Soho Square. Committee Minutes, 1873; 1880–7 (Middlesex Hospital Group Archives).
  Hospital Reports, 1842–1890 (MHGA).
  Smith, P., Case-book, July 1869–Dec. 1870 (MHGA).
Middlesex Hospital. Prudhoe Ward, Case-book, June 1863–Oct. 1866 (MHGA).
  West, C., Letter to the Medical Committee, 5 Nov. 1846, Fair Minute Book, Feb. 1845–Apr. 1847 (MHGA).

ROYAL COLLEGE OF OBSTETRICIANS AND GYNAECOLOGISTS
Bell, W. B., 'The history of the origin and rise of the Royal College of Obstetricians and Gynaecologists', 2 vols. Unpublished MSS., 1934.
Examination Committee Correspondence, B1/1–8.
Examination Committee Minutes, Nov. 1929–Nov. 1935.
Correspondence Relating to the Foundation of the College, A1/1–7; A1/8–10.
Correspondence Following First Council, A1/11–13; A1/14–18.
General Correspondence, 1929–1934, A1/29–31.
Gynaecological Visiting Society, Correspondence Relating to the Foundation of the College, 1926.
Minute Book of the Executive Committee of the Proposed College of

Obstetricians and Gynaecologists of Great Britain, July 1926–September 1929, A1/1.
Minutes of Council, Sept. 1929–Dec. 1932, A2/1.

SOCIETIES

British Gynaecological Society. Minutes of Council Meetings, I 41 (Royal Society of Medicine).
  Minutes of General Meetings, I 43 (RSM).
  Secretarial Correspondence, I 51 (RSM).
Obstetrical Society of London. Minutes of Council, I 71 (RSM).

GOVERNMENT DOCUMENTS

Report from the Select Committee on Medical Education, PP. 1834, vol. XIII.
Special Report from the Select Committee on the Medical Act (1858) Amendment Bill, PP. 1878–9, vol. XII.

PRIMARY SOURCES

Alexander, W., *The History of Women, from the Earliest Antiquity, to the Present Time; Giving Some Account of Almost Every Interesting Particular Concerning That Sex, among All Nations, Ancient and Modern*, 2 vols. London: T. Strahan and T. Cadell, 1779.
Allan, J. McGrigor, 'On the real differences in the minds of men and women', *Journal of the Anthropological Society*, 7 (1869), 195–221.
Anderson, E. G., 'Sex in mind and education, a reply', *Fortnightly Review*, 21 (1874), 582–94.
'Andrology as a specialty', *Journal of the American Medical Association*, 17 (1891), 631.
Apostoli, G. *Sur un nouveau traitement de la métrite chronique et en particulier de l'endométrite par la galvano-caustique chimique intra-utérine*. Paris: O. Doin, 1887.
Atlee, W. L., 'A table of all the known operations of ovariotomy from 1701 to 1851, comprising 222 cases, and giving a synoptical history of each case', *Transactions of the American Medical Association*, 4 (1851), 286–314.
'The authorities of the Hospital for Women and their honorary medical officers', *Medical Times and Gazette*, 1 (1874), 374–5.
Aveling, J. H., 'British gynaecology, past and present', *British Gynaecological Journal*, 1 (1885–6), 72–95.
  'The College of Surgeons of England, and Obstetric medicine', *Obstetrical Journal of Great Britain and Ireland*, 3 (1875–6), 732–6.
  English Midwives: Their History and Prospects, ed. J. L. Thornton. 1872; London: H. K. Elliott, 1967.
  'Instruction of midwives' (letter), *British Medical Journal*, 1 (1874), 252–3.
Aveling, J. H., 'Instruction of midwives' (letter), *British Medical Journal*, 1 (1874), 433.

Balls-Headley, W., *The Evolution of the Diseases of Women*. London: Smith, Elder and Co., 1894.

Bantock, G. G., 'Table of 238 cases of completed ovariotomy (163 to 400 inclusive) with remarks', *British Gynaecological Journal*, 5 (1889–90), 343–76; 430–7.

Barnes, R., 'An address on obstetric medicine and its position in medical education', *Obstetrical Journal of Great Britain and Ireland*, 3 (1875–6), 289–99.

'On the correlations of the sexual functions and mental disorders of women', *British Gynaecological Journal*, 6 (1890–1), 390–413; 416–30.

'The foundation of the British Gynaecological Society', *British Gynaecological Journal*, 1 (1885–6), 233–8.

'Lectures on the diseases of women', *Lancet*, 1 (1880), 4–6; 155–7; 2 (1880), 121–3; 923–5.

'Lumleian lectures on the convulsive diseases of women', *British Medical Journal*, 1 (1873), 391–4; 421–5; 453–5; 483–5.

On the Relations between Medicine, Surgery, and Obstetrics in London. New York: W. Wood and Co., 1884.

'On vicarious menstruation', *British Gynaecological Journal*, 2 (1886–7), 151–83.

'Women, diseases of', in Quain, R. (ed.), *A Dictionary of Medicine: Including General Pathology, General Therapeutics, Hygiene, and the Diseases Peculiar to Women and Children*, 2 vols. London: Longmans, Green, and Co., 1882.

Barnes, R. and Barnes, R. S. F., *A System of Obstetric Medicine and Surgery*. 2 vols. London: Smith, Elder and Co., 1884.

Battey, R., 'Is there a proper field for Battey's operation?' *Transactions of the American Gynaecological Society*, 2 (1877), 279–305.

Bell, W. B., *The Sex Complex: A Study of the Relationships of the Internal Secretions to the Female Characteristics and Functions in Health and Disease*. London: Baillière, Tindall and Cox, 1916.

Bernard, C., *Introduction à l'étude de la médecine éxperimentale*. Paris: J.-B. Baillière et Fils, 1865.

Bertillon, A., et al., *Dictionnaire des sciences anthropologiques: anatomie, craniologie, archéologie préhistorique, ethnographie*. Paris: O. Doin, 1884.

Blackwell, E., *Essays in Medical Sociology*. 1902; New York: Arno Press and the New York Times, 1972.

Blair, A., 'The general practitioner and the maternity service' (letter), *British Medical Journal*, 2 (1924), 1177–8.

Bland-Sutton, Sir J., *The Story of a Surgeon*. London: Methuen and Co., 1930.

Bonney, V., 'The continuing high mortality of childbearing', *Proceedings of the Royal Society of Medicine*, 12 (1919), pt. III, 75–107.

Bourgeois, L., *Observations diverses sur la stérilité, perte de fruit, foecondité, accouchements, et maladies des femmes et enfants nouveaux naiz*. Paris: M. Mondiere, 1642.

Brown, I. B., *On the Curability of Certain Forms of Insanity, Epilepsy, Catalepsy, and Hysteria in Females*. London: R. Hardwicke, 1866.

Bucknill, J. C., and Tuke, D. H., *A Manual of Psychological Medicine: containing the History, Nosology, Description, Statistics, Diagnosis, Pathology, and Treatment of Insanity*. London: J. Churchill, 1858.

Burdett, H. C., 'Home hospitals: their scope, object, and management', *British Medical Journal*, 2 (1877), 243–5.

Hospitals and Asylums of the World: Their Origin, Construction, Administration, Management, and Legislation, 4 vols. London: J. and A. Churchill, 1891–3.

Cadogan, W., *An Essay on the Management of Children, from Their Birth to Three Years of Age*. 6th edn. 1748; London: The Foundling Hospital, 1753.

Cappe, C., *Thoughts on the Desirableness and Utility of Ladies Visiting the Female Wards of Hospitals and Lunatic Asylums*. London: n.p., 1816.

Carter, R. B., *On the Pathology and Treatment of Hysteria*. London: J. Churchill, 1853.

'Casey vs. Imlach', *Lancet*, 2 (1886), 304.

'Censor' (pseud.), 'Use of the speculum vaginae', *Lancet*, 1 (1845), 105.

'Use of the speculum vaginae', *Lancet*, 1 (1845), 223.

Chadwick, E., *Report on the Sanitary Condition of the Labouring Population of Great Britain*. London: W. Clowes and Sons, 1842.

'The Chelsea Hospital for Women', *Lancet*, 1 (1894), 365; 631–2; 709; 2 (1894), 160–1; 200–1; 214; 462–3; 595–7.

Chéreau, A., *Memoires pour servir à l'étude des maladies des ovaires*. Paris: Jortin, Masson et Cie, 1844.

Clarke, E. H., *Sex in Education: Or, a Fair Chance for the Girls*. Boston: J. R. Osgood and Co., 1873.

'Clay on *Extirpation of Diseased Ovaria*' (review article), *British and Foreign Medical Review*, 16 (1843), 387–402.

'Clinical review of *Clinical Midwifery, with the Histories of Four Hundred Cases of Difficult Labour*, by R. Lee', *Medico-Chirurgical Review and Journal of Practical Medicine*, n.s., 38 (1843), 241–8.

Cobbe, F. P., 'The little health of ladies', *Contemporary Review*, 31 (1877), 276–96.

Craig, J., *A New Universal Etymological, Technological, and Pronouncing Dictionary of the English Language, Embracing all the Terms Used in Art, Science and Literature*, 2 vols. London: H. G. Collins, 1849.

Curling, T. B., 'Testicles', in Todd, R. B., *The Cyclopaedia of Anatomy and Physiology*, 5 vols. London: Longman, Brown, Green, Longman and Roberts, 1835–59, IV, 976–1016.

Darwin, C., *The Descent of Man and Selection in Relation to Sex*. 1871; 2nd edn. London: J. Murray, 1909.

The Variation of Animals and Plants under Domestication, 2 vols. London: J. Murray, 1868.

van Deventer, H., *The Art of Midwifery Improv'd. Fully and Plainly Laying down Whatever Instructions are Requisite to make a Compleat Midwife . . . Also a New Method, demonstrating, how Infants Ill Situated in the Womb*

. . . May, by the Hand Only . . . be Turned into Their Right Position . . . To Which is Added a Preface Giving Some Account of This Work, by an Eminent Physician. London: Curll, J. Pemberton, and W. Taylor, 1716.

'On the diagnosis and treatment of ovarian disease, with the history of one hundred and fifty-six cases, by Robert Lee', *Lancet*, 2 (1851), 536–40.

'Discussion on Robert Lee's "Analysis of one hundred and eight cases of ovariotomy which have occurred in Great Britain"', *Lancet*, 2 (1850), 584–7.

'Discussion sur les kystes ovariques', *Bulletin de l'Académie Impériale de Médecine*, 22 (1856–7), 20–323.

Dolan, T. M., 'Gynaecological specialism and general practice', *British Gynaecological Journal*, 5 (1889–90), 284–304; 327–31.

Douglas, J., *Short Account of the State of Midwifery in London, Westminster, &c.* London: For the Author, 1736.

Edis, A. W., 'On the relations of gynaecology to general therapeutics', *British Gynaecological Journal*, 4 (1889–90), 7–23.

Ellis, H., *Man and Woman: A Study of Human Secondary Sexual Characters.* 1894; 4th edn. London: Walter Scott Publishing Co., 1904.

Engels, F., *The Condition of the Working Class in England.* 1845; Oxford: Blackwell, 1958.

Farre, A., 'Uterus and its appendages', in Todd, R. B. (ed.), *The Cyclopaedia of Anatomy and Physiology.* 5 vols. London: Longman, Brown, Green, Longman and Roberts, 1835–59, V, 545–725.

Gamgee, S., *The Influence of Vivisection on Human Surgery.* London: J. and A. Churchill, 1881.

Garson, J. G., 'Pelvimetry', *Journal of Anatomy and Physiology*, 16 (1881–2), 106–34.

Gegenbaur, C., *Elements of Comparative Anatomy.* London: Macmillan and Co., 1878.

'Gratuitous medical services: special hospitals', *British Medical Journal*, 2 (1861), 261–3.

Hall, E., 'Gynaecology among the insane in private practice', *British Gynaecological Journal*, 14 (1898), 571–6.

Hall, M., 'On a new and lamentable form of hysteria', *Lancet*, 1 (1850), 660–1.

Hegar, A., 'Castration in mental and nervous disease: a symposium', *American Journal of Medical Science*, 92 (1886), 455–90.

Hicks, J. B., 'On the difference between the sexes in regard to the aspect and treatment of disease', *British Medical Journal*, 1 (1877), 318–20; 347–9; 377–9; 413–15; 447–9; 475–6.

'Notes of cases in obstetric jurisprudence', *Lancet*, 2 (1885), 198–9; 243–4; 285–6.

Hobbs, A. T., 'Surgical gynaecology in insanity', *British Medical Journal*, 2 (1897), 769–70.

'The hospital for ladies', *The Times*, 22 May 1865, 9.

Hull, R., 'On the speculum vaginae', *London Medical Gazette*, 13 (1851), 493–5.

Inman, T., 'Tables of the mortality after operations', *Lancet*, 2 (1844), 39–40.

'Inquisitor' (pseud.), 'The speculum question' (letter), *Medical Times and Gazette*, 25 (1852), 196–7.

'Is ovariotomy justifiable?' *Monthly Journal of Medical Science*, 41 (1846), 53–67.

Jamieson, J., 'Sex, in health and disease', *Australian Medical Journal*, n.s., 9 (1887), 145–58.

Johnson, J. 'Extirpation of the ovaria', *Medico-Chirurgical Review*, n.s., 2 (1825), 215–17.

Jones, W., *Practical Observations on Diseases of Women*. London: H. Baillière, 1839.

Julien M., 'Recherches sur les suites eloignées de l'opération de la castration chez la femme et sur la valeur de l'opothérapie ovarienne'. Lille University M.D. thesis. Lille: H. Morel, 1899.

King, V. O., 'Case of menstruation in the male', *Canada Medical Journal*, 2 (1867), 472–3.

Lane, W. A., 'Which are the chief factors which determine the differences which exist in the form of the male and the female pelves?' *British Medical Journal*, 2 (1887), 832.

Laycock, T., 'On annual vital periods, being a fifth contribution to vital proleptics', *Lancet*, 1 (1843–4), 85–9.

'Evidence and arguments in proof of the existence of a general law of periodicity in the phenomena of life', *Lancet*, 1 (1842–3), 124–9; 160–4.

'Further development of a general law of vital periodicity; being a second contribution to proleptics', *Lancet*, 1 (1842–3), 423–7.

'On the influence of the moon on the atmosphere of the earth, and on the pathological influence of the seasons', *Lancet*, 2 (1842–3), 826–30.

'On lunar influence; being a fourth contribution to proleptics', *Lancet*, 2 (1842–3), 438–44.

'On the major periods of development in man, being a sixth contribution to proleptics, *Lancet*, 1 (1843–4), 253–8.

'On some of the causes which determine the minor periods of vital movements', *Lancet*, 1 (1842–3), 929–33.

A Treatise on the Nervous Diseases of Women: Comprising an Inquiry into the Nature, Causes and Treatment of Spinal and Hysterical Disorders. London: Longman, Orme, Brown, Green and Longman, 1840.

Leake, J., *Introduction to the Theory and Practice of Midwifery*. London: Baldwin and Murray, 1787.

Lee, R., 'An analysis of one hundred and eight cases of ovariotomy which have occurred in Great Britain', *Medico-Chirurgical Transactions*, 16 (1851), 10–35.

'An estimate of the extent to which human life has been prolonged or abridged by ovariotomy', *Proceedings of the Royal Medical and Chirurgical Society of London*, 4 (1861–4), 186–7.

'Lectures on the structure and physiology of the ovaria', *Medical Times and Gazette*, 14 (1857), 305–7; 329–30; 637–8.

'On the diagnosis and treatment of ovarian disease, with the history of one hundred and fifty-six cases, by Robert Lee', *Lancet*, 2 (1851), 536–40.

'On the use of the speculum in the diagnosis and treatment of uterine diseases', *Medico-Chirurgical Transactions*, 33 (1850), 261–78.

'The legal aspects of sterilisation', *Lancet*, 1 (1929), 988.

'Legality of sterilisation', *British Medical Journal*, 1 (1970), 704–5.

Litchfield, T., 'On the use and abuse of the speculum' (letter), *Lancet*, 1 (1850), 705.

Lizars, J., 'Observations on extirpation of the ovaria, with cases', *Edinburgh Medical and Surgical Journal*, 22 (1824), 247–56.

Locock, C., 'Amenorrhoea', in J. Forbes, A. Tweedie and J. Conolly (eds.), *The Cyclopaedia of Practical Medicine*, 4 vols. London: Sherwood, Gilbert, and Piper, and Baldwin and Cradock, 1833–5, I, 68.

'A London surgeon' (pseud.), 'Special hospitals' (letter), *Lancet*, 1 (1858), 20–1.

Lycett, J. A., 'Gynaecology in general practice', *British Gynaecological Journal*, 6 (1890–1), 208–20.

Martin, W., 'Special hospitals', *British Medical Journal*, 2 (1861), 301–4; 326–7.

Macnaughton-Jones, H., 'A gynaecological question of importance in forensic medicine relating to the hymen', *British Gynaecological Journal*, 10 (1894–5), 38–48.

Maubray, J., *Midwifery Brought to Perfection by Manual Operation*. London: J. Holland, 1723.

Maudsley, H., *Body and Mind: An Inquiry into Their Connection and Mutual Influence, Specially in Reference to Mental Disorders*. London: Macmillan and Co., 1870.

'Sex in mind and in education', *Fortnightly Review*, 21 (1874), 446–83.

Mayhew, H., *London Labour and the London Poor: A Cyclopaedia of the Condition and Earnings of Those That Will Work, Those That Cannot Work, and Those That Will Not Work*, 4 vols. London: Griffin, Bohn and Co., 1861.

Meadows, A., 'On certain obstetric and gynaecological operations', *British Medical Journal*, 2 (1886), 356–8.

Morant, G., *Hints to Husbands: A Revelation of the Man-Midwife's Mysteries*. London: Simpkin, Marshall, and Co., 1857.

Mundé, P., 'Mental disturbances in the female produced and cured by gynaecological operations', *American Gynaecological and Obstetrical Journal*, 12 (1898), 51–5.

Murphy, J., 'The influence of surgery on gynaecology', *Provincial Medical Journal*, 10 (1891), 403–4.

Newman, H. P., 'Woman and her diseases vs. gynaecology', *American Gynaecological and Obstetrical Journal*, 2 (1896), 417–22.
Nicholls, F., *The Petition of the Unborn Babes to the Censors of the Royal College of Physicians*. London: M. Cooper, 1751.
'Normal ovariotomy: Battey's operation: Tait's operation', *British Medical Journal*, 1 (1887), 576–7.
'The Obstetrical and Gynaecological Section of the Royal Society of Medicine', *Lancet*, 2 (1907), 1831.
'The Obstetrical Society's charges and Mr. Baker Brown's reply', *Lancet*, 1 (1867), 427–41.
Oliver, J., 'Woman physically and ethically considered', *Liverpool Medico-Chirurgical Journal*, 9 (1889), 219–26.
'Ovariotomy', *British Medical Journal*, 2 (1862), 494.
'Ovariotomy in the Royal Medical and Chirurgical Society', *British Medical Journal*, 2 (1862), 521–2.
Oxley, W. H. F., 'Prevention of puerperal sepsis in general practice', *British Medical Journal*, 1 (1934), 1017–19.
Palmer, C. D., 'Gynaecology and general medicine: their reciprocal relations', *American Journal of Obstetrics and the Diseases of Women and Children*, 34 (1896), 375–9.
Pears, C., 'The case of a full grown woman in whom the ovaria were deficient', *Philosophical Transactions of the Royal Society of London*, 115 (1805), 225–7.
Pila, D., 'Etude critique de la castration chez la femme: ses résultats thérapeutiques, ses abus et ses conséquences sociales'. M.D. thesis, University of Paris. Paris: J. Rousset, 1901.
Ploss, H., Bartels, M., and Bartels, P., *Woman: An Historical, Gynaecological, and Anthropological Compendium*, ed. E. J. Dingwall. 3 vols. 1885; London: Heinemann, 1935.
'The Plymouth speculum case', *Medical Times and Gazette*, 26 (1852), 294.
Pott, P., *The Chirurgical Works*. London: Hawes, Clarke and Collins, 1775.
Power, J., *Essays on the Female Economy*. London: Burgess and Hill, 1821.
Priestly, W. O., 'On over-operating in gynaecology', *British Medical Journal*, 2 (1895), 284–7.
'Pudor' (pseud.), 'The speculum committee' (letter), *Medical Times*, 22 (1850), 45.
Radford, T., *Observations on the Caesarean Section and on Other Obstetric Operations*. Manchester: n.p., 1855.
  On the Value of Embryonic and Foetal Life, Legally, Morally, and Socially Considered. n.p., 1848.
Rentoul, R. R., 'The training of the medical student in midwifery', *Lancet*, 1 (1891), 875–6.
'Replies to correspondents', *Lancet*, 1 (1842), 664.
' Report of the Infantile Mortality Committee of the Obstetrical Society of London', *Transactions of the Obstetrical Society of London*, 12 (1870), 132–49; 13 (1871), 388–403.

'Restrictions on the practice of midwifery', *London Medical Gazette*, n.s., 1 (1845), 779–82.

Ridenbaugh, M. R., *The Biography of Ephraim McDowell, M.D.* New York: C. L. Webster and Co., 1890.

Rigby, E., *On the Constitutional Treatment of Female Disorders*. London: H. Renshaw, 1856.

　On Dysmenorrhea and other Uterine Affections in Connection with Derangements of the Assimilating Functions, London: H. Renshaw, 1844.

　'Reports on uterine diseases', *Medical Times*, 10 (1844), 505–6; 547–9. 11 (1844–5), 14–6; 29–31; 72–4; 112–15; 153–4; 195–7; 269–70; 293–5; 338–9; 378–80; 416–17; 475–6. 12 (1845), 4–6; 93–4; 176–7; 217–18; 263–4; 343–4; 402–3; 465–6. 15 (1846–7), 9–10; 82–3.

Roberton, J., *Essays and Notes on the Physiology and Diseases of Women, and on Practical Midwifery*. London: J. Churchill; Manchester: Simms and Dinham, 1851.

　'On the period of puberty in Esquimaux women', *Edinburgh Medical and Surgical Journal*, 63 (1845), 57–65.

Rochard, J., *Histoire de la chirurgie française au XIXᵉ siècle*. Paris: Baillière et Fils, 1875.

Romanes, G. J., *Essays*, ed. C. L. Morgan. London, New York and Bombay: Longmans and Co., 1897.

'Royal Medico-Chirurgical Society: the speculum in uterine disease', *Lancet*, 1 (1850), 701–5.

'The sanitary condition of the milliners and dressmakers of London', *Lancet*, 1 (1853), 519–20.

Saundby, R., *Medical Ethics: A Guide to Professional Conduct*. 1902; 2nd edn. London: C. Griffin and Co., 1907.

Schurig, M., *Gynaecologia historico-medica hoc est congressus muliebris consideratio physico-medico-forensis. Qua utriusque sexus salacitas et castitas deinde coitus ipse eiusque voluptas et varia circa hunc actum occurrentia nec non coitus ob atresiam seu vaginae uterinae imperforationem et alias causas impeditus et denegatus, item nefandus et sodomiticus raris observationibus et aliquot casibus medico-forensibus exhibentur*. Leipzig and Dresden: Hekel, 1730.

'Sex in occupation', *Obstetrical Journal of Great Britain and Ireland*, 2 (1874–5), 157–9.

Shaw, T. C., 'The sexes in lunacy', *St. Bartholomew's Hospital Reports*, 24 (1888), 1–15.

Shaw, W. F., 'The birth of a College', *Journal of Obstetrics and Gynaecology of the British Empire*, 57 (1950), 876–90.

Shaw, W. F., 'The College: its past, present and future. The William Meredith Fletcher Shaw Memorial Lecture', *Journal of Obstetrics and Gynaecology of the British Empire*, 61 (1954), 557–66.

　Twenty-Five Years: The Story of the Royal College of Obstetricians and Gynaecologists 1929–1954. London: Churchill, 1954.

Simpson, Sir J. Y., *Obstetric Memoirs and Contributions*, ed. W. O. Priestley and H. R. Storer. 2 vols. Edinburgh: A. and C. Black, 1871.

The Works of Sir James Y. Simpson, Bart, ed. Sir W. G. Simpson, 3 vols. Edinburgh: A. and C. Black, 1871.

Smith, P., *Scriptural Authority for the Mitigation of the Pains of Labour by Chloroform and other Anaesthetic Agents*. London: S. Highley, 1848.

Smith, W. T., 'On the abolition of craniotomy from obstetric practice, in all cases where the foetus is living and viable', *Transactions of the Obstetrical Society of London*, 1 (1859), 21–50.

'Introductory lecture to a course of lectures on obstetricy (delivered at the Hunterian School of Medicine) 1847–8', *Lancet*, 2 (1847), 371–4.

'Lectures on parturition, and the principles and practice of obstetricy', *Lancet*, 2 (1848), 117–20.

Society for the Total Abolition of Vivisection, *Correspondence with T. Spencer Wells, F.R.C.S., on Ovariotomy*. 3rd edn. London: Pickering and Co., 1882.

'Special hospitals', *British Medical Journal*, 1860, 625–9.

'Special hospitals', *British Medical Journal*, 2 (1861), 124–8.

'Spectator' (pseud.), 'The use and abuse of the speculum' (letter), *Medical Times*, 22 (1850), 45.

Spencer, H., 'A College of Obstetrics and Gynaecology' (letter), *British Medical Journal*, 1 (1929), 523.

Stevens, J., *Man-Midwifery Exposed, or the Danger and Immorality of Employing Men in Midwifery Proved; and the Remedy for the Evil Found*. London: W. Horsell, 1850.

Stone, S., *A Complete Practice of Midwifery*. London: T. Cooper, 1737.

Tait, R. L., 'The antiseptic theory tested by the statistics of one hundred cases of successful ovariotomy', *Medico-Chirurgical Transactions*, 63 (1880), 161–80.

'Cases treated antiseptically on Lister's method', *Lancet*, 1 (1871), 45–6.

'Clinical lecture on the details necessary in the performance of abdominal section', *Lancet*, 2 (1891), 597–9.

Diseases of Women. Birmingham: Cornish Brothers, 1887.

Diseases of Women and Abdominal Surgery. Vol. I (No further vols. publ.) Leicester: Richardson and Co.; Philadelphia: Lea Brothers, 1889.

'One hundred and thirty-nine consecutive ovariotomies performed between January 1st 1884 and December 31st 1885 without a death', *British Medical Journal*, 1 (1886), 921–4.

Two Essays on the Law of Evolution. Birmingham: Cornish Brothers, 1885.

The Uselessness of Vivisection as a Method of Scientific Research. London: Victoria Street Society, 1882.

Tardieu, A., *Question médico-légale de l'identité*. Paris: J. B. Baillière et fils, 1874.

Taylor, C. B., *The Contagious Diseases Acts (Women), from a Sanitary Point of View; Showing How and Why Such Despotic Measures not Only Fail to Repress Disease, but Tend to Increase Its Most Serious Manifestations*. Part II. London: Tweedie, 1870.

Observations on the Contagious Diseases Acts (Women, not Animals), Show-

ing *How the New Law Debases Women, Debauches Men, Destroys the Liberty of the Subject, and Tends to Increase Disease.* Nottingham: F. Banks, n.d. (*c.*1870).

'The teaching of midwifery and Mr. Syme's Committee on Medical Education', *Lancet*, 2 (1868), 708–9.

Thicknesse, P., *Man-Midwifery Analysed.* London: R. Davies, 1764.

Turner, W., 'The index of the pelvic brim as a basis for classification', *Journal of Anatomy and Physiology*, 20 (1885–6), 125–43.

Underhill, J. W., 'The female generative organs in their medico-legal relations', *American Journal of Obstetrics*, 12 (1879), 91–111.

Vrolik, G., *Considerations sur la diversité des bassins de differentes races humaines.* Amsterdam: J. Van Der Hay et Fils, 1826.

Walker, A., *Beauty Illustrated by an Analysis and Classification of Beauty in Woman.* London: H. G. Bohn, 1852.

Walker, K., *Diseases of the Male Organs of Generation.* London: H. Frowde, and Hodder and Stoughton, 1923.

Waller, C., 'Lectures on the functions and diseases of the womb', *Lancet*, 1 (1839–40), 393.

Wells, Sir T. S., *Modern Abdominal Surgery: The Bradshaw Lecture Delivered at the Royal College of Surgeons of England. With an Appendix on the Castration of Women.* London: J. and A. Churchill, 1891.

'The revival of ovariotomy, and its influence on modern surgery', *British Medical Journal*, 2 (1884), 893–6.

West, C., *Lectures on the Diseases of Women.* 3rd edn. London: J. Churchill and Sons, 1864.

Wilkinson, J. J. G., *The Forcible Introspection of the Women for the Army and Navy by the Oligarchy Considered Physically.* London: n.p., 1870.

Williams, S. W. D., 'Cases illustrating the action of amenorrhoea as a cause of insanity', *Journal of Mental Science*, 9 (1863–4), 344–53.

Williams, W. R., *The Influence of Sex in Disease.* London: J. and A. Churchill, 1885.

Willughby, P., *Observations in Midwifery*, ed. H. Blenkinsop. Warwick: H. T. Cooke and Sons, 1863.

Wiltshire, A., 'Clinical lecture on vicarious or ectopic menstruation, or menses devii', *Lancet*, 2 (1885), 513–17.

'Lectures on the comparative physiology of menstruation', *British Medical Journal*, 1 (1883), 395–400; 443–8; 500–2.

'Woman in her psychological relations', *Journal of Psychological Medicine and Mental Pathology*, 4 (1851), 18–50.

'Woman in her social relations, past and present', *Journal of Psychological Medicine and Mental Pathology*, 9 (1856), 521–44.

Zola, E., *Fécondité.* 1899; 2 vols. Paris: Fasquelle Editeurs, 1925.

SECONDARY SOURCES

Abel-Smith, B., *The Hospitals, 1800–1948: A Study in Social Administration in England and Wales.* London: Heinemann, 1964.

Albury, W. R., 'Experiment and explanation in the physiology of Bichat and Magendie', *Studies in the History of Biology*, 1 (1977), 47–131.

Alexander, S., 'Women's work in nineteenth-century London: a study of the years 1820–1850', in Mitchell, J. and Oakley, A. (eds.), *The Rights and Wrongs of Women*. Harmondsworth: Penguin Books, 1976, pp. 59–111.

Armstrong, D., *Political Anatomy of the Body: Medical Knowledge in Britain in the Twentieth Century*. Cambridge: Cambridge University Press, 1983.

Barker-Benfield, B., 'Sexual surgery in late nineteenth-century America', *International Journal of the Health Services*, 5 (1975), 279–98.

Bell, E. M., *Storming the Citadel: The Rise of the Woman Doctor*. London: Constable, 1953.

Berger, J., *Ways of Seeing*. London: B.B.C. Publications; Harmondsworth: Penguin Books, 1972.

Bett, W. R., *Sir John Bland-Sutton 1855–1936*. Edinburgh and London: E. and S. Livingstone, 1956.

Blanckaert, C., 'Médecine et histoire naturelle de l'homme: l'anthropologie française dans la seconde moitié du XIX siècle', in Poirier, J. and Poirier, J. L. (eds.), *Médecine et philosophie à la fin du XIXᵉ siècle*. Paris: Université Paris-Val de Marne, 1981, pp. 101–16.

Bloch, M. and Bloch, J. H., 'Women and the dialectics of nature in eighteenth-century French thought', in MacCormack, C. and Strathern, M. (eds.), *Nature, Culture, and Gender*. Cambridge: Cambridge University Press, 1980, pp. 25–41.

Bolt, C., *Victorian Attitudes to Race*. London: Routledge and Kegan Paul; Toronto: University of Toronto Press, 1971.

Borell, M. E., 'Origins of the hormone concept: internal secretions and physiological research, 1889–1905', Ph.D. thesis, Yale University, 1976.

Boss, B. and Boss, J., 'Ignorant midwives – a further rejoinder', *Society for the Social History of Medicine Bulletin*, 32 (1983), 71.

Bourne, A., *A Doctor's Creed: The Memoirs of a Gynaecologist*. London: Gollancz, 1962.

Buck, P., 'People who counted: political arithmetic in the eighteenth century', *Isis*, 73 (1982), 28–45.

Bullough, V. and Voght, M., 'Women, menstruation and nineteenth-century medicine', *Bulletin of the History of Medicine*, 47 (1973), 66–82.

Burrow, J. W., *Evolution and Society: A Study in Victorian Social Theory*. Cambridge: Cambridge University Press, 1966.

Bynum, W., 'The great chain of being after forty years: an appraisal', *History of Science*, 13 (1975), 1–28.

Calder, J., *Women and Marriage in Victorian Fiction*. London: Thames and Hudson, 1976.

Canguilhem, G., *Etudes d'histoire et de philosophie des sciences*. Paris: Librairie Philosophique J. Vrin, 1968.

Cianfrani, T., *A Short History of Obstetrics and Gynaecology*. Springfield: Thomas, 1960.

Clark, A., *Working Life of Women in the Seventeenth Century*. London: Routledge and Sons; New York: E. P. Dutton and Co., 1919.

Clark, G., *A History of the Royal College of Physicians of London*, 2 vols. London: Oxford University Press, 1966.

Coleman, W., *Death is a Social Disease: Public Health and Political Economy in Early Industrial France*. Madison WI: University of Wisconsin Press, 1982.

Collins, E. T., *The History and Tradition of Moorfields Eye Hospital*. London: H. K. Lewis and Co., 1929.

Compston, H. F. B., *The Magdalen Hospital: The Story of a Great Charity*. London: SPCK, 1917.

Cooke, A. M., *A History of the Royal College of Physicians of London*, vol. III. Oxford: Clarendon Press, 1972.

Cope, Z., *The Royal College of Surgeons of England: A History*. London: A. Blond Ltd., 1959.

Cowen, D. L., 'Liberty, laissez-faire and licensure in nineteenth-century Britain', *Bulletin of the History of Medicine*, 43 (1969), 30–40.

Das, K., *Obstetric Forceps: Its History and Evolution*. Calcutta: The Art Press, 1929.

Davidoff, L., 'Class and gender in Victorian England', in Newton, J. L., Ryan, M. P. and Walkowitz, J. R. (eds.), *Sex and Class in Women's History*. London: Routledge and Kegan Paul, 1983, pp. 17–71.

'Mastered for life: servant and wife in Victorian and Edwardian England', *Journal of Social History*, 7 (1974), 406–28.

'The separation of home and work? Landladies and lodgers in nine-teenth- and twentieth-century England', in Burman, S. (ed.), *Fit Work for Women*. London: Croom Helm, 1979, pp. 64–93.

Davies, C., 'The health visitor as mother's friend: a woman's place in public health, 1900–14', *Social History of Medicine*, 1 (1988), 39–59.

Davin, A., 'Imperialism and motherhood', *History Workshop Journal*, 5 (1978), 9–65.

Delaporte, F., *Le second règne de la nature: essai sur les questions de la végétalité au XVIIIᵉ siècle*. Paris: Flammarion, 1979.

Deloyers, L., *François Magendie: précurseur de la médecine expérimentale*. Brussels, 1970.

Dingwall, R. and Lewis, P. (eds.), *The Sociology of the Professions*. London and Basingstoke: Macmillan Press, 1983.

Donnison, J., *Midwives and Medical Men: A History of Inter-Professional Rivalries and Women's Rights*. London: Heinemann, 1977.

Douglas, A., '"The fashionable diseases": Women's complaints and their treatment in nineteenth-century America', *Journal of Interdisciplinary History*, 4 (1973), 25–52.

Eccles, A., *Obstetrics and Gynaecology in Tudor and Stuart England*. London and Canberra: Croom Helm, 1982.

Edwards, S., *Female Sexuality and the Law: A Study of Constructs of Female*

Sexuality as They Inform Statute and Legal Procedure. Oxford: Martin Robertson, 1981.

Elliott, P., 'Vivisection and the emergence of experimental physiology in nineteenth-century France', in Rupke, N. A. (ed.), *Vivisection in Historical Perspective.* London, New York and Sydney: Croom Helm, 1987, pp. 48–77.

Elshtain, J. B., *Public Man, Private Woman: Women in Social and Political Thought.* Oxford: Martin Robertson, 1981.

Elston, M. A., 'Women and anti-vivisection in Victorian England', in Rupke, N. A. (ed.), *Vivisection in Historical Perspective.* London, New York and Sydney: Croom Helm, 1987, pp. 259–94.

Eyler, J. M., 'Mortality statistics and Victorian health policy: program and criticism', *Bulletin of the History of Medicine*, 50 (1976), 335–55.

Fee, E., 'Nineteenth-century craniology: the study of the female skull', *Bulletin of the History of Medicine*, 53 (1979), 415–33.

'Science and the "Woman Question", 1860–1920: a study of English scientific periodicals', Ph.D. thesis, Princeton University, 1978.

Figlio, K., 'Chlorosis and chronic disease in nineteenth-century Britain: the social constitution of somatic illness in a capitalist society', *Social History*, 3 (1978), 167–97.

'The historiography of scientific medicine: an invitation to the human sciences', *Comparative Studies in Society and History*, 19 (1977), 262–86.

'The metaphor of organisation: an historiographical perspective on the bio-medical sciences of the early nineteenth century', *History of Science*, 14 (1976), 17–53.

Foucault, M., *Discipline and Punish: The Birth of the Prison.* Harmondsworth: Penguin Books, 1979.

(ed.), *Hérculine Barbin.* Brighton: Harvester Press, 1980.

Histoire de la sexualité, 3 vols. Paris: Gallimard, 1977–84.

French, R. D., *Antivivisection and Medical Science in Victorian Society.* Princeton: Princeton University Press, 1975.

Fox-Genovese, E., 'Placing women's history in history', *New Left Review*, 133 (1982), 5–29.

Gelfand, T., 'The origins of a modern concept of medical specialization: John Morgan's *Discourse* of 1765', *Bulletin of the History of Medicine*, 50 (1976), 511–35.

Professionalising Modern Medicine: Paris Surgeons and Medical Science and Institutions. Westport CT: Greenwood Press, 1980.

Girouard, M., *The Return to Camelot: Chivalry and the English Gentleman.* New Haven and London: Yale University Press, 1981.

Glaister, J., *Dr William Smellie and His Contemporaries: A Contribution to the History of Midwifery in the Eighteenth Century.* Glasgow: Maclehose, 1894.

Gordon, L., *Woman's Body, Woman's Right: A Social History of Birth Control in America.* Hardmondsworth: Penguin, 1977.

Gorham, D., 'The "Maiden Tribute of Modern Babylon" re-examined:

child prostitution and the idea of childhood in late-Victorian England', *Victorian Studies*, 21 (1978), 353–79.

de Groot, J., ' "Sex" and "race": the construction of language and image in the nineteenth century', in Mendus, S. and Rendall, J. (eds.), *Sexuality and Subordination: Interdisciplinary Studies of Gender in the Nineteenth Century*. London and New York: Routledge, 1989.

Hall, C., 'The early formation of Victorian domestic ideology', in Burman, S. (ed.), *Fit Work for Women*. London: Croom Helm, 1979, pp. 15–32.

Haller, J. S., and Haller, R. M., *The Physician and Sexuality in Victorian America*. Urbana, Chicago and London: University of Illinois Press, 1974.

Hamilton, D., *The Healers: A History of Medicine in Scotland*. Edinburgh: Canongate, 1981.

Hannaway, C., 'From private hygiene to public health: a transformation in Western medicine in the eighteenth and nineteenth centuries', in Ogawa, T. (ed.), *Public Health*. Tokyo: Saikon Pub. Co., 1981, pp. 108–28.

Harley, D., 'Ignorant midwives: a persistent stereotype', *Society for the Social History of Medicine Bulletin*, 28 (1981), 6–9.

Helsinger, E. K., Sheets, R. L. and Veeder, W. (eds.), *The Woman Question: Social Issues, 1837–1883*, 3 vols. Manchester: Manchester University Press, 1983.

Hewitt, M., *Wives and Mothers in Victorian Industry*. Westport CT: Greenwood Press, 1958.

Himmelfarb, H., 'The culture of poverty', in Dyos, H. J. and Wolff, M. (eds.), *The Victorian City: Images and Reality*, 2 vols. London and Boston. Routledge and Kegan Paul, 1973, II, 707–36.

Hirsin, J., *Policing Prostitution in Nineteenth-Century Paris*. Princeton: Princeton University Press, 1985.

Honigsbaum, F., *The Division in British Medicine: A History of the Separation of General Practice from Hospital Care 1911–1968*. London: Kogan Page, 1979.

Hoolihan, C., 'Thomas Young, M.D. (1726?–1783) and obstetrical education at Edinburgh', *Journal of the History of Medicine and Allied Sciences*, 40 (1985), 327–45.

Jeffcoate, T. N. S., 'The precious ovary', *Transactions and Report of the Liverpool Medical Institution*, 1966, pp. 15–31.

Jones, G. S., *Outcast London: A Study of the Relationship between Classes in Victorian Society*. Oxford: Clarendon Press, 1971.

Jordanova, L., 'Earth science and environmental medicine: the synthesis of the late Enlightenment', in Jordanova, L. and Porter, R. (eds.), *Images of the Earth*. Chalfont St Giles: The British Society for the History of Science, 1979, pp. 119–46.

'Medicalisation and modernisation: some problems in the historical sociology of medicine', unpublished paper, April 1980.

'Natural facts: a historical perspective on science and sexuality', in

MacCormack, C., and Strathern, M. (eds.), *Nature, Culture, and Gender*. Cambridge: Cambridge University Press, 1980, pp. 42–67.

'Naturalizing the family: literature and the bio-medical sciences in the late eighteenth century', in Jordanova, L. (ed.), *Languages of Nature: Critical Essays on Science and Literature*. London: Free Association Books, 1986, pp. 86–116.

'Policing public health in France, 1780–1815', in Ogawa, T. (ed.), *Public Health*. Tokyo: Saikon Pub. Co., 1981.

Jorion, P., 'The downfall of the skull', *Royal Anthropological Institute Newsletter*, 48 (1982), 8–11.

Kerr, J. M. M., Johnstone, R. W. and Phillips, M. H. (eds.), *Historical Review of British Obstetrics and Gynaecology 1800–1950*. Edinburgh and London: E. and S. Livingstone, 1954.

van Keuren, D. K., 'Human science in Victorian Britain: anthropology in institutional and disciplinary formation, 1863–1908', Ph.D. thesis, University of Pennsylvania, 1982.

Knibiehler, Y., 'Les médecins et la "nature feminine" au temps du code civil', *Annales: E.S.C.*, 31 (1976), 824–45.

Lansbury, C., *The Old Brown Dog: Women, Workers, and Vivisection in Edwardian England*. Madison, Wisconsin: University of Wisconsin Press, 1985.

Laqueur, T., 'Orgasm, generation, and the politics of reproductive biology', *Representations*, 14 (1986), 1–41.

Leonardo, R. A., *History of Gynaecology*. New York: Froben Press, 1944.

Lewis, J., *The Politics of Motherhood: Child and Maternal Welfare in England, 1900–1939*. London: Croom Helm, 1980.

Lloyd, G., *The Man of Reason: 'Male' and 'Female' in Western Philosophy*. London: Methuen, 1984.

Lomas, P., 'An interpretation of modern obstetric practice', in Kitzinger, S. and Davis, J. A. (eds.), *The Place of Birth: A Study of the Environment in which Birth Takes Place with Special Reference to Home Confinements*. Oxford: Oxford University Press, 1978.

Loudon, I. S. L., 'The concept of the family doctor', *Bulletin of the History of Medicine*, 58 (1984), 347–62.

'Deaths in childbed from the eighteenth century to 1935', *Medical History*, 30 (1986), 1–41.

Medical Care and the General Practitioner 1750–1850. Oxford: Clarendon Press, 1986.

'Nature vs. intervention in obstetrics: a historical survey', unpublished paper, May 1986.

'The origins and growth of the dispensary movement in England', *Bulletin of the History of Medicine*, 55 (1981), 322–42.

McHugh, P., *Prostitution and Victorian Social Reform*. London: Croom Helm, 1980.

McKay, W. J. S., *The History of Ancient Gynaecology*. London: Baillière, Tindall, and Cox, 1901.

McLaren, A., *Birth Control in Nineteenth-Century England*. London: Croom Helm, 1978.

Maclean, I., *The Renaissance Notion of Woman: A Study in the Fortunes of Scholasticism and Medical Science in European Intellectual Life*. Cambridge: Cambridge University Press, 1980.

Manton, J., *Elizabeth Garrett Anderson*. London: Methuen and Co., 1965.

Medvei, V. C., *A History of Endocrinology*. Lancaster, Boston, The Hague: MTP Press Ltd, 1982.

Morantz, R., 'The lady and her physician', in Hartman, M. S., and Banner, L. (eds.), *Clio's Consciousness Raised: New Perspectives on the History of Women*. New York, Evanston, San Francisco: Harper Colophon Books, 1974, pp. 38–51.

Morantz-Sanchez, R. M., *Sympathy and Science: Women Physicians in American Medicine*. New York and Oxford: Oxford University Press, 1985.

Moravia, S., *Filosofia e scienze umane nell'età dei lumi*. Florence: Sansoni Editori Nuova S.p.A., 1982.

La scienza dell'uomo nel Settecento. Bari: Laterza, 1970.

Morson, C., *St Peter's Hospital for Stone, 1860–1960*. Edinburgh and London: E. and S. Livingstone, 1960.

Moscucci, O., *The Royal College of Obstetricians and Gynaecologists, 1929–1989: A History*. Forthcoming.

Newman, C., *The Evolution of Medical Education in the Nineteenth Century*. London: Oxford University Press, 1957.

Newton, J., Ryan, M. P. and Walkowitz, J. R. (eds.), *Sex and Class in Women's History*. London: Routledge, 1983.

Olmstead, J. M. D., *Claude Bernard, Physiologist*. London, Toronto, Melbourne and Sydney: Cassell and Co., 1939.

Orr, L., *Jules Michelet: Nature, History and Language*. Ithaca, New York: Cornell University Press, 1976.

Oxford, A. W., *History of the Samaritan Free Hospital*. Cambridge: W. Heffer, 1931.

Pearce, S. B. P., *An Ideal in the Working: The Story of the Magdalen Hospital 1758 to 1958*. London: Magdalen Hospital, 1958.

Pearson, M., *The Age of Consent: Victorian Prostitution and Its Enemies*. Newton Abbot: David and Charles, 1972.

Peel, J., *The Lives of the Fellows of the Royal College of Obstetricians and Gynaecologists 1929–1969*. London: Heinemann Medical Books, 1976.

Pelling, M., 'Surgeons, Barbers and Barber-Surgeons: an occupational group in an English provincial town, 1550–1640', *Society for the Social History of Medicine Bulletin*, 28 (1981), 14–16.

'Medical practice in the early modern period: trade or profession?', *Society for the Social History of Medicine Bulletin*, 32 (1983), 27–30.

Pernick, M. S., *A Calculus of Suffering: Pain, Professionalism, and Anesthesia in Nineteenth-Century America*. New York: Columbia University Press, 1985.

Peterson, M. J., *The Medical Profession in Mid-Victorian London*. Berkeley, Los Angeles and London: University of California Press, 1978.

'The Victorian governess: status incongruence in family and society', in Vicinus, M. (ed.), *Suffer and Be Still: Women in the Victorian Age*. Bloomington and London: Indiana University Press, 1972, pp. 3–19.

Pinker, J., *English Hospital Statistics 1861–1938*. London: Heinemann, 1966.

Plowden, E., *The Case of Eliza Armstrong: 'A Child of 13 Bought for £5'*. London: BBC Publications, 1974.

Poovey, M., '"Scenes of an indelicate character": the medical "treatment" of Victorian women', *Representations*, 14 (1986), 137–68.

Porter, R., 'William Hunter: a surgeon and a gentleman', in Bynum, W. and Porter, R. (eds.) *William Hunter and the Eighteenth-Century Medical World*. Cambridge: Cambridge University Press, 1985, pp. 7–34.

'Female quacks', unpublished paper, November 1988.

Prochaska, F. K., *Women and Philanthropy in Nineteenth-Century England*. Oxford: Clarendon Press, 1980.

Pundel, J. P., *Histoire de l'opération césarienne*. Brussels: Presses Académiques Européennes, 1969.

Radcliffe, W., *Milestones in Midwifery*. Bristol: J. Wright, 1967.

Ramsey, M., 'The politics of professional monopoly in nineteenth-century medicine: the French model and its rivals', in Geison, G. L. (ed.), *Professions and the French State, 1700–1900*. Philadelphia: University of Pennsylvania Press, 1984, pp. 225–305.

Reiser, S., *Medicine and the Reign of Technology*. Cambridge: Cambridge University Press, 1978.

Ricci, J. V., *The Genealogy of Gynaecology: History of the Development of Gynaecology Throughout the Ages*. Philadelphia: The Blakiston Co., 1943.

One Hundred Years of Gynaecology 1800–1900. Philadelphia: The Blakiston Co., 1945.

'The vaginal speculum and its modifications throughout the ages', *Contributions from the Department of Gynaecology of the City Hospital, New York, 1848–1949*, n.p., pp. 1–55.

Rich, A., *Of Woman Born*. London: Virago Press, 1977.

Roberts, R. S., 'The personnel and practice of medicine in Tudor and Stuart England, Part I. The Provinces', *Medical History*, 6 (1962), 363–82.

'The personnel and practice of medicine in Tudor and Stuart England, Part II. London', *Medical History*, 8 (1964), 217–34.

Roger, J., *Les sciences de la vie dans la pensée Française du XVIIIᵉ siècle: la génération des animaux de Descartes à l'Encyclopédie*. Paris: A. Colin, 1963.

Rose, L., *The Massacre of the Innocents: Infanticide in Britain 1800–1939*. London: Routledge and Kegan Paul, 1986.

Rosen, G., *From Medical Police to Social Medicine: Essays on the History of Health Care*. New York: Science History Publications, 1974.

The Specialization of Medicine, with Particular Reference to Ophthalmology. New York: Froben Press, 1944.

Rosenberg, C., 'Florence Nightingale on contagion: the hospital as moral universe', in Rosenberg, C. (ed.), *Healing and History: Essays for George Rosen.* New York: Science History Publications; Folkestone: Dawson and Sons, 1979, pp. 116–36.

and Smith-Rosenberg, C., 'The female animal: medical and biological views of woman and her role in nineteenth-century America', *Journal of American History*, 60 (1973), 332–56.

Rosenberg, R., *Beyond Separate Spheres.* New Haven: Yale University Press, 1982.

Schiebinger, L., 'Skeletons in the closet: the first illustrations of the female skeleton in eighteenth-century anatomy', *Representations*, 14 (1986), 42–82.

Schiller, J., *Claude Bernard et les problèmes scientifiques de son temps.* Paris: Editions du Cèdre, 1967.

La notion d'organisation dans l'histoire de la biologie. Paris: Maloine S.A., 1978.

Schoenwald, R. L., 'Training urban man: a hypothesis about the sanitary movement', in Dyos, H. J. and Wolff, M. (eds.), *The Victorian City: Images and Reality*, 2 vols. London and Boston: Routledge and Kegan Paul, 1973, II, 669–92.

Scott, J. W. and L. A. Tilly, *Women, Work and Family.* New York: Holt, Reinhart and Wilson, 1978.

Shepherd, J. A., *Lawson Tait: The Rebellious Surgeon (1845–1899).* Lawrence, Kansas: Coronado Press, 1980.

Spencer Wells: The Life and Work of a Victorian Surgeon. Edinburgh: E. and S. Livingstone, 1965.

Shorter, E., *A History of Women's Bodies.* London: Allen Lane, 1983.

Showalter, E., *The Female Malady: Women, Madness and English Culture, 1830–1980.* London: Virago Press, 1987.

Simmer, H. H., 'Pflüger's nerve reflex theory of menstruation: the product of analogy, teleology and neurophysiology', *Clio Medica*, 12 (1977) 57–90.

Skegg, P. D. G., *Law, Ethics, and Medicine: Studies in Medical Law.* Oxford: Clarendon Press, 1984.

Smith, F. B., *The People's Health, 1830–1910.* London: Croom Helm, 1979.

Smith, R., 'Scientific thought and the boundary of insanity and criminal responsibility', *Psychological Medicine*, 10 (1980), 15–23.

Trial by Medicine: Insanity and Responsibility in Victorian Trials. Edinburgh: Edinburgh University Press, 1981.

Smith-Rosenberg, C., 'The hysterical woman: sex roles conflict in nineteenth-century America', *Social Research*, 39 (1972), 652–78.

'Puberty to menopause: the cycle of femininity in nineteenth-century America', in Hartman, M. S. and Banner, L. (eds.), *Clio's Consciousness Raised: New Perspectives on the History of Women.* New York,

Evanston and San Francisco: Harper Colophon Books, 1974, pp. 23–37.

Soloway, R. A., *Birth Control and the Population Question in England, 1877–1930*. Chapel Hill: University of North Carolina Press, 1982.

Speert, H., *Obstetric and Gynaecologic Milestones*, New York: The Macmillan Co., 1958.

Spencer, H. R., *A History of British Midwifery from 1650 to 1800*. London: J. Bale and Sons, and Danielsson, 1927.

Staum, M. S., 'Cabanis and the science of Man', Ph.D. thesis, Cornell University, 1971.

Stepan, N., *The Idea of Race in Science: Great Britain 1800–1960*. London and Basingstoke: Macmillan Press, 1982.

Stevens, R., *Medical Practice in Modern England: The Impact of Specialization and State Medicine*. New Haven and London: Yale University Press, 1966.

Stevenson, L. G., 'The siege of Warwick Lane, together with a brief history of the Society of Collegiate Physicians, 1767–98', *Journal of the History of Medicine*, 7 (1952), 105–21.

Stocking, G. W., Jr., 'French anthropology in 1800', *Isis*, 5 (1964), 134–50.

Race, Culture, and Evolution: Essays in the History of Anthropology. 1968; New York: Free Press; London: Collier-Macmillan, 1982.

Sulloway, F. J., *Freud, Biologist of the Mind: Beyond the Psychoanalytic Legend*. New York: Basic Books, 1979.

Summers, A., 'A home from home: women's philanthropic work in the nineteenth century', in Burman, S. (ed.), *Fit Work for Women*. London: Croom Helm, 1979, pp. 33–63.

'Pride and prejudice: ladies and nurses in the Crimean War', *History Workshop Journal*, 16 (1983), 32–56.

Taylor, B., 'The Woman-Power', in Lipshitz, S. (ed.), *Tearing the Veil: Essays on Femininity*. London, Henley and Boston: Routledge and Kegan Paul, 1978, pp. 119–44.

Teitelbaum, M. S. and Winter, J. M., *The Fear of Population Decline*. Orlando: Academic Press, 1985.

Temkin, O., 'The role of surgery in the rise of modern medical thought', *Bulletin of the History of Medicine*, 25 (1951), 248–59.

Thompson, E. P., 'Time, work-discipline, and industrial capitalism', *Past and Present*, 35 (1967), 56–97.

Tröhler, U., 'Quantification in British medicine and surgery 1750–1830, with special reference to its introduction into therapeutics', Ph.D. thesis, University of London, 1978.

Vaughan, P., *Doctors' Commons: A Short History of the British Medical Association*. London, Melbourne and Toronto: Heinemann, 1959.

Verbrugge, M., 'Women and medicine in nineteenth-century America', *Signs: Journal of Women in Culture and Society*, 1 (1976), 957–72.

Versluysen, M. C., 'Midwives, medical men and "poor women labouring of child": lying-in hospitals in eighteenth-century London', in

Roberts, H. (ed.), *Women, Health, and Reproduction*. London: Routledge and Kegan Paul, 1981, pp. 18–49.

Vicinus, M. (ed.), *Suffer and Be Still*. Bloomington and London: Indiana University Press, 1972.

A Widening Sphere: Changing Roles of Victorian Women. London: Methuen and Co., 1977.

Virtanen, E., *Claude Bernard and His Place in the History of Ideas*. Lincoln: Nebraska University Press, 1960.

Waddington, I., 'General practitioners and consultants in early nineteenth-century England: the sociology of an intra-professional conflict', in Woodward, J. and Richards, D. (eds.), *Health Care and Popular Medicine in Nineteenth-Century England*. London: Croom Helm, 1977, pp. 164–88.

The Medical Profession in the Industrial Revolution. Dublin: Gill and Macmillan Humanities Press, 1984.

'The struggle to reform the Royal College of Physicians, 1767–1771: a sociological analysis', *Medical History*, 17 (1973), 107–26.

Walkowitz, J. R., *Prostitution and Victorian Society: Women, Class, and the State*. Cambridge: Cambridge University Press, 1980.

Wall, C., *The History of the Surgeons' Company 1745–1800*. London: Hutchinson Scientific and Technical Publications, 1937.

A History of the Worshipful Society of Apothecaries of London. Vol. I, 1617–1815. (No further vols. publ.) Abstracted and arranged by H. C. Cameron, rev., annotated and edited by E. A. Underwood. London: Oxford University Press, 1963.

Wangensteen, O. H., and Wangensteen, S. D., *The Rise of Surgery: From Empiric Craft to Scientific Discipline*. Folkestone: Dawson and Sons, 1978.

Warner, M., *Alone of All Her Sex: The Myth and the Cult of the Virgin Mary*. London: Weidenfeld and Nicolson, 1976.

Weber, G., 'Science and society in nineteenth-century anthropology', *History of Science*, 12 (1974), 260–83.

Weideger, P., *History's Mistress: A New Interpretation of a Nineteenth-Century Ethnographic Classic*. Harmondsworth: Penguin Books, 1985.

Weindling, P., 'The British Mineralogical Society: a case study in science and social improvement', in Inkster, I. and Morrell, J. (eds.), *Metropolis and Province: Science in British Culture, 1780–1850*. London, Melbourne and Sydney: Hutchinson, 1983, pp. 120–50.

Wertz, R. W. and Wertz, D. C., *Lying-In: A History of Childbirth in America*. New York: Schocken Books, 1979.

Williams, E. A., 'The science of Man: anthropological thought and institutions in nineteenth-century France', Ph.D. thesis, Indiana University, 1983.

Williams, R., *The Country and the City*. St Albans: Paladin Books, 1975.

Wilson, A., 'Participant or patient? Seventeenth century childbirth from the mother's point of view', in Porter, R. (ed.), *Patients and Prac-*

titioners: Lay Perceptions of Medicine in Pre-Industrial Society. Cambridge: Cambridge University Press, 1985.

A Safe Deliverance: Conflict and Ritual in British Childbirth, 1600–1750. Cambridge: Cambridge University Press, forthcoming.

'William Hunter and the varieties of man-midwifery', in Bynum, W. and Porter, R. (eds.), *William Hunter and the Eighteenth-Century Medical World*. Cambridge: Cambridge University Press, 1985, pp. 343–69.

Wilson, L. B., 'Les maladies des femmes: women, charlatanry, and professional medicine in eighteenth-century France', Ph.D. thesis, University of Stanford, 1982.

Winterton, W. R., 'The story of the London gynaecological hospitals', *Proceedings of the Royal Society of Medicine*, 54 (1961), 191–8.

Wohl, A. S., *Endangered Lives: Public Health in Victorian Britain*. London: J. M. Dent and Sons, Ltd., 1983.

Wright, P. and Treacher, A., *The Problem of Medical Knowledge: Examining the Social Construction of Medicine*. Edinburgh: Edinburgh University Press, 1982.

Wyman, A. L., 'The surgeoness: the female practitioner of surgery 1400–1800', *Medical History*, 28 (1984), 22–41.

Young, J. H., *Caesarean Section: The History and Development of the Operation from the Earliest Times*. London: Lewis and Co., 1944.

Young, S., *The Annals of the Barber Surgeons*. London: Blades, East and Blades, 1890.

Youngson, A. J., *The Scientific Revolution in Victorian Medicine*. London: Croom Helm, 1979.

Index